PAYING THE DOCTOR

Systems of Remuneration and Their Effects

WILLIAM A. GLASER

Bureau of Applied Social Research
Columbia University

THE JOHNS HOPKINS PRESS
BALTIMORE AND LONDON

Manufactured in the United States of America

The Johns Hopkins Press, Baltimore, Maryland 21218
The Johns Hopkins Press Ltd., London

Library of Congress Catalog Card Number 72–97054
Standard Book Number 8018–1083–3

For James

ACKNOWLEDGMENTS

I am particularly indebted to Arthur Seldon and James Hogarth for very thorough readings of the entire manuscript. Valuable comments on successive drafts were also provided by Odin Anderson, Keith Taylor, Amitai Etzioni, James Price, Edwin F. Daily, and Charles Kadushin. Nancy Middleton Gallienne contributed exceptional editorial help.

The gathering of data overseas was made possible by Grants RG-7934 and CH-00027 of the National Institutes of Health, United States Public Health Service. Preparation of a preliminary report was supported by Contract PH-86-63-118 of the Division of Community Health Services, United States Public Health Service. This book was prepared under a grant from the Health Information Foundation, Center for Health Administration Studies, University of Chicago.

The study was administered at the Bureau of Applied Social Research by Clara Shapiro and Madeline Simonson. As usual, Nelson Glover made an invaluable contribution to my work by his accurate typing of all drafts.

I am most indebted to the many medical administrators and scholars abroad who were so generous with their time and information. The numerous persons who granted me interviews and allowed me to visit their organizations are listed in the appendix.

The epigraph by R. H. Tawney preceding the text is taken from *The Acquisitive Society* (London: G. Bell and Sons, 1921), pp. 108–9. Quoted by permission of Harcourt, Brace & World, Inc.

CONTENTS

PAYING THE DOCTOR

And did you ever observe that there are two classes of patients in states, slaves and freemen; and the slave doctors run about and cure the slaves, or wait for them in the dispensaries—practitioners of this sort never talk to their patients individually, or let them talk about their own individual complaints? The slave-doctor prescribes what mere experience suggests, as if he had exact knowledge; and when he has given his orders, like a tyrant, he rushes off with equal assurance to some other servant who is ill; and so he relieves the master of the house of the care of his invalid slaves. But the other doctor, who is a freeman, attends and practises upon freemen; and he carries his enquiries far back, and goes into the nature of the disorder; he enters into discourse with the patient and with his friends, and is at once getting information from the sick man, and also instructing him as far as he is able, and he will not prescribe for him until he has first convinced him; at last, when he has brought the patient more and more under his persuasive influences and set him on the road to health, he attempts to effect a cure. Now which is the better way of proceeding in a physician and in a trainer?

PLATO
The Laws

We trust our health to the physician; our fortune and sometimes our life and reputation to the lawyer and attorney. Such confidence could not safely be reposed in people of a very mean or low condition. Their reward must be such, therefore, as may give them that rank in the society which so important a trust requires. The long time and the great expense which must be laid out in their education, when combined with this circumstance, necessarily enhance still further the price of their labour.

ADAM SMITH
The Wealth of Nations

The essence of [a profession], is that, though men enter it for the sake of livelihood, the measure of their success is the service which they perform, not the gains which they amass. They may, as in the case of a successful doctor, grow rich; but the meaning of their profession, both for themselves and for the public, is not that they make money but that they make health, or safety, or knowledge, or good government or good law. They depend on it for their income, but they do not consider that any conduct which increases their income is on that account right.

R. H. TAWNEY
The Acquisitive Society

I

THE EFFECTS OF PAYMENT SYSTEMS

A profession applies scientific knowledge to the solution of society's problems. Expert personnel and facilities should be available at the right places at times of need. The professionals should be fully qualified and should be motivated to give sufficient insight and effort. Exploitative, destructive, or erroneous actions should be discouraged.

Professional services, like all human action, are performed through a particular form of social organization. Every social institution provides incentives and rewards for its participants. The problem in any social institution is to organize social relationships in ways that will promote fulfilment of that institution's goals. Professional institutions and their incentive systems therefore are supposed to make possible rather than obstruct the realization of the profession's mission.

During the twentieth century, medical care has changed in both technique and in organization, in response to public demands for wider coverage and improved quality. Nation-wide systems of organizing and paying doctors have sprung up in association with many governments. But if older methods of medical organization fell short of producing a sufficient quantity and quality of medical care, the new trends are examined critically as well. Are they improving medical care; do gaps remain; do the new arrangements produce unexpected disadvantages?

Payment systems existing under older forms of medical practice in America and abroad aroused numerous complaints. It was said that patients of limited means often failed to obtain medical care because of inability to pay, that doctors gravitated to the more affluent cities and away from the countryside, that doctors entered the more remunerative rather than the more needed specialities, that doctors performed the more profitable rather than the more beneficial procedures, and so on.

The reorganization of medical practice during this century has extended to payment systems: instead of the direct and private relationship between doctor and patient, governments and health insurance funds are more involved as third parties in paying the doctor on behalf of the patient; earlier forms of prepayment have been reorganized and expanded; new procedures have been adopted for calculating the pay rates. But if older payment systems fell short of encouraging the best supply and use of medical services, the same defects might remain or increase under newer circumstances. Therefore, any planner seeking to manipulate a payment system must guess whether changes will help realize the profession's goals or whether they will introduce new barriers and distortions. But before a planner can decide, he must examine the available evidence.

Purpose of This Book

This volume will analyze the principal methods of paying doctors in several countries. I will describe the administrative mechanisms for distributing money to doctors. The book will convey the dynamics of each system: it will summarize how the various payment systems take their present forms and how decisionmakers set the fees or salaries of the medical profession. My principal aim is to summarize the evidence about the effects of each payment system upon medical care and upon the medical profession.[1] Rather than reporting the structure and events in each individual country, the general principles common to the chief types of payment method will be summarized.[2]

The basic task of this book is to answer a central question in medical economics and medical administration: If doctors are paid by one or another method, what is the difference in how the public is treated? More generally, the book is part of the growing literature in the economics and administration of social insurance and of government social services.

But the book also is written from the perspective of wider interests in the social sciences. First, it is addressed to the political economist's interest in

[1] In selecting these research problems, my thinking was influenced by several recent publications. My interest in why particular fees or salary rates are adopted in each country was derived from reading the analysis of the criteria for fixing paramedical wages in the British National Health Service in, H. A. Clegg and T. E. Chester, *Wage Policy and the Health Service* (Oxford: Basil Blackwell, 1957). When asking questions about the effects of each payment system, I kept in mind the hypotheses in, Franz Goldmann, "Methods of Payment for Physicians' Services in Medical Care Programs," *American Journal of Public Health*, vol. 42, no. 2 (February 1952), pp. 131–41; and Milton I. Roemer, "On Paying the Doctor and the Implications of Different Methods," *Journal of Health and Human Behavior*, vol. 3, no. 1 (Spring 1962), pp. 4–14.

[2] Many books and articles describe the medical services of each country, and some examine the administrative structure of the payment systems. They will be cited throughout this book. An excellent summary of the formal organization of general practitioners' pay in several European countries is, James Hogarth, *The Payment of the General Practitioner* (Oxford: Pergamon Press, 1963). For a valuable overview of medical costs and expenditures in many countries—including half the nations in this book—see Brian Abel-Smith, *An International Study of Health Expenditure* (Geneva: World Health Organization, 1967).

how the adoption of one or another mechanism for rewarding labor affects the recruitment of labor in that specialty, and affects the satisfaction of wants in the market.

Second, the book deals with many issues in political sociology—how certain national decisions are made by the interaction of officials and pressure groups, how these decisions are affected by the diverse values held by the public and by members of a profession. Examples are given of how social institutions evolve and become stabilized through struggles among interested parties and through the implementation of customs.

Finally, the book is a contribution to the literature in the new field of comparative administration. It describes how different governments in the world organize procedures to cope with comparable problems. And much of the book revolves around the central themes of variations and consistencies in institutional arrangements: If organization varies from one country to another, what are the different effects upon the public and upon the staffs; and, if different countries have similar arrangements, are different results nevertheless generated by some other variations in national social structures?

The book is an analysis and not a polemic. The payment of doctors is an impassioned issue throughout the world. But a visitor to many countries is struck by the complexities, the dependence of medical services on many administrative conditions besides pay alone, and the fact that evil and unselfish virtue are never completely isolated on opposite sides. By discussing these complexities, I hope to shift the debate to the more sober plane of research findings and pragmatic administrative experimentation.

I make no attempt to discredit doctors by emphasizing their self-interested behavior to the exclusion of their social services. A book about the payment of any occupation necessarily must concentrate on how individuals increase their incomes and on how the occupation collectively presses to improve the reward system. Since doctors behave like any other professionals, this reasoning applies to them as well, despite their defensiveness on the subject. This sensitivity has various sources: the common rhetoric among the medical profession and among the public that treatment is and should be motivated by nonpecuniary humanitarian impulses; the polemics over payment systems; and the embarrassing fact that doctors strive further to raise incomes that already are among society's highest. But every professional pursues society's interests as well as his own, and the problem of social organization is to create a reward system enabling him to maximize both.

I do not present any pet scheme about how health services should be run and how doctors should be paid. One's preconceptions soon fade after investigating the great variety of systems and outcomes abroad. Instead of telling America—or any other country—how it should organize itself, this manuscript will describe numerous pitfalls, conditions under which medical goals are not fulfilled, and conditions that result in greater satisfaction. No simple administrative technique can be adopted with automatic success.

Each country's planners must fit a system to their own conditions, and only trial-and-error will reveal its potential for success.

Methods of Research

This book is one product of a study of the social organization of medical care in a number of countries.[3] From May 1961 through August 1962 I visited the following countries and interviewed informants about medical organization: England, Sweden, the Netherlands, West Germany, France, Switzerland, Spain, Italy, Greece, Poland, the Soviet Union, Turkey, Cyprus, Lebanon, Egypt, and Israel. Also, I visited the World Health Organization's main headquarters, its European Regional Office, and its Eastern Mediterranean Regional Office. In each country I interviewed some or all of the following persons: the international relations officer, the chief medical officer, and other officials of the principal national health insurance fund; secretaries and presidents of the medical, nursing, and hospital associations; professors in medical and nursing schools; lay administrators, medical directors, and matrons of some hospitals; doctors in polyclinics and in office practice; private office practitioners; young house officers and undergraduate medical students; and scholars who have done research about the medical profession. Some of my informants were participants in the official meetings that fixed doctors' pay. In each country, I visited between two and ten hospitals for information about the entire hospital organization. I reinterviewed some of my German, Dutch, and French informants during 1966. Most interviews were conducted in English or French. Interpreters were used in a few interviews in the U.S.S.R. and Germany. Usually the informant and I were alone. My principal informants are listed in the appendix.

In addition to interviews and examination of organizational files, the research has included an extensive review of the literature. Many footnotes are annotated bibliographies, and therefore no single bibliography will be presented at the back of the book.

For simplicity in presentation, I shall focus on the principal public method of paying clinicians in each country. In practice, most countries have several payment methods, but I shall not attempt a complete discussion of how every technique operates in every country. Rather, the purpose is to analyze how the chief systems of payment—fee-for-service, salary, and capitation—work in practice in the countries that I visited. Examining the same system in several countries makes it possible to distinguish the effects inherent in the payment method from the effects associated with the national setting.

[3] The other principal publication is a cross-national comparison of the social structure of hospitals. William A. Glaser, *Medical Organization and the Social Setting* (New York: Atherton Press, 1969). For an overview of the workings and consequences of the national health insurance schemes and national health services described in this book, see William A. Glaser, "Socialized Medicine in Practice," *Public Interest*, vol. I, no. 3 (Winter 1966), pp. 90–106.

Although data are drawn from national health insurance and national health services, this does not mean I consider these systems normal or preferable. Only organized programs have produced systematic evidence about how they work. Hardly any data have been collected anywhere about completely private transactions between doctor and patient.

Of the sixteen countries I visited, only Lebanon at that time lacked any system of national health insurance or a national health service. While my interviews elicited many speculations about how the almost completely private delivery and payment of medical care worked in practice, and while I obtained reports by practicing doctors about their own work, no reliable evidence existed about general patterns.[4] But although I could not present Lebanon as a case example, implicitly it underlies many pages in this book: I often thought of this medical "state of nature" when speculating about the effects of the introduction of any organized system of medical care.

A book must go to press at a fixed time, but pay rates are always under revision. In order to describe fee schedules and salary scales, I have given examples in local currencies at the time this book was prepared, during the late 1960's. These lists of numbers are designed merely to show the structure of the payment system. By the time the reader sees them, the rates in most cases will have been raised, but the structure of the system will probably not have changed.

Because we are interested in the structure of payment systems rather than in the international equivalence of incomes and services, the text will deal entirely in local currencies. However, I present here a convenient summary of the figures in mid-1969:

Country	Unit of Currency	Value of One Unit Is $
Cyprus	Pound (£)	$2.40
Egypt	Pound (EL)	2.30
England	Pound (£)	2.40
France	Franc (F)	0.18
Germany (Federal Republic)	Deutsche Mark (DM)	0.25
Greece	Drachma	0.03
Israel	Pound (IL)	0.29
Italy	Lira	0.0016
Lebanon	Pound (LL)	0.32
The Netherlands	Guilder (f.)	0.28
Poland	Zloty	0.04
Spain	Peseta (pta.)	0.017
Sweden	Krona (Kr.)	0.19
Switzerland	Franc (Fr S)	0.23
Turkey	Lira (TL)	0.09
U.S.S.R.	Ruble	1.10

[4] The speculations were summarized in one of the rare publications about Lebanese medical practice, François Dupré La Tour, "Médecins et malades au Liban," *Travaux et jours*, no. 3 (October–December 1961), pp. 21–39.

II

ORGANIZED SYSTEMS OF MEDICAL CARE

Before the modern development of nationwide organized systems of financing and paying for medical care, medicine was practiced in several ways. A particular country might present all or a few. Some were more common than others, and patterns changed from time to time. One was the free practitioner whose relationships with the patient were exclusive and private in both the delivery and payment of care. Another was the contract physician, with some sort of relationship with an association of consumers who prepaid costs by a subscription fee. A third type of doctor was an employee or officer of the governing authority. An individual physician might specialize in one of these roles or might divide his time among several.

The Free Practitioner

The independent entrepreneur has existed in the actual history of all countries, as well as in the folklore of the medical profession. But, like any entrepreneur, he has been able to survive only if market conditions enabled him to cover his costs. As long as medicine used intuitive diagnostic techniques and treatments that were few, portable, and cheap, the free practitioner could treat patients with minimum expense in his own home or in the patient's home. For many centuries in Europe and elsewhere numerous physicians could work in this manner and meet their costs from fees paid directly by patients according to the individual doctor's price schedule.

The fee in private practice is set according to some combination of the following factors:[1]

[1] Adapted from, Jules Backman, "Factors Affecting Fee Setting in the Professions," *Journal of Accountancy*, vol. 95, no. 5 (May 1953), pp. 554–66. On the decisionmaking and effects of the "sliding scale"—i.e., fixing fees according to the patients' ability to pay, see Herbert Klarman, *The Economics of Health* (New York: Columbia University Press, 1965), pp. 20–22, and sources cited therein.

1. Cost of service rendered:
    a. Expenses incurred—office expense, capital equipment, etc.
    b. Time involved
2. Patient demand:
    a. Number of patients
    b. Each patient's ability to pay
3. Value of service rendered:
    a. Success or failure
    b. Importance of the disease to the survival of the patient
    c. Complexity of the treatment
4. Customary fees in the community
5. Whether the client is the doctor's regular patient
6. Limitations under the law or under the rules of professional associations

The existence of criteria other than simple market competition reflects the presence of monopolistic restrictions and bargaining advantages in every medical market. Sellers can pass on their costs to buyers and can vary prices according to each buyer's ability to pay only if they regulate competition among themselves and only if buyers lack knowledge about alternative sellers.[2] National health insurance and national health services are attempts to organize the buyers.

An entrepreneurial model cannot fit situations where services are rendered most efficiently on a large scale. For this reason, the classical free practitioner has been unable to dispense all kinds of care for several centuries, and the limitation—if not obsolescence—of the role has become increasingly evident since the scientific innovations of the nineteenth and twentieth centuries. Many years ago the isolation, housing, and feeding of patients with acute infectious illnesses were clearly more efficient in large hospital buildings with nursing staffs and with kitchens than in scattered private homes. The traditional custodial and housing functions of hospitals were combined with newer diagnostic and therapeutic functions, as the buildings acquired the equipment, chemicals, electric power, and technical staffs demanded by modern science. The economies of scale applied to ambulatory as well as inpatient care: the most economical arrangement and the best guarantees of high-quality care in many countries have been to use the hospital's facilities in an outpatient department or to create special facilities in a polyclinic for ambulatory patients. Thus doctor and patient meet on a site and use materials that neither owns. Even the personal doctor-patient relationship has been altered in many of these encounters: instead of being retained by an individual patient, the doctor might be called upon by an organization to treat

[2] How private professional markets deviate from perfect competitive markets is described by D. S. Lees, *Economic Consequences of the Professions* (London: Institute of Economic Affairs, 1966).

a number of patients who merely happened to be in a building at the same time.

In Europe, and in other countries experiencing these developments, medical professions that prized the model of the free practitioner found it difficult to reconcile their traditional payment systems with the essentially new working conditions in hospitals and polyclinics. In many countries, payment was not made; for several centuries doctors categorized their hospital work as a charitable donation of their time. As the hospital became the experimental laboratory of modern clinical science, many specialists welcomed the opportunity to learn new techniques in return for their donated services. Another formula during the twentieth century was a barter of time for privileges: in return for treating hospital or polyclinic patients whom he did not know, the doctor was given the right to treat his private patients in the building, with the aid of the facilities and staff that he could not buy and manage himself. Paid nothing for several hours of hospital work each week, many doctors continued to earn all their income from fees of private patients, and thus the traditional model of free practitioner was preserved. In a few countries, the organization owning the hospital or polyclinic paid the doctors small sums for their time, but, significantly, these were called "honoraria"—gifts—and the physicians clearly were not receiving salaries or fees commensurate with their normal income, nor did they incur any obligations.[3]

The increasingly complex and expensive forms of medical care could be integrated with the entrepreneurial model of medical practice only if the doctor could afford to buy and manage his own hospital. But this was possible only if the doctor had enough patients capable of paying high fees. In most countries, proprietary hospitals (private clinics) arose during the twentieth century, owned by fashionable specialists with predominantly wealthy clienteles. The more affluent the country—such as the United States and France—the greater the number of private clinics. But this has been a precarious basis for independent medical practice: private clinics could not exist if scientific progress and government regulatory standards raised their costs beyond the patients' purchasing power.

Besides the tendency of modern care to require expensive collectivized facilities, the model of the free practitioner has encountered another fundamental challenge. Small businessmen merchandising most goods and services need not be troubled by customers without means: they are obligated to sell only to those who can pay. But a fundamental and growing belief in modern times is that medical care is a humanitarian right and should be provided

[3] At any one time, of course, several different payment arrangements were being used in each country, according to the character of the hospitals and the roles of the doctor. The use of honoraria in British voluntary hospitals and the use of salaries for some staff members of public hospitals are described in, Brian Abel-Smith, *The Hospitals 1800–1945* (London: William Heinemann, 1964), chaps. 1, 3, 4, 9, and 19 passim.

regardless of ability to pay and without a sliding scale of fees. Therefore, the basic conception of medical care as the purchase of doctors' services by individual patients has been challenged.[4]

The often-quoted Preamble to the Constitution of the World Health Organization states:

> The States Parties to this Constitution declare, in conformity with the Charter of the United Nations, that the following principles are basic to the happiness, harmonious relations and security of all peoples:
>
> Health is a state of complete physical, mental and social well-being and not merely the absence of disease or infirmity.
>
> The enjoyment of the highest attainable standard of health is one of the fundamental rights of every human being without distinction of race, religion, political belief, economic or social condition. . . .
>
> Governments have a responsibility for the health of their peoples which can be fulfilled only by the provision of adequate health and social measures.

Contractual Relations with an Association

For centuries the European population has understood the economic risks of illness: at times when considerable expenditures might be necessary to pay practitioners or hospitals, the patient's purchasing power diminishes. Therefore, many countries have long had private associations designed to spread risks and prepay costs by regular subscriptions. Some of these associations were specially organized for medical care alone; others were guilds, trade unions, social clubs, or religious societies that added medical insurance to their other functions. Often these "sick funds" established regular arrangements with particular physicians, whereby the doctors would charge reasonable fees—perhaps according to the funds' schedules—and they alone would care for the subscribers.

In Germany, for example, guilds and other associations survived long after the Middle Ages. In the absence of a strong state, these associations multiplied and provided many social welfare functions for the working classes. Some associations consisted of persons in the same occupation in several localities; others recruited persons only from the same community. A variety of service benefits arrangements were made between local funds and local doctors: salaried, capitation, and fee-for-service schemes could be found

[4] How changing conditions throughout medical practice altered the entrepreneurial model in the United States is described in, Odin W. Anderson, "The Medical Profession and the Public: An Examination of Interrelationships" (Chicago: Center for Health Administration Studies, University of Chicago, 1966). The resultant changes in the market for medical care are discussed in, Manuel Gottlieb, "Some Aspects of the Pricing Problem in Medical Care" (unpublished paper presented at the meetings of the American Association for the Advancement of Science, 1963).

in different localities and often among different funds in the same community. A few funds, particularly those whose members were wealthier and who patronized higher-priced private office practitioners, gave their members cash benefits as a partial contribution to the doctors' bills.[5]

As I shall explain in greater detail later, "capitation" is the method of paying a doctor a fixed annual sum for each person on a list, regardless of whether they become ill. The doctor usually is expected to give all necessary care without extra charges.

Benefit societies of many kinds existed in England after the Reformation. Some were antecedents of trade unions, but also collected and distributed money for members' welfare; some were social clubs with supplementary welfare functions; others were bureaucratic insurance organizations that did nothing but collect and distribute money for the subscribers' welfare. Many were called "Friendly Societies," and Parliament passed several laws regulating them for the members' protection and encouraging their growth. Some offered medical benefits, although the services varied according to the affluence of each Society's membership and treasury. Many Friendly Societies sponsored closed panel medical practice on the basis of capitation fees—i.e., one or more doctors would contract with a Society to provide all necessary general practitioner care to the members for a fixed annual fee per member, and members could seek their benefits only from those doctors. Some Societies provided medical benefits under different arrangements, such as salaried doctors, but the capitation system spread widely as the result of voluntary agreement between Societies and doctors, particularly in working class districts.[6]

Perhaps no country has had so long and continuous a history of health insurance as Holland. Medical clubs have existed in Holland since the Middle Ages, with only a brief interruption during the Napoleonic occupation. Some were sponsored by medieval guilds and modern trade unions, some resembled commercial insurance funds, some were part of the religious movements that have always been central forces in Dutch organizational life, and others were sponsored by other groups. By 1940 about 650 sick funds existed, with a great range in affluence, membership, administrative procedure, and benefits. Many doctors were retained by "sick clubs" on the latter's terms. In addition, many free practitioners after 1800 organized their own prepayment funds as a method of protecting their incomes. By establishing their own prepayment schemes, the doctors earned higher fees and avoided de-

[5] The history of German sick funds before the national health insurance law of 1883 appears in, Horst Peters, *Die Geschichte der Sozialversicherung* (Bad Godesberg: Asgard-Verlag, 1959), pp. 17–37; and Walter Vogel, *Bismarcks Arbeiterversicherung* (Brunswick: Georg Westermann Verlag, 1951), chap. 3, and sources cited therein.

[6] R. W. Harris, *National Health Insurance in Great Britain 1911–1946* (London: George Allen & Unwin, 1946), chaps. 3, 4, and 10.

pendence on the lay-dominated, sometimes penny-pinching, and sometimes unfriendly organizations run by labor unions and churches.

By joining any of these groups Dutch patients obtained better doctors and more services. Members' weekly subscriptions often were passed directly on to the doctor in the form of capitation fees. For the city doctor with a predominantly lower-class clientele, these funds and the capitation system solved his collection problems; for other city doctors, the system enabled them to salvage some payment from their lower-class patients, but basically their income came from private practice paid for by fee-for-service. In many Dutch villages, where cash incomes were generally low, such prepayment methods became common. Many small towns had one or two doctors who agreed to give all necessary care to anyone who prepaid costs by a weekly contribution. Thus all or most of the villagers constituted the doctors' lists, and most of the doctors' incomes might come from capitation.[7]

Officers of the Governing Authority

Many governments in the past retained physicians full-time or part-time for a variety of tasks. Some gave care to the poor in public hospitals. Others practiced in remote parts of the country. Some were sanitary inspectors or performed other medical tasks of a public and nonclinical sort. All received substantial salaries. Usually their status was somewhat above that of a salaried government employee. Even in the unusual instances when they shared the same salary scale as other civil servants—as in the British and French colonial services—physicians fell into the higher pay groups.

Sweden, for example, has had a long tradition of physicians receiving salaries from the government, but the doctors are not considered on a par with other civil servants. For many centuries the monarchy has been conceived as a benevolent force in Swedish life, as the organizer of social welfare and of other programs benefiting the people. Before the Reformation, the Roman Catholic Church had sponsored medical services, as it had elsewhere in Europe, but these disappeared when the Church was banished. The Crown then had to create new secular medical services. During the sixteenth century, and later, many foreign doctors were invited to enter "the King's service," to give medical care to the army, the Court, and the public, and to give medical courses at the universities. Young Swedes studied at medical schools, first on the continent and later at home, and they returned to take jobs in the King's service. All these jobs were salaried. At the end of the

[7] Historical information about Dutch health insurance appears in, L. V. Ledeboer, "Medical Care Insurance in the Netherlands," *Bulletin of the International Social Security Association*, vol. 11, no. 9 (September 1958), pp. 397–99; and Arthur Newsholme, *International Studies on the Relation between the Private and Official Practice of Medicine* (London: George Allen & Unwin, 1931), 1: 23–26.

eighteenth century, a network of district medical officers was nominally appointed by the King (actually in the King's name by the Royal Medical Board) to care for the poor and to oversee health conditions in individual districts of the country.

Types of National Medical Systems

Pressures to improve the organization and financing of medical care through public action have come from several sources. In many countries for the past century, workers, farmers, and the aged in certain regions have complained about maldistribution of doctors, hospitals, and facilities; or they have complained that the available doctors and installations were too expensive. Within governments, the political parties of the Left and the trade unions often have campaigned for reforms of medical organization and for better planning; sometimes authoritarian governments of the Right have reorganized and expanded medical services in order to gain the favor of the hostile lower classes. Administrators in public health and hospital administration have also initiated proposals to create more integrated systems of installations and of personnel who were formerly independent, on the grounds that modern clinical techniques can be used most effectively and economically on a larger scale, with differentiation and specialization of units and people, and with better coordination.

The two forms of large-scale medical organization that have spread during the twentieth century are national health insurance and national health services. National health insurance schemes exist in most European countries and in the more affluent nations elsewhere, such as Australia, New Zealand, and the United States. National health services are still rare—Great Britain, the Soviet Union, and China are the only large countries in which they function—but they are bound to spread in the world because they are the nuclei for medical care in many underdeveloped countries.[8] The central differences between the two systems are the methods of financing and the extent of coverage. Under national health insurance, taxes are levied on employees and their employers, the proceeds are deposited in special funds, and the funds pay for medical care. Under national health services, medical care is financed from the national treasury. Usually only payers of payroll taxes and their dependents can draw health insurance benefits, but every citizen by right can use a national health service.[9]

[8] The proportions of all doctors in government service are low in most Western countries but are very high in Asia and Africa. *World Health Statistics Annual 1962* (Geneva: World Health Organization, 1966), 3: 18–42.

[9] Good descriptions of national health insurance in many countries appear in *Social Security Programs throughout the World* (Washington: Division of Research and Statistics, Social Security Administration, U.S. Department of Health, Education, and Welfare, revised ed., 1969); "Volume and Cost of Sickness Benefits in Kind and Cash," *Bulletin of*

National Health Insurance

Germany

The first national health insurance law was enacted by the *Reichstag* in 1883, on Chancellor Otto von Bismarck's recommendation. Administrative rationality might dictate creation of a single government insurance fund, since overhead costs and conflicts would be reduced, but in Germany, as in other countries later, a number of voluntary sick funds already existed. Among the numerous concessions made by nearly every government to implement the inauguration of a new system has been the régime's agreement to allow the existing funds to survive and to acquire official status. Another motive of the government is to save the trouble of setting up completely new machinery. In practice, the pre-existing sick funds become the depositories for money collected by government taxation, and they pay for their members' disability allowances, medical care, hospitalization, and drugs in accordance with statutes and public regulations. This was the German plan.

At present, health insurance is compulsory for all workers with annual incomes of 10,800 DM or less, for most pensioners, and for many self-employed persons. Some groups may join voluntarily. The insured person is fully covered and all his dependents get limited coverage. About 85 per cent of the population is covered. As in nearly all other countries with national health insurance, the upper income groups and certain self-employed persons must rely on private medical care—perhaps supported by private health insurance—and most of those that are unemployed must rely on public charity. One of the differences among countries is inclusion of the farm population; they are covered in Germany. The German system is financed by equal taxes on workers' earnings and on employers' earnings. The taxes do not fall disproportionately on employers, nor does the government offer subsidies, two facts that severely limit the resources of the funds and the fees of the doctors.

Legislation requires the individual to join one of the sick funds. Formerly as many as 20,000 funds existed concurrently, but today about 2,000 remain, after consolidations required by legislative reforms. Two-thirds of the funds

---

the International Social Security Association, vol. 16, nos. 3–4 (March–April 1963), plus the series of mimeographed reports under the same title; *Évolution et tendances de la sécurité sociale* (Geneva: International Social Security Association, 1959); K. C. Charron, *Health Services, Health Insurance, and Their Inter-Relationship* (Ottawa: Department of National Health and Welfare, 1963); John Simpson, "European Medical Care Systems," *Medical World*, vol. 95, no. 1 (July 1961), pp. 11–15; G. Teeling-Smith, "Health Services in Western Europe," *Medical Care*, vol. 3, no. 2 (April–June 1965), pp. 103–14; J. F. Follmann, Jr., *Medical Care and Health Insurance* (Homewood, Ill.: Richard D. Irwin, 1963), chaps. 2 and 3; and "Medical Care Protection under Social Security Schemes: A Statistical Study of Selected Countries," *International Labour Review*, vol. 89, no. 6 (June 1964), pp. 570–93.

are small ones for individual factories or for groups of business firms. Over half the population belongs to the *Ortskrankenkassen*, serving persons in a specific geographical area, and the proportion of their subscribers will probably continue to grow. Since the law requires persons to join a fund without specifying the type, sixteen *Ersatzkassen* (substitute funds) have developed, offering higher benefits in return for higher tax contributions. Many white-collar and some industrial workers not committed to employer-sponsored funds have joined *Ersatzkassen;* their subscribers number about one-fifth of the population, and their popularity may be growing. Because of Germany's tradition of local autonomy and because of the federal structure of the government the local sick funds and the *Land* (i.e., provincial) federations of funds have considerable power in prescribing their own benefits and in making their own arrangements with local medical societies and with hospitals. Even Hitler did not completely centralize and standardize the funds, and the *Land* offices of the funds and medical societies have regained most of the power they temporarily lost during his régime. Some national uniformity is achieved through laws and the central offices of each type of fund. For example, the practices of the geographical sick funds are co-ordinated (but, of course, not completely standardized) by a national office called the *Bundesverband der Ortskrankenkassen.*

The insured patient may go to any doctor who has been admitted to insurance practice. The patient gets a ticket (called a *Krankenschein*), either from his local sick fund office or from his employer, which he presents to the doctor. The ticket performs several functions. It notifies the doctor that the patient is currently covered by health insurance. It bears a calendar upon which the doctor notes all treatments, and it becomes his bill submitted to the Insurance Doctors' Association. During the depression, when there were large deficits in the sick funds, charges were made for the tickets, and they were a vital source of revenue and a check upon excessive use of doctors. This charge is no longer levied. During each quarter of the year, the patient gets one ticket. He may change his doctor at any time, but the red-tape of getting a second ticket probably holds him until the quarter ends. The patient may go directly either to a G.P. or to a specialist. Supplementary documents cover referrals. The insurance doctor is obligated to care for every insured patient who visits his office or requests a medically legitimate house call. Accepting this obligation is a condition for the doctor's admission into insurance practice. It is illegal for him to charge the patient for medically necessary work, since he is paid in full when he sends his tickets for the quarter to the office that administers payment. If the patient requests a home or office visit that the doctor deems medically unnecessary, he may charge the patient a private fee, but he cannot send a ticket listing that procedure to the payment office.

Amid the variety of sick funds, co-ordination is achieved by several public bodies. The *Bundestag* enacts legislation and the Ministry of Labor and Social Affairs announces general guidelines. Federal, state, and regional insurance offices directly supervise the sick funds and the federal and state co-ordinating offices. The organization of the medical profession also brings about some unity. As we shall see, all doctors in insurance practice belong to special associations that bargain with the various sick funds and remunerate the doctors according to standardized fee schedules.[10]

Other Countries with Numerous Sick Funds

A melange of sick funds with their attendant administrative complexity is the rule rather than the exception under national health insurance, because of the success of the private funds in gaining official status after the enactment of the statute. Over one hundred sick funds exist in Holland at present, and most insured persons have the opportunity to choose among several in their locality. Most funds have evolved out of earlier schemes organized by medical societies and by individual doctors, sometimes in collaboration with laymen. Other funds are sponsored by trade unions, religious associations, and industrial firms. As in most national health insurance schemes, coverage is based on employment and thus is not universal. Income limits change by law from time to time. In the late 1960's, all employees with annual incomes of no more than 12,400 guilders (abbreviated f.) a year must be covered; elderly persons with incomes of no more than f. 6,260 and persons other than employees with incomes of no more than f. 12,400 may join voluntarily. The payroll tax is paid partly by the employee and partly by the employer, for persons insured compulsorily, and is paid in full by those persons insured voluntarily. Benefits extend to the insured person's spouse and minor children. About half the population is insured compulsorily and about twenty per cent voluntarily. Amendments to the original law of 1941 have expanded coverage by including new groups and raising the income ceiling. The very poor, the very rich, and many farmers are not covered by national health insurance and must seek care by private fees, through commercial health insurance, or from charity.

Sufficient uniformity is achieved in Holland by several co-ordinating bodies, as in Germany. Laws of the Parliament set forth general principles

[10] Descriptions of German national health insurance at present can be found in *Évolution et tendances de la sécurité sociale: Allemagne* (Geneva: International Social Security Association, 1959); Rolf Schlögell, *Bundesrepublik Deutschland* (Cologne: Kassenärztliche Bundesvereinigung, 1962); and Reimer Schmidt and Walter Bogs, "Krankenversicherung," *Handwörterbuch der Sozialwissenschaften* (Stuttgart: Gustav Fischer, 1959), 6: 276–96. The organization of the principal sick funds is described in the special issue of the periodical *Die Ortskrankenkasse*, vol. 42, nos. 9–10 (1–15 May 1960). The laws and administrative regulations governing the sick funds can be found in several volumes in the series "Fortbildung und Praxis," published by Asgard Verlag in Bad Godesberg.

and are administered by the Ministry of Social Affairs and Public Health. Each sick fund of a certain type belongs to a national association—for example, all the sick funds originally created by the medical profession—and these associations in turn belong to a co-ordinating body with a secretariat called the *Ziekenfondsraad* (Sick Funds Council). All tax collections and medical payments are administered by a single office—the State Insurance Bank. The Royal Dutch Medical Association represents doctors throughout the country in dealings with the sick funds and takes a special interest in the funds which doctors founded and which still include medical representation on their governing boards.[11]

Italy is an example of a country with many largely unco-ordinated sick funds. Since 1927, the promotion of health insurance has been public policy, but the numerous pre-existing sick funds were allowed to administer the program. Through subsequent laws and decrees more categories of the population were encouraged or required to subscribe to a fund, taxes were levied on workers and employers, and the funds were obligated to follow certain official procedures. Compulsory health insurance was made law in 1943, and the separate sick funds for workers in industry, agriculture, commerce, banking, and the insurance business were merged into an official body, called the *Istituto Nazionale per l'Assistenza Malattie ai Lavoratori* (INAM); subsequently the name was changed to the *Istituto Nazionale per l'Assicurazione contro le Malattie*, but the initials for the original title are still used. Over 80 per cent of the population now is covered by some form of compulsory health insurance, and half belong to INAM. The rest subscribe to funds for particular medical problems (such as tuberculosis and industrial accidents) and for special occupations (such as seamen, journalists, independent farmers, etc.). Each sick fund has its own procedures and scale of benefits; since equalization accounts are not provided by the government from general taxation, some funds are wealthier than others. INAM itself has not unified the separate programs from which it originated; some groups continue to have separate accounts, benefits, and fee schedules.

The number of organizations is criticized by many Italian leaders on the grounds of conflicting policies, unnecessary duplication of services, scattered responsibility for the same patient, and excessive costs; and many hope all health insurance eventually will be merged and truly unified under INAM, or some other body. Meanwhile, the separate funds continue to exist as autonomous public bodies outside the government structure, and they have enough money and political allies to resist reorganization. Democratic legis-

[11] Dutch health insurance is described in, L. V. Ledeboer, *De Ziekenfondsverzekering in Nederland* (Amsterdam: Ziekenfondsraad, 1965); and Ledeboer, "Medical Care Insurance in the Netherlands," *Bulletin of the International Social Security Association*, vol. 11, no. 9 (September 1958), pp. 397–413; "Medical Care Insurance in the Netherlands," *International Labour Review*, vol. 79, no. 4 (April 1959), pp. 418–39.

latures shrink from making drastic changes in the organization of medical care, and Italy's coalition Cabinets are too precarious to overcome such powerful vested interests.[12]

Unified Funds

A few countries united their sick funds either at the time national health insurance was first manifested, or shortly thereafter. This is possible only if the state need not cope with a legacy of extensive private health insurance and church-related social welfare programs; and it is possible only if the government is strong. In practice, the administration of the fund is decentralized.

Like many other countries, France between 1928 and 1945 had national health insurance that was basically a legislative support for the numerous formerly private sick funds: certain categories of employee were required to enroll in any of the available funds, and the subscription payments were converted into taxes levied on wages and on the employer. Pledged to reform the social system, the new government in 1945 used its powers to decree the merger of nearly all the sick funds—and certain other social security bodies—into a single hierarchy with "primary funds" at the *département* level and a National Social Security Fund at the top. Only a few special sick funds survive under national health insurance—those for miners, railwaymen, agricultural workers, and a few other groups. Unlike the insurance systems of other countries, for over twenty years the French funds combined collection and payment for maternity, death, and old age, as well as the benefits for medical care, hospitalization, drugs, and disability. Total unification was amended in 1967, in large part to control medical expenditures and to discourage the constant payment of medical deficits from the social security programs with surpluses. Three separate hierarchies of funds were created—for health insurance, family allowances, and old age benefits—under a Central Agency of Social Security Organs. Health insurance remains unified—unlike most other countries—in the sense that only one system of sick funds is official, and only one fund exists in an area.

[12] Italian health insurance is described in, Umberto Borsi and Ferruccio Pergolesi (editors), *Trattato di diritto del lavoro* (Padua: Casa Editrice Dott. Antonio Milani, 1954), vol. 4, esp. pt. 1, pp. 420–40, and pt. 2, pp. 3–164 and 199–219; *Evolution et tendances de la sécurité sociale: Italie* (Geneva: International Social Security Administration, 1959); Comitato di studio per la sicurezza sociale, *Per un sistema di sicurezza sociale in Italia* (Bologna: Societa Editrice Il Mulino, 1965); and *The Italian System of Social Insurance* (Rome: Istituto Nazionale della Previdenza Sociale, 1959). A mixed commission of employers, union representatives, government officials, and experts proposed unification of health insurance and other reforms of the social services in *Relazione preliminare sulla riforma della previdenza sociale* and *Osservazioni e proposte sulla riforma della previdenza sociale* (Rome: Consiglio nazionale dell'economica e del lavoro, 1963). A history of Italian social insurance appears in *Relazione preliminare sulla riforma*, Appendix A.

As in nearly all other countries using the insurance principle, eligibility in France is determined by a statutory list of occupations. All employed and self-employed persons are covered by social security, either by requirement or voluntarily. Although not all enjoy complete social security benefits, all subscribers and their dependents participate in health insurance. Taxes fall heavily on the employer: the employee pays 3.50 per cent of his wage for health insurance up to 14,400 F annually, and the employer adds 11.50 per cent. (For the other social security programs, the employee pays an additional 3 per cent, and the employer an extra 18 per cent.) Like German health insurance, the fund pays the hospital directly for all the patient's costs. But unlike the predominant method elsewhere, the patient first pays the doctor and is reimbursed subsequently by his fund.

The task of co-ordination is simplified by the fact that only one sick fund exists in each area, the funds are organized in a hierarchy leading to Paris, and the laws and supervisory guidelines of the Ministry of Social Affairs apply to all equally. The National Health Insurance Fund is authorized to make transfers in accounts, so that less affluent regions receive benefits comparable to richer areas. A special association, the National Federation of Social Security Organs (FNOSS), supplies advice and information to all funds and acts as common bargaining agent in negotiations with the medical profession and the government.[13]

Sweden too has a simple network of sick funds, with only one to a locality. All are governed by the Sickness Insurance Act of 1953 and come under the regulation of a National Insurance Office. As in France, co-ordination is facilitated by a National Federation of Sickness Funds. Numerous funds arose in the nineteenth century, but duplication was discouraged, before the enactment of compulsory coverage in 1953, by earlier laws requiring all the funds in a specific locality to merge as a condition for receiving government subsidies.

An unusual feature of the Swedish system is that the entire population belongs to the funds and can draw benefits, regardless of employment status. Normally this is possible only in a national health service financed out of general taxation. Usually the insurance principle is based on employment and a small proportion of the population inevitably stays out—the wealthy self-employed who voluntarily abstain and the unemployed who are ineligible. But two-thirds of the Swedish population were already covered under voluntary health insurance, and the purpose of the 1953 statute was to

[13] Information about French health insurance can be found in, Jacques Doublet and Georges Lavau, *Sécurité sociale* (Paris: Presses Universitaires de France, 1957); Pierre Laroque et al., *Les institutions sociales de la France* (Paris: La Documentation Française, 2d ed., 1963); *La sécurité sociale en France* (Paris: La Documentation Française, revised ed., 1965); and Pierre Grandjeat, "L'assurance-maladie en France," *Révue économique*, no. 2 (March 1967), pp. 251–91. Organizational changes after 1967 are described in "La réforme de la sécurité sociale," *Notes et études documentaires*, no. 3452 (5 January 1968).

achieve universality without enacting the national health service that the medical profession opposed. In this respect, Sweden's experience may foreshadow America's in the future: in both countries a large proportion of the population had purchased voluntary health insurance, and the funds were given official status and statutory power in order to accomplish full coverage.[14]

National Health Service

National health insurance is solely a method of collecting money to pay doctors and hospitals. It differs from voluntary insurance only in that it spreads subscriptions over a wider base and can drive more advantageous bargains with the suppliers of services. In practice, as we shall see later in this book, legislators and sick funds adapt the system to please the doctors.

National health services are a more fundamental innovation. The national treasury assumes a much larger share of the country's medical care and thus confronts far higher expenses than do the sick funds under health insurance. The very poor patients are often omitted from health insurance, but must be treated by a health service. Usually more basic changes are made in the working conditions of doctors and in the organization of hospitals. National health services are adopted because national health insurance is incomplete or cannot be financed adequately through payroll taxes.

Soviet Union

The bureaucratic type of national health service organizes medical care like any other department of the government. Hospitals and polyclinics are nationalized. Physicians become employees or officials of a branch of the civil service. Any citizen may use the medical facilities regardless of his status as employee or taxpayer, with no charge or with nominal charges. Doctors and medical installations receive their money from the Treasury.

The Soviet Union has the world's most extensive national health service, but it evolved gradually. Before the Revolution, Russian medical care was administered by a variety of public and private medical plans, small sick funds, and a limited amount of private office practice. The new government expanded the salaried service, both by necessity and conviction. It assumed power in a country ruined by war and depression, disorganized, and beset by epidemics. As any other government would have had to do, it established a salaried public medical service to cope with the emergency. As zealous Marxists, the new leaders were probably predisposed toward organizing the

[14] For accounts of Swedish national health insurance, see Ernst Michanek, *Sjukförsäkring för Alla* (Stockholm: Tidens Forlag, 2d ed., 1960); *Social Sweden* (Stockholm: Social Welfare Board, 1952); and Konrad Persson, *Social Welfare in Sweden* (Stockholm: Föreningen för Främjande av Folkpensionering och Annan Allmän Försäkring, 2d ed., 1961).

entire economy into a series of salaried and centrally directed public bureaucracies. Eventually the Soviet medical service became a comprehensive national structure characterized by national ownership of all facilities, salaried public employment of virtually all medical personnel, and central direction pursuant to plans. But the growth of the system was spasmodic.

Economic histories of the early years of Soviet Russia reveal much uncertainty over how the economy would be organized. Since Russia was the first socialist country, the leaders had no guiding precedents. The Revolution had occurred in an overwhelmingly agricultural country whose population lacked rational skills and Marxist loyalties, which made the problem particularly baffling. For many years there were debates and conflicting programs—e.g., whether factories should be part of State bureaucracies or owned by autonomous workers' councils; whether trade unions had any place in a Socialist society—until Stalin with characteristic decisiveness created new industrial installations and made them units of a centrally directed bureaucracy. Likewise, many years passed before the medical services were fixed in their present form.

Within a year of the Revolution, the government created a Commissariat of Health to plan and direct all medical work in the country. The national health service of later years was not fully envisioned, and the system of the 1920's had many features of a more limited health insurance program. Europeans of this period were already familiar with health insurance, and the name and some of the administrative details were used in the Russian system. All factories and employing organizations—whether owned by the government, by trade union councils, or by private persons—were supposed to give up to 20 per cent of their wage bill to the government to pay for social insurance. The workers and their dependents—but not the more numerous peasants and other self-employed persons—were entitled to receive free medical care from the salaried doctors employed by health departments or by other government agencies. In 1937 health was taken out of the social insurance program and made a public service available to all and financed out of general tax revenues.[15]

From its beginning the new government has consisted of a hierarchy of Soviets (i.e., councils), with each following directives from the higher level. At the top was the Supreme Soviet of Russia—since reorganized and renamed the Supreme Soviet of the U.S.S.R. At the bottom of the hierarchy was (and is) the soviet of the city, town, or rural district. The local soviet administers public facilities, including all medical services. The departments of health of local soviets thus are the principal employers of doctors in the country.

[15] Much of Soviet social welfare continues to operate on insurance principles with respect to finance, coverage, and size of benefits. For a description, see Charles I. Schottland et al., *A Report on Social Security Programs in the Soviet Union* (Washington: Social Security Administration, 1960); and Bernice Madison, *Social Welfare in the Soviet Union* (Stanford: Stanford University Press, 1968).

In addition, some doctors have salaried jobs with factories, railroads, the armed forces, and other government agencies. The administrative and technical hierarchy is staffed by doctors, and therefore the physician can rise from the ranks into posts with more skill, authority, and pay.

From the start, the Soviet medical services have given general medical care in an organized setting. The average doctor does not see patients in a private office but in a polyclinic or hospital constructed by the government. Although Westerners often think of the polyclinic as a novelty and as a special peculiarity of the U.S.S.R., it is neither. The provision of general medical care by salaried doctors working in polyclinics had been common in Poland, Hungary, and some other parts of the Austro-Hungarian Empire for decades before the Russian Revolution. If doctors lack the resources to equip properly their personal offices, the Ministry of Health or sick funds may have to guarantee adequate facilities by building polyclinics; thus polyclinics are now spreading through some of the less wealthy European countries and may eventually become common in the underdeveloped countries. The Bolsheviks simply adopted a pre-existing Eastern European institution well suited to their needs.

Then, as now, a physician giving general medical care (the *vrach*) was assigned to a small district (an *uchastok*); all residents of the district automatically were assigned to him; several *uchastok* doctors had their offices in a polyclinic for a larger district (a *rayon*). The numerous factory doctors also work in government-owned clinics. An employed person often consults the doctor in his factory or place of employment, instead of staying home and visiting his *uchastok* doctor. The general practitioner on his own still exists in rural areas, but his status is not unlike that of an urban *vrach*, since his house may be owned by the collective farm and some of his equipment may be supplied by the government. Few rural medical officers were appointed during the 1920's, since the limited number of doctors were hired to care for the city dwellers covered by health insurance, since most peasants were not covered, and since the government and the peasants were enemies. Because coverage is now universal, numerous solo *vrach* jobs are available in the countryside, but many remain unfilled, since doctors prefer polyclinic or hospital jobs in the cities.[16]

[16] Detailed descriptions of contemporary Soviet medical organization have been published by Mark G. Field, *Soviet Socialized Medicine: An Introduction* (New York: Free Press, 1967); Ksemja V. Maistrakh, *The Organization of Public Health in the U.S.S.R.* (Washington: National Institutes of Health, 1959); S. A. Podolnyi, *Organizatsiya Raboty Poliklinik Gorodskikh Bol'nits* (Moscow: MEDGIZ, 1955). The early years of Soviet medicine are reported in, Anna J. Haines, *Health Work in Soviet Russia* (New York: Vanguard Press, 1928). The daily work of polyclinics and practicing physicians is described in R. S. Saxton, "Soviet General Practitioners and Polyclinics," *British Medical Journal Supplement* (17 August 1957), pp. 95–97; T. F. Fox, "Russia Revisited: Impressions of Soviet Medicine," *Lancet* (9 and 16 October 1954), pp. 748–53, 803–7; and C. Fraser Brockington, "Public Health in Russia," ibid. (21 July 1956), pp. 138–41.

Underdeveloped Countries

The Soviet Union adopted a national health service after national health insurance proved inadequate to meet the needs of the people for medical care. This trend may be followed by all other countries of limited means, because they lack the economic base for successful insurance. Since insurance usually covers only those in salaried occupations, a large proportion of the population remains unprotected—e.g., farmers, farm laborers, the urban unemployed, peddlers, handicraftsmen, and their numerous dependents. Because wages are low, accidents are common, and dependents are numerous and disease-ridden, the yield from payroll taxes is inadequate to pay for subscribers' medical care. Hospitals and polyclinics usually are incapable of providing services to the insured without drastic improvement and reorganization.

Usually an underdeveloped country inherits from its departing colonial master a salaried medical service of doctors who work in urban hospitals and in urban and rural polyclinics. Private practitioners are available to those who can pay fees; often the salaried government doctors have a part-time private practice. The private practitioners are patronized regularly by the wealthier classes and occasionally by the urban masses. The urban and rural public usually is treated free or for a nominal charge by the salaried doctor at publicly owned facilities, by folk practitioners charging low private fees, or by no-one. When the public becomes accustomed to seeking scientific modern medicine, the public health services are soon overwhelmed by masses of patients. The Ministry of Health then tries to expand the national health service, to the limits of the available money and personnel.[17]

Great Britain

Even a nation as wealthy as England turned to a national health service when its national health insurance was inadequate to arrest a decline in medical care. Between 1912 and 1948, Britain had National Health Insurance. Basically, this was a regularization and extension by Act of Parliament of the pre-existing medical programs of the Friendly Societies. The statute made

[17] On the economic difficulties confronting social insurance in underdeveloped countries, see J. Henry Richardson, *Economic and Financial Aspects of Social Security* (London: George Allen & Unwin, 1960), chap. 11. For an example of a troubled health insurance scheme, see S. S. Kulkarni, "Evolution of State Medical Aid," *Indian Journal of Medical Science*, vol. 11, no. 12 (December 1957), pp. 973–82. For reports of the early development and problems of a national health service in one underdeveloped country, see John R. McGibony, "Health Care in India: Its Patterns and Problems," *Hospitals* (*J.A.H.A.*), vol. 35, no. 10 (16 May 1961), pp. 40–44, 126, and no. 11 (1 June 1961), pp. 47–52; Reginald E. Rewell, "Medicine in the New India," *Lancet* (13 September 1958), pp. 574–77; E. D. Churchill, "Reflections on the Challenge to the Medical Profession in India," *New England Journal of Medicine*, vol. 259, no. 12 (18 September 1958), pp. 551–57; and "Medical Needs of India," *Lancet* (3 January 1960), pp. 265–66.

coverage compulsory for certain occupational groups, prescribed the rates of payment by subscriber to sick fund and from sick fund to doctor, and specified the administrative procedures and benefits. The Friendly Societies, existing insurance firms, and comparable private organizations were designated as "Approved Societies" to administer the program—the political concession that statutory health insurance programs commonly make to the existing private organizations. As before, the system was basically a way to prepay workers' costs for medical care. Manual workers and some others with low annual incomes were required by law to join an approved society. Middle and upper income groups, many nonmanual workers, and the dependents of insured persons were not covered. One-third of the population was insured. The country's hospitals became antiquated because National Health Insurance did not pay for inpatient care and because their owners—primarily voluntary associations and local governments—could not afford modernization.[18]

The goals of the National Health Service were to universalize coverage and to resuscitate the hospitals. Nearly all hospitals were nationalized. The costs of general practitioner care, outpatient hospital care, inpatient treatments, drugs, other prescriptions, and preventive services were to be met by annual appropriations of Parliament from general tax revenue. Unlike the Soviet Union, Britain's National Health Service does not arrange doctors and installations in a hierarchy ruled from the Ministry of Health. Rather, the Service is a loose hierarchy of committees representing lay and medical groups, following guidelines issued by the Ministry of Health. Physicians sign contracts with these committees to give general or specialized care, but the doctors remain independent professionals rather than members of an administrative command structure. The general practitioners' contracts are with regional Executive Councils; the specialists' contracts designate them "officers" of the Regional Hospital Boards. The more detailed supervision of hospitals rests with the Boards' subordinates, the Hospital Group Management Committees.

In response to the pressures of the medical societies, the working conditions of doctors are much like those under National Health Insurance, or in a well-financed private practice. The principal differences for the doctor are the source of his pay and the greater demand resulting from complete coverage of the population. The general practitioner sees patients in a private office which he has financed or which was financed by a group that he has freely joined. The National Health Service does not own polyclinics employing doctors. The specialist sees patients upon referral by their general practitioners in either the outpatient department or the wards of the hospital.

[18] Hermann Levy, *National Health Insurance* (Cambridge: University Press, 1944); R. W. Harris, *National Health Insurance in Great Britain, 1911–1946* (London: George Allen & Unwin, 1946).

The patient can be treated by any general practitioner who will register. In practice, patients see the specialists whom the general practitioners request or whom the hospital assigns, but patients can obtain transfers, if they do not like the specialists.[19]

To place each country in a total picture, the following chart presents an overview of the principal ways of delivering medical care and paying doctors in the countries I visited. Most countries have a great variety of arrangements, but the chart gives the principal one in each country. The type of system is either national health insurance covering some or all of the population or a national health service with complete coverage. The unit of payment is either fee-for-service, salary, capitation, or case payments. The method is either direct payment to the doctor by the sick funds or government (service benefits) or reimbursement of the patient after he has paid the doctor (cash benefits).

	Type of System	Payment of Specialists		Payment of General Practitioners	
		Unit	Method	Unit	Method
Cyprus	Service	Salary	Direct	Salary	Direct
Egypt	Service	Salary	Direct	Salary	Direct
France	Insurance	Fee	Reimbursement	Fee	Reimbursement
Germany (Federal Republic)	Insurance	Fee	Direct	Fee	Direct
Great Britain	Service	Salary	Direct	Capitation	Direct
Greece	Insurance	Salary	Direct	Salary	Direct
Israel	Insurance	Salary	Direct	Salary	Direct
Italy	Insurance	Salary	Direct	Capitation, fee	Direct
Lebanon (until late 1960's)	None	Fee	Private	Fee	Private
The Netherlands	Insurance	Salary, Fee, Case	Direct	Capitation	Direct
Poland	Service	Salary	Direct	Salary	Direct
Spain	Insurance	Capitation	Direct	Capitation	Direct
Sweden	Insurance	Salary, Fee	Reimbursement	Fee	Reimbursement
Switzerland	Insurance	Fee	Direct, reimbursement	Fee	Direct, reimbursement
Turkey	Insurance	Salary	Direct	Salary	Direct
U.S.S.R.	Service	Salary	Direct	Salary	Direct

[19] Many authoritative books describe the National Health Service, among them, James Stirling Ross, *The National Health Service in Great Britain* (London: Oxford University Press, 1952); Harry Eckstein, *The English Health Service* (Cambridge: Harvard University Press, 1958); Almont Lindsey, *Socialized Medicine in England and Wales* (Chapel Hill: The University of North Carolina Press, 1962); Rosemary Stevens, *Medical Practice in Modern England* (New Haven: Yale University Press, 1966); and Charles Allan Birch, *Medicine in Britain: A Guide for Overseas Doctors* (London: Ballière, Tindall, & Cassell, 1966).

III

TYPES OF PAYMENT: FEE-FOR-SERVICE

The possible ways of paying doctors for medical care are fee-for-service, salary, capitation, and case payment. None are linked inextricably to any way of organizing a country's medical services. National health insurance systems and national health services can be found using each of the payment methods, but national health services tend to use the more predictable device of salary and to avoid fee-for-service. As we shall see in chapter VI, the adoption of a particular payment mechanism results from national tradition and from political maneuvers.

Fee-for-service is payment for each medical procedure. Under "service benefits" or "direct payment" methods, the third party—i.e., the sick fund or the health service—pays the doctor directly, and the patient usually pays him nothing. Under "cash benefits" or "reimbursement" methods, the patient pays the doctor and subsequently regains all or most of the fee from the third party.

Capitation is a fixed annual payment for each person on a list regularly assigned to a doctor. The physician gives all necessary care to the members on the list who come to him. Even if a person never visits him, the doctor automatically collects the capitation fee; even if a person has many medical problems, the doctor usually can collect no more than the capitation fee. Patients usually pay nothing to the doctor.

Salary is a fixed amount of money scaled according to the rank of the job and paid according to the amount of time the doctor gives. Patients usually pay the doctor nothing. Some arrangements allow the doctor to collect fees from the third party, in addition to the salary given for basic care.

Case payments are fixed sums given the doctor for giving a patient all necessary care. They differ from capitation fees, which are paid for persons on a list regardless of illness. Case payments differ from fee-for-service in that payments are not itemized by procedure and totaled. The few case payment systems use the service benefits principle: the third party pays the doctor, and the patient pays nothing.

Service Benefits: The Netherlands

The general sick funds of Holland (*algemene ziekenfondsen*) use the service benefits principle. A subscriber's taxes are deposited in his sick fund, which then pays his physician. Patients pay doctors nothing for care under national health insurance, but any person may see any physician privately outside the scheme and may then pay directly. For patients under national health insurance, specialists work on the basis of fee-for-service and case payments, while general practitioners receive capitation fees.

The patient is regularly assigned to a general practitioner and can see a specialist under health insurance only by referral. The patient must present to the specialist a transfer card (*verwijskaart*) issued by his general practitioner. Senior specialists in the largest Dutch hospitals receive part-time salaries for their teaching, administration, and therapy. Specialists in most hospitals receive all their income from private fees, social security fees, and case payments, earned from both inpatients and outpatients. As in England, most Dutch specialists have hospital affiliations. Those who see private and insured ambulatory patients in the hospital outpatient department are expected to pay an hourly rental to the hospital. The rental is usually so low—perhaps 6 or 8 guilders—that many hospital specialists conduct their entire practice in the hospital and maintain no private offices.

The Dutch fee schedule is longer, more detailed, and more precisely constructed than any other I have seen.[1] Thousands of entries appear under eight classifications or "tariffs." Lessons have been taken from the controversies over health insurance payments in neighboring Germany: many of the specific formulae in the fee schedule are designed to prevent overperformance; other entries aim to prevent or discourage anyone but a fully qualified specialist from collecting a fee.

More than half the fee schedule's pages are occupied by Tariff III, a list of nearly one thousand procedures paid for on a fee-for-service basis. These are chiefly surgical interventions, but some included are in the fields of orthopedics, otorhinolaryngology, ophthalmology, gynecology, and obstetrics. The list includes for each procedure the specialist's fee, the fee for the anesthesiologist (if any), and the fee for the specialist's assistant (if any). Table 1 presents a few very general examples. All entries are in guilders, the exchange rate of which on the free market is currently f. 1 = $0.28.

Most procedures in Tariff III are customarily performed on hospital inpatients, although some are done in the hospital outpatient department. The

[1] The fee schedule in effect at the time of writing is *Tarievan voor de Honorering van Specialistische Hulp en voor de Honorering van Tandheelkundig-Specialistische Hulp door Algemene Ziekenfondsen* (Amsterdam: Ziekenfondsraad, 1966). That monograph's thorough explanatory notes describe the logic of the payment system in detail. New editions with new rates are issued periodically, but usually the schedule retains the same structure.

TABLE 1. EXCERPTS FROM THE FEE SCHEDULE OF THE NETHERLANDS

Specialty and Procedure	Specialist	Anesthe-siologist	Specialist's Assistant
Surgery:			
Appendectomy	68.50	21.50	
Extensive plastic operation	171.00	51.50	42.75
Gastrectomy	155.00	55.50	38.75
Diagnostic gastroscopy	34.25	17.00	
Embolectomy	111.00	42.75	
Intra-cardial operation with use of "artificial heart" equipment	391.00	257.00	98.00 and 49.00
Orthopedics:			
Nonoperative reduction of fracture of femur	103.00	11.50	
Operative reduction of fracture of femur	137.00	51.50	34.25
Nonoperative reduction of fracture of tibia	68.50	11.50	
Operative reduction of fracture of tibia	103.00	34.25	
Otorhinolaryngology:			
Septum resection	60.00	21.50	
Conchotomy	31.25	12.75	
Plastic correction of nasal deformity	120.00	42.75	
Tonsillectomy by age of patient:			
10 and younger	25.75	11.50	
11 through 15	34.25	17.00	
16 and older	51.50	17.00	
Neurology:			
Electroshock treatment	8.50	11.50	
Electro-corticogram	34.25		
Diagnostic intracranial puncture	30.25	17.00	

basic fee includes all necessary preoperative and postoperative care. If the specialist performs several procedures on the same patient at the same time, he collects only fractions of the lower paid ones, according to formulae specified by the fee schedule.

Only major procedures allow employment of an assistant at the expense of the sick funds. Of course a hospital, such as a teaching hospital, can assign one of its salaried junior doctors to assist at any unpaid procedure, but only the specialist and anesthesiologist collect bills from the local offices of the sick funds. Of course, in private practice, the specialist might charge an extra fee for his assistant for a procedure where the funds made no extra payment.

The present fee schedule has been used since 1949. Each year's negotiations make only a few revisions in structure and usually raise the monetary rates generally. The fees for each specialty are negotiated by conferences between representatives of the six principal sick funds and representatives of the specialists' association in that field. Each year's fee schedule—including the capitation payments to general practitioners—must formally be approved by a committee responsible both to the governing board of the *Ziekenfondsraad* and to the government.

The negotiators must make two decisions, the ratio among procedures within the fee schedule and the general financial level of fees. The relative cost of the procedure depends entirely on the time spent in its performance. The negotiating committees pick the appendectomy, the tonsillectomy, the gastrectomy, and the herniorrhaphy as four basic procedures, and the fees for all other procedures are set in ratio to them as the amount of time differs. For example, it is assumed that the operation for an appendectomy takes about twenty minutes, the surgeon has four consultations before and after the operation, and therefore he devotes about an hour to that case. A tonsillectomy for a teenager takes about half the time, and therefore is scheduled at half the fee for an appendectomy. The negotiators usually retain the same ratios each year, but the relative value of a procedure is changed if the time to perform it has increased or decreased substantially.

The criterion of time is used to fix the fees in specialties besides surgery. A procedure costs the same as an appendectomy if it takes an hour; the relative costs of procedures within a specialty's list depend on the time spent on each. The criterion of time makes fees among specialties similar in Holland, more so than in most countries. Elsewhere, the surgeons seem more glamorous and powerful, and surgical fees under national health insurance are much higher than those in other fields. Surgery and obstetrics are believed to be the best-paid fields in Holland too, because of the inherent effects of fee schedules, but their superiority over the medical specialties is narrower.

Several considerations determine the decisions about the general monetary level of fees. The negotiating committees try to fix both the ratio among procedures and their monetary value so that a specialist with an average practice will have a reasonable income. For example, the committee members might postulate that a surgeon should earn f. 350 in a five-hour day devoted to health insurance cases. During these five hours, he would do five appendectomies; or he would do one appendectomy, two hours of cases in the outpatient clinic (paid by the case method described later in this chapter), and two hours of other procedures (paid by the itemized tariff in the fee schedule). Therefore the committee tries to set fees for procedures and for case payments so that the surgeon will earn f. 350 in a day.

The state of the economy affects the payment of both specialists and general practitioners. All fees and case payments must be set within the financial prospects of the sick funds during the coming year. The sick funds' accountants thus have an important influence over what their medical representatives can grant in the negotiating sessions. Rises in the cost of living result in correspondingly higher fees for both specialists and general practitioners. Increases in prices and wages in the rest of the economy are supposed to make the money available automatically, since the sick funds would collect more from payroll taxes. The theory has worked well when the economy expanded only gradually. But the sudden increase in prices and wages during the mid-1960's led the doctors—and particularly the general practitioners—to feel they were underpaid, resulting in demands beyond the sick funds' offers. For a time, Holland experienced the vociferous conflict between doctors and sick funds that has been far more common elsewhere.

The negotiators are not under pressure to guarantee very high incomes for specialists. Even more than in general practice, it is assumed that the specialist will have much time and opportunity for private practice. No Dutch doctor can become rich through insurance alone, because of the controls over excessive performance of procedures, because of the limiting effects of the capitation and case systems of payment, and because of the ceilings on general practitioners' lists.

Another fee schedule (Tariff IV) lists a few complex diagnostic tests not involving surgical intervention. These can be done either to hospital inpatients or to outpatients. For example:

Procedure	Guilders (1966 rates)
Electroencephalogram	12.75
Bronchoscopy	28.00
Heart catheterization	120.00

The pathologist is paid f. 18.10 for each examination referred to him by a specialist (Tariff V).

Another fee schedule lists hundreds of laboratory examinations and their costs (Tariff VII). The basic rate is calculated to pay for the materials and employee's time needed for each procedure. In addition, each basic fee per test is increased by a certain percentage, and this increment is the fee for the doctor who is the laboratory manager. The increment for some tests in 1962 was as high as 108 per cent or 142 per cent. If the laboratory manager is a clinician who devotes only part of his time to the laboratory, his increment is lower.

There is yet another long fee schedule (Tariff VIII) for diagnostic and therapeutic tasks by radiologists. As we shall see, particularly in the later discussion of case payment, the Dutch system contains formulae to discourage excessive performance of procedures, and this principle is extended into the radiology fee schedule. (In the other countries I visited, the precautions against overperformance seemed concentrated in other fields.) If an X-ray examination is repeated within two months, the second examination is worth only 75 per cent of the full fee. For radiotherapy, a radiologist may earn no more than f. 152 annually for each patient and no more than f. 65.75 if he is the owner of the equipment.

Service Benefits: West Germany

National health insurance in Germany differs from Holland's in that fee-for-service is supposed to cover all medical procedures. In Holland, the fee schedule under Tariff III applies to surgical and technical work, case payments cover other specialties, and capitation is used in general practice. Some countries follow the German practice of a single comprehensive fee schedule, while a few use the Dutch pattern of differentiating payment methods by type of practice and by the nature of the work.

The German system is unique in that the medical profession itself has been incorporated into the structure of setting the fees and distributing money. The sick funds' counterpart at present is the Association of Insurance Doctors. The basic unit is the Association in each *Land*, called the *Kassenärztliche Landesvereinigung*, and occasionally abbreviated KLV. The Land Associations are united in the *Kassenärztliche Bundesvereinigung*, sometimes abbreviated KBV.

The four parties to the clinical and financial relationship are the doctor, the patient, the sick fund, and the KLV. Once the sick funds paid the doctor, but now they make no direct contact. Some individual sick funds delegated payments to associations of their doctors early in the twentieth century, and the practice became universal by law in 1933. Now the patient pays the sick fund through his payroll tax, the sick funds in each *Land* pay their *Kassenärztliche Landesvereinigung*, the doctors in that *Land* send their patients' tickets to the KLV office, and the KLV alone pays the doctor his fees under insurance.

The general monetary level of the fees depends on the money given by the sick funds to the KLV's.[2] These lump sums are negotiated within each *Land* by the KLV secretariat and the *Land* association of each type of sick fund. The negotiations include the biennial renewal of the entire contract between the sick funds and the KLV, but the money payment almost always is the principal issue. The rest of the *Land* contract tends to follow the *Bundesmantelvertrag*,[3] a model contract issued jointly by the *Kassenärztliche Bundesvereinigung* and the *Bundesverband der Ortskrankenkassen*. The negotiations occur in a series of separate sessions: all sick funds cannot join together, since their budgetary capacities and the medical costs of their patients differ; instead, for example, the *Landesverband der Ortskrankenkassen* negotiates its own payment with the *Kassenärztliche Landesvereinigung*. The conversations are now conducted on a technical basis with much less acrimony than one might expect after the many decades of bitter conflict between doctors and sick funds. The contracts and payment agreements must not violate the law, but otherwise the State may not interfere in the decisions of the sick funds and the Insurance Doctors' Associations, since these bodies are legally autonomous and are not governmental subdivisions.

The criteria determining the size of each sick fund's payment to the KLV

[2] The following paragraphs do not apply to the *Ersatzkassen*, who have their own fee schedule governing the flow of money from fund to KLV to doctor.

[3] The text is "Bundesmantelvertrag über den allgemeinen Inhalt der Gesamtverträge," *Ärztliche Mitteilungen*, vol. 44, no. 33 (12 September 1959).

are the sick fund's ability to pay and the costs of medical care for its members in recent years. Two kinds of detailed documents are the basis of discussions: publicly known figures on the membership and income of the sick fund; and records submitted by the KLV secretariat showing the per capita costs of treating that fund's patients in recent years. The discussion of patient costs may extend to the number of acts performed under the fee schedule applying to that sick fund during the last year.[4] Various formulae are used by negotiators when trying to combine past medical costs with anticipated future trends to produce an equitable and adequate sum for the two years after the contract is signed: estimates are made of probable future trends in medical procedures for the fund's members and in the fund's income, to increase the last biennial lump sum by a reasonable amount.[5] Usually the payment is expected only to pay the costs of the fund's members at a level related to the fund's affluence, but juggling sometimes occurs: if a KLV has very rich and very poor funds in its *Land*, it may charge differentially as if it were a private practitioner using a sliding scale, thereby allowing the poor funds to pay less than their members' total costs, while asking the rich funds to pay extra. Probably the rich funds resist, because of the high and rising costs of the drugs, sick leaves, and hospital charges that they must pay directly from the money they do not give the KLV's.

The sick funds cannot economize at the expense of the doctors' fees, as they once did, because of the somewhat automatic procedures for arriving at the payment of the KLV's. So they underpay the hospitals, or so the displeased hospital administrators and nursing associations believe. Also, they try to control the granting of disability allowances and the prescribing of drugs.

Because industrial areas have higher incomes and higher per capita use of doctors, the Insurance Doctors' Association in urban *Länder* (such as Hamburg) have much more money than those in rural *Länder* (such as neighboring Schleswig-Holstein). Insurance Doctors' Associations in very mixed *Länder* (such as North-Rhine-Westphalia) must keep complicated accounts, with rich industrial funds paying per capita rates nearly double those of the poor agricultural funds.

Each KLV distributes the lump sum among doctors in the *Land* according to the doctors' procedures, the relative values of which are laid down in a fee schedule entitled *Gebührenordnung für Ärzte* (literally "Fee Schedule for Doctors").[6] The *Gebührenordnung* is a decree of the Executive Branch of the

[4] Summaries of these figures on a nationwide basis can be found in the annual reports of the *Kassenärztliche Bundesvereinigung*, published in the periodical *Ärztliche Mitteilungen*.

[5] Examples of the reasoning used by negotiators are given by James Hogarth, *The Payment of the General Practitioner* (Oxford: Pergamon Press, 1963), pp. 233–34.

[6] The edition in effect at the time of writing was published in the *Bundesgesetzblatt*, 1965, pt. 1, pp. 123ff., and in a pamphlet by the Deutscher Ärzte Verlag, Cologne, 1965. The definitive commentary and guide to its use is, Dietrich Brück, *Kommentar zur Gebührenordung für Ärzte vom 18 Marz 1965* (Cologne: Deutscher Ärzte-Verlag, 1965 et seq.).

Republic, based on authority from the Insurance Doctors' Act of 1961. It would guide the courts in the awarding of fees in law suits involving doctors, patients, and sick funds if no contracts were signed between the KLV's and the sick funds. It has not been needed for this purpose and has been used only to guide the KLV's when paying doctors for the patients' tickets. *Gebührenordnung* replaced an antiquated and widely denounced fee schedule colloquially called *Preugo*, that had first been issued by the Prussian government in the nineteenth century and that had not been modernized since 1924.[7] In practice, *Preugo* also had been used only as a guide to the relative costs of medical services when the KLV's and their predecessors distributed money for doctors' treatments. The more affluent sick funds paid more than the rates published in *Preugo*, while poor funds paid less.[8]

Gebührenordnung lists over one thousand procedures and fills nearly one hundred pages. Table 2 gives a few entries to give the reader a general impression. All costs are in Deutsche Marks, which at the time of writing have a free market exchange rate of 1 DM = $0.25.

Besides those in the table, other procedures are listed in all the medical specialties. The fee schedule emphasizes technical procedures using equipment, or physical interventions. At the time *Gebührenordnung* replaced *Preugo* it was hoped that doctors would always be paid the full fee listed in the schedule. But deviations have occurred, since some funds have more money than others, just as in the past. But in the payments by the same fund, if *Gebührenordnung* lists three procedures at 12 DM, 6 DM, and 3 DM, the doctor is always paid for these procedures at the ratio of 4:2:1.

The list of fees for visits and for the writing of certificates is more detailed than in most countries with official fee schedules. Many special circumstances are given different costs. An office visit during scheduled visiting hours may not be charged in addition to a particular procedure performed during the visit; but the doctor may charge for both an office visit performed outside regular hours and for a procedure performed during the visit, and he may

[7] Since it survived throughout the history of German national health insurance, *Preugo* was the fee schedule that was described by all previous authors and that was the target of all controversies. The last edition was *Amtliche Gebührenordnung für approbierte Ärzte und Zahnärzte* (*Die "PREUGO"*) (Cologne: Deutscher Ärzte-Verlag, 1961). A partial English translation appears in, Hogarth, *Payment of General Practitioner* (note 5), pp. 609–18. The leading commentary was, Dietrich Brück, *Kommentar zur amtlichen Gebührenordnung für approbierte Ärzte und Zahnärzte* (*PREUGO*) (Cologne: Deutscher Ärzte-Verlag, 3d ed., 1963). Since *Preugo* omitted all recent developments in medicine, the House of Delegates of the KBV occasionally issued a supplementary fee schedule itemizing these additional procedures, such as *Analoge Bewertungen* (Cologne: Deutscher Ärzte-Verlag, 1962). The new *Gebührenordnung* replaced both these fee schedules, and is supposed to be kept up to date.

[8] Differences among the funds in relation to *Preugo* are listed in *Statistisches Jahrbuch der Kassenärztlichen Bundesvereinigung* (Cologne: Kassenärztliche Bundesvereinigung, 1965), p. 49.

TABLE 2. EXCERPTS FROM THE FEE SCHEDULE OF GERMANY

	DM
Office visits:	
Daytime	3.00
Night	7.50
Sunday, holiday	6.00
Day telephone call	3.00
Night telephone call	7.50
Home visits:	
Daytime	6.00
Emergency day visit	9.00
Evening	12.00
Night	20.00
Sunday, holiday	12.00
Filling out certificates and reports	Between 2.00 and 30.00
Most microscopic, chemical, bacteriological, serological and other tests	Between 3.50 and 30.00
Injections, in addition to cost of drugs:	
Subcutaneous	3.00
Intravenous, intra-arterial	4.00
Intraneural, intra-articular	6.00
Into the aorta or heart	12.00
Surgery:	
Opening a superficial abscess	4.00
Removal of superficial foreign bodies	8.00
Ligature and resection of a large blood vessel in a single operation	25.00
Extensive skin transplant	40.00
Embolectomy on peripheral vessels	60.00
Probing larynx	25.00
Major thoracic operation	250.00
Hernia of diaphragm	150.00
Internal and thoracic medicine:	
Electrocardiogram	17.50
Schellong's heart function test	5.00
Vasogram	15.00
Laying out of pneumothorax	46.00
Obstetrics and gynecology:	
Pelvic examination	7.00
Normal delivery	30.00
Artificial interventions during delivery	Between 8.00 and 120.00
Caesarean section	125.00

charge for both a home visit and for a procedure performed in the course of the visit. If the doctor treats several persons during the same visit to a hospital, nursing home, or private home, he may charge the full rate for the first patient but only half rates for the others. Visits by several doctors are more profitable for each individual than a visit by one. The fee schedule includes formulae for paying doctors' traveling expenses and travel time for home visits.

The *Ersatzkassen*, like the statutory funds, pay the KLV's, which in turn pay the individual doctors who treat the *Ersatzkassen* patients, but the calculations are simpler because no lump sums are paid by the funds. Rather, the *Ersatzkassen* pay the KLV's on a fee-for-service basis, corresponding to the procedures performed by each doctor. The KLV simply transmits the money from each *Ersatzkasse* to each doctor, but it performs the very important function of controlling overperformance by doctors Since the *Ersatzkassen's* members have higher incomes and pay higher social security taxes than the persons covered by the statutory funds, the *Ersatzkassen* offer more benefits to their subscribers and pay higher fees to the doctors. These are the attractions inducing eligible persons to elect coverage by the *Ersatzkassen* instead of by the statutory funds. Since they are not agencies in public law, the *Ersatzkassen* have much more freedom and flexibility than the statutory funds in adopting their own fee schedules. New schedules are announced every few years, after consultation with medical associations.[9]

Fee-for-Service with Cost-Sharing: Switzerland

One of the recurring controversies in service benefits schemes is whether the patient should contribute any part of the sick fund's payment to the doctor. Arguments for cost-sharing are that contributions by the patient will defray the funds' expenses, will deter unnecessary visits to the doctor, and will inform the patient more completely about the doctor's bills. But once a national health insurance scheme is on a full service benefits basis, resistance by the political parties of the Left and by the trade unions makes changes to a partially paid arrangement rare. For example, the government of West Germany proposed, but ultimately abandoned during the 1960's a plan to introduce patient charges. Not only did the Social Democrats and trade unions oppose this infringement on the welfare principle, but many doctors feared a reduction in work.[10]

Most cantons in Switzerland have an official insurance system that pays the doctors in full, but the patients are required to reimburse the sick funds for part of the cost. The reason is financial need rather than a belief that patients should participate in their own care: the tax basis of health insurance is inadequate to provide enough money. Switzerland never has had compulsory national health insurance, in general because proposals for any

[9] The schedule in effect at the time of writing is *Ersatzkassen Adgo* (Cologne: Deutscher Ärzte-Verlag, 1966). The leading commentary is, Dietrich Brück and S. Guillemet, *Kommentar zur Ersatzkassen—ADGO* (Cologne: Deutscher Ärzte-Verlag, 1961). The *Ersatzkassen* antedate national health insurance, and their history is reported in Werner Friederici, *Die Ersatzkassen in der Krankenversicherung: Ihre Entwicklung und Würdigung* (Pasewalk: Buchdruckerei Willy Herholz, 1932).

[10] The full story is reported in, William Safran, *Veto Group Politics: The Case of Health Insurance Reform in West Germany* (San Francisco: Chandler Publishing Co., 1967).

national programs usually lose in Swiss popular referendums, but in particular because the opponents always warn against a repetition of the un-Swiss turbulence that has beset health insurance in neighboring Germany. Instead of national health insurance, Switzerland has a law authorizing the national government to subsidize local sick funds, provided these funds offer minimum benefits and follow certain procedures. Bills to establish national compulsory insurance passed the Federal Assembly twice—for medical care generally in 1899 and for tuberculosis in 1949—but were defeated in national referendums.

The federal law of 1911 allowed each canton to make its own decision. As a result, there are twenty-five systems, according to the various political pressures in Switzerland's nineteen cantons and six half-cantons. No canton has compulsory insurance for the entire population; only five have *compulsory* health insurance covering any part of the population, and they give their member communes power to expand coverage further; nine cantons pass along the entire decision to their local communes, and in only two cantons have a majority of the communes made insurance compulsory; five cantons have no compulsory health insurance, although most have voluntary insurance. In those cantons and communes with compulsory health insurance, a great range can be found in coverage, benefit, and procedure.[11]

Despite the plethora of rules and funds, over 80 per cent of the population is covered under compulsory or voluntary health insurance for some medical conditions. Employers are not required to contribute money to their employees' coverage. Unless the 1911 law had exempted them, the powerful Swiss employers would have blocked its passage; the danger of payroll taxes like those abroad is a reason why Swiss employers' associations oppose compulsory national health insurance today. But a few employers contribute voluntarily to their employees' medical coverage, under the terms of contracts exacted by trade unions. Thus medical benefits are paid primarily from the contributions of the persons covered—a principal reason why patients must make additional payments to the sick funds. The federal government subsidizes the approved sick funds—this is the principal accomplishment of the 1911 law—but for many years the contributions were only a

[11] Good summaries appear in, Marcel Grossmann, "Switzerland, Where the Voluntary Insurance Principle Prevails," in, Helmut Schoeck (editor), *Financing Medical Care* (Caldwell, Ida.: Caxton Printers, 1962); Hogarth, *Payment of General Practitioner* (note 5), chap. 7; Arnold Saxer et al., "Social Security in Switzerland," *Bulletin of the International Social Security Association*, vol. 14, no. 9 (September 1961), pp. 457–520; and Paul Biedermann, *Die Entwicklung der Krankenversicherung in der Schweiz* (Zurich: Buchdruckerei Davos, 1955). The annual statistical report about health insurance published by the Federal Office of Social Insurance appears regularly in the *Schweizerische Ärztezeitung*. An interesting comparison of German and Swiss health insurance was written by Rolf Schlögell, "Vergleichende Darstellung der Krankenversicherung Osterreichs, der Schweiz, und der Bundesrepublik Deutschland," *Ärztliche Mitteilungen*, vol. 40, nos. 32–34 (November–December 1955), pp. 943–46, 967–74, 995–1001.

fraction of the funds' incomes. A new law in 1964 raised the federal contributions and was intended to improve the situation. But since the employers' contributions continue to remain low—and they are an essential basis of a generously financed social security system—the Swiss system seemed destined to continue with limited income and restricted benefits.

Before 1964, each fund set its own policy on cost-sharing and other matters, and patients in different cantons paid between 10 and 25 per cent of the full fees. The federal law made the federal subsidy a proportion of the funds' expenses. Thus it increases as medical costs rise. Previously, the absolute sum was limited by law, and the federal subsidy became a steadily diminishing proportion of the funds' income as costs rose. By the time of the new law, the federal subsidy covered little more than the funds' administrative expenses. The law also standardized the rate of cost-sharing.

Under the first year of the expanded federal contributions, the money for national health insurance came from the following sources:

Subscribers' premiums	68%
Patients' cost-sharing	9
Federal subsidy	14
Cantonal and communal subsidies	5
Employers' contributions	2
Other	2
	100%

The employers' principal burden is to continue part of the worker's pay during illness, thereby relieving funds of the considerable sickness allowances falling on them in other countries.[12]

Cost-sharing by the patient occurs both before and after treatment. As in Germany, the insured patient must present a treatment ticket (*Krankenschein* or *feuille de maladie*) to the doctor. The ticket is issued by the sick fund, and the patient must pay a "franchise" charge for it, as did some members of German sick funds several decades ago. Like the fees themselves, the franchise varies according to the patient's income class: 15 fr. for the poorest patient, 25 fr. for the middle income patient, and 150 fr. for the rich patient—a rate that discourages many wealthier people from seeking care under insurance. The doctor itemizes his treatments on the ticket and collects his fee either from the patient or the sick fund, depending on the procedure in that canton. The patient is reimbursed or the doctor is paid directly according to a fee schedule previously negotiated between the cantonal medical society and the fund. If the fund pays the doctor under a service benefits system, it then bills the patient 10 per cent of the doctor's fee. Usually a bill is sent by

[12] Rates for cost-sharing by patients before 1964 are quoted in *The Cost of Medical Care* (Geneva: International Labour Office, 1959), p. 25. The statute of 1964 is summarized in "Was bringt das revidierte KUVG?" *Schweizerische Ärztezeitung*, vol. 45, no. 37 (1964). The sources for funds during 1964 are listed in "Die Krankenversicherung im Jahre 1964," ibid., vol. 47, no. 37 (16 September 1966), p. 970.

mail; in the past some funds deducted the shared cost from the patient's disability allowance. If the canton has a cash benefits procedure, the fund reimburses the patient at 10 per cent less than the official fee schedule.

Cash Benefits

All but the lowest income patients under the American Blue Shield insurance are paid by cash benefits (or, as it is customarily called in the United States, "indemnity insurance"): the patient pays the doctor at the latter's normal fee, and the fund reimburses the patient according to its own fee schedule.[13] Americans have come to take this arrangement for granted, but it is rare abroad. National health insurance has been established on a cash benefits basis in a few countries with militant medical professions and affluent populations: the doctors wish a free hand to charge the wealthier patients according to ability to pay, and they fear the standardized rates and financial controls that govern direct dealings with sick funds. The leading examples are France and Scandinavia.

Switzerland has a mixed system that gives the profession freedom from State controls at the present time and that enables it to collect higher fees from wealthier patients. If the cantonal medical association cannot agree to a contract with the sick funds, cash benefits prevail in that canton for all patients. Some cantons have contracts explicitly providing reimbursement arrangements for all patients; others have double systems with service benefits for the lower income groups and cash benefits for the more affluent.[14]

Cash Benefits: France

A central position in the payment system is occupied by the *Commission Nationale Tripartite*, consisting of representatives from the national office of the federation of medical associations (the *Confédération des Syndicats Médicaux Français*), from the national federation of social security agencies (the *Fédération Nationale des Organismes de Sécurité Sociale* or FNOSS), and from the government (the Ministries of Social Affairs, Economic Affairs, Finance, and Agriculture).[15] The Tripartite Commission is concerned with all relations

[13] Herman M. Somers and Anne R. Somers, *Doctors, Patients, and Health Insurance* (Washington: The Brookings Institution, 1961), chap. 16.

[14] The varied cantonal arrangements under the new law are summarized in "Vertragliche Verständigung im Vordergrund—Übersicht über die Beziehungen zwischen Ärzten und Krankenkassen am Jahreswechsel," *Schweizerische Ärztezeitung*, vol. 48, no. 2 (13 January 1967), pp. 27–31.

[15] The health insurance system and the procedure for paying doctors—as they stood several years ago—are described in, Hogarth, *Payment of General Practitioner* (note 5), chap. 5; and Henry Galant, "France: A Comprehensive Health Plan," *Current History*, vol. 44, no. 262 (June 1963), pp. 351–58, 368. I shall include the changes announced in "Rapport de la Commission de l'Article 24 du Décret du 12 Mai 1960," *Notes et documents*, no. 17

between the medical profession and national health insurance, and particularly the payment of doctors. The Commission adopts a list of medical acts reimbursed under social security, called the *Nomenclature*. It is a list of relative weights among the items and descends from a fee schedule proposed by the *Confédération* during the 1930's. In addition to issuing the *Nomenclature*, the Commission prescribes the maximum monetary fees that shall prevail in various regions of the country.

In each *département* and in a few subdivisions the local medical society and the local social security fund negotiate a collective agreement setting the fee schedule and other administrative matters for treatment of insured persons. Their decisions are largely predetermined by the actions of the Tripartite Commission: the relative weights are binding throughout France; the local agreement fixing the money value of fees may not exceed the ceilings set for that region by the Commission, and in practice the medical society demands and the social security fund grants the amount specified by the ceiling. If there is a collective agreement, all insured patients treated in that area can be reimbursed 70 per cent of the fees they paid the doctor. If there is no collective agreement, the local social security fund asks the Commission to prescribe a fee schedule governing its payments; usually the schedule is the one prevailing for that region of the country. If a doctor in such an area signs an individual agreement with the local fund binding him to charge no more than the fee schedule, his insured patients will be reimbursed at 70 per cent, just as if they resided in areas with collective agreements. If an insured patient goes to a doctor covered by neither a collective nor an individual agreement, the fund reimburses him at a much lower proportion (in practice about 40 per cent) of the official fees, regardless of what the doctor charged him. Thus the system allows the social security agencies and the Ministries of Social Affairs and Finance to control the fees charged insured persons by doctors and to control the reimbursement of patients by funds. Since over 85 per cent of the French population has medical coverage under some form of social security and since over 70 per cent of the persons in the main program are covered by collective or individual agreements between doctors and funds, most of the charges for doctors' services in France are regulated.

At the time of writing, eighty *départements* and ten districts with 70 per cent of the insured have collective agreements. Eight *départements* have no collective agreements between medical society and sick fund, but most of their doctors have signed individual agreements. Nearly 90 per cent of all French doctors are covered by collective or individual agreements. The holdouts include many physicians in Paris, Lyons,

(First Trimester, 1965) and "Soins médicaux dispensés aux assurés sociaux: Le régime conventionnel après la réforme du décret 60–451 du 12 mai 1960," *Révue de la sécurité sociale*, no. 173 (December 1965), supplement. A good summary of the changes is in, Jean Mignon, "La réforme du régime conventionnel par le décret du 7 janvier 1966," *Droit social*, vol. 28, nos. 7–8 (July–August 1966), pp. 434–42.

and Nice with upper-class clienteles that were not covered by social security until recently.[16]

The fee schedule governs the specialist and the general practitioner in his office practice and home visits, in private clinics and in the private services of public hospitals. (Many specialists serve in public hospitals for a few hours a day but are paid salaries by the hospital instead of fees by the patient. During the rest of their day, they conduct a regular office practice, including insured patients who pay the usual fees.) The fees may be exceeded only in exceptional circumstances: if the patient is unusually wealthy, if the patient is unusually demanding (e.g., if he requests several medically unnecessary home visits), or if the doctor has been admitted to a special list of meritorious practitioners.

After approval by the Tripartite Commission, the *Nomenclature* is issued by the Prime Minister as a decree with the force of law. It serves the double function of listing the relative values of all the medical acts covered by insurance and providing the code letters and numbers for communication to the social security fund. One of the traditions of French medicine is the virtually unlimited confidentiality of the doctor-patient relationship. After the patient pays the doctor, the doctor gives a receipt on a form issued by social security: the upper half contains full information about the treatment and charges and is kept by the patient; the lower half gives the specialty field, the code letters and the numbers for the procedures according to the *Nomenclature*. The letters and numbers are so devised that, after the patient forwards the lower half of the receipt to the social security fund, the laymen in the fund know the payment and the general character of the medical procedures, but they cannot infer the precise treatments. Mention of the specialty in which the procedures fall is designed to enforce the rule that only a licensed specialist can perform the procedures in his field.

The preoccupation with professional secrecy appears much greater in France than in any other country. It results from the long traditions of personal privacy and secretive proprietor-customer relationships throughout French society. The threat to professional secrecy was one of the arguments long used against national health insurance, and a considerable philosophical and legal literature accumulated about the preservation of secrets in the light of the numerous certificates required by modern methods of organizing and financing care. In most other countries, fee schedules are expressed directly in money, and receipts sent to sick funds specify the medical procedures.[17]

[16] The figures for successive years during the 1960's can be found in "Rapport de la Commission . . ." (note 15), pp. 10–12.

[17] French medical secretiveness has been so extreme that the profession long objected to stating the causes of death on death certificates and resisted the obligatory reporting of infectious diseases, according to Arthur Newsholme, *International Studies on the Relation between the Private and Official Practice of Medicine* (London: George Allen & Unwin, 1931), 2: 86–88.

The basic units of medical care are identified by key letters:[18]

C = office visit
C_s = office visit with a qualified specialist
C.NPSY = office visit with a qualified neuropsychiatrist
V = daytime home visit
V_s = daytime home visit by a qualified specialist
V.NPSY = daytime home visit by a qualified neuropsychiatrist
VD = Sunday home visit
VN = night home visit
PC = simple medical procedure, minor surgical procedure
K = procedure by a surgeon or by another specialist
R = procedure by a radiologist

other key letters refer to services performed by dentists, midwives, and others.

The value of each procedure depends on a numerical coefficient, and the *Nomenclature* is basically a list of over 2,000 procedures and their coefficients. (The cash value of each procedure is a decision separate from the fixing of coefficients, and I shall discuss it later.) The largest variations are for procedures with key letters *PC* and *K*. Numerous operations in neurosurgery and thoracic surgery are listed between *K* 150 and *K* 300: for example, a "thoracic gastro-esophagectomy or thoracic-abdominal surgery with immediate re-establishment of the connection" is listed as *K* 250 and thus is paid 250 times the cash value of *K*. Minor medical acts also vary in weight: for example, an intratracheal injection is *PC* 1.5, a single intravenous infusion is *PC* 2, incision of a deep abscess is *PC* 5. Even visits can be weighted differently, depending on the status of the doctor: for example, an office visit to a G.P. is *C* 1, to a specialist it was once *C* 2, to a professor or a leading hospital service chief it is still *C* 3.

Minor medical and surgical procedures (*PC*) and radiological procedures performed in the patient's home are paid at higher rates, compensating the doctor for his time and trouble. Fees for the more expensive procedures—*K* 15 and above—include preoperative care, any local anesthetics, work of the physician's assistants, and postoperative care for up to twenty days. If several distinct procedures are performed at the same time, the most important one is paid in full, and the others at half rates.

Specialists and some distinguished doctors normally would collect higher fees than general practitioners and, in order to make participation in social security attractive to them, they get higher rates for office and home visits.

[18] The following discussion is based on the version in effect at the time of writing: *Soins dispensés aux assurés: nomenclatures* (Paris: Ministère du Travail, Textes Officiels, série B: Sécurité Sociale, no. 4, 1962). For a convenient publication of the *Nomenclature* incorporating amendments to the 1962 edition, see the Supplement to *Concours médical*, vol. 86, no. 45 (7 November 1964).

For example, *C* 3 and *V* 3 are allowed to medical school professors and to specialists in regional hospital centers. Until 1962, neuropsychiatrists were allowed to collect *C* 3 and *V* 3, and other specialists were paid *C* 2 and *V* 2; in 1962 these two groups got special rates, slightly below triple and double pay respectively. The rate for psychiatrists attempts to solve a common dilemma in national health insurance fee schedules: other specialties can collect high fees because their procedures can easily be itemized and given high value in a fee schedule, but the psychiatrist's work often consists of long conversations rather than technical procedures. Psychiatrists in some countries are dissatisfied with the ordinary rates for office visits, but psychiatrists have enjoyed somewhat higher status in France.

The decisions about the structure of the *Nomenclature* concern the relations among the technical procedures in medical care, and these judgments about the value and importance of medical procedures are made by the profession itself. The Tripartite Commission follows the recommendations of an advisory Committee on Nomenclature consisting of doctors from the *Confédération*, the Ministry of Social Affairs, and FNOSS. Although the Committee members' different organizational loyalties cause them to disagree about certain questions, the Committee meetings concern the technical medical problem of rating medical procedures and are conducted in a spirit of amity and professional courtesy. The difficult and contentious task of creating a new schedule of relative values no longer arises: each year the Committee tends to preserve the bulk of the coefficients from the previous years, and since the *Nomenclature* has been in use for decades, most of the problems have long since been settled. The first official *Nomenclature* was adopted by the *Confédération* and the Ministry of Labor in 1934, its original form was strongly influenced by the *Confédération*, each of the annual reviews ever since has made only slight changes, and its present form is remarkably like its first.[19]

Each year the Committee must decide whether to change the existing coefficients among the medical procedures in the same specialty and among the medical procedures in different specialties. The first is a technical decision and is easier to make. If a specialty has acquired new procedures, the Commitee must rate them in relation to that specialty's existing procedures; if a particular procedure has become more or less difficult as a result of technical change in that specialty, the Committee may raise or lower its coefficient in relation to the specialty's other coefficients. As a guide to reasoning, the Committee often selects one procedure in each field as basic. For example, an appendectomy often is picked as a basic surgical procedure. Since an appendectomy is *K* 50, it seems reasonable that a gastrectomy should be

[19] The *Nomenclature* and the monetary equivalents for 1936 are described in, Barbara N. Armstrong, *The Health Insurance Doctor: His Role in Great Britain, Denmark, and France* (Princeton: Princeton University Press, 1939), pp. 175–88 passim.

worth *K* 150. Once an appendectomy was *K* 50 and a herniorrhaphy *K* 40, but during the early 1960's the Committee decided that the two operations had become of equal difficulty and rated them both *K* 50.

Fixing relative coefficients *among* fields is more puzzling. Although many of their acts are intrinsically difficult to compare, the payment system requires rating all in coefficients of *K* or *PC*. Unlike the relative values within an individual field, this issue involves the internal politics of the medical profession. Everyone can pick up a copy of the *Nomenclature* and see how every procedure is evaluated, and specialties often complain their procedures are underpaid, particularly in comparison with the surgeons. Surgery has long been the most glamorous field in French medicine—many of the profession's celebrities during the nineteenth century were surgeons, today the ablest young doctors (as evidenced by internships in university hospitals) still gravitate into surgery—and the *Nomenclature* always has treated surgery well.

The Committee members from the *Confédération* are often under cross-pressures: the better-paid specialties favor the *status quo* while their other constituents press for higher coefficients for one or many procedures. Sometimes the *Confédération* leaders have been criticized by a specialty or by general practitioners for not having gotten high enough coefficients. For many years general practitioners complained that the *Nomenclature* coefficients and the monetary values of *PC* and *K* gave undue preference to the technical specialties. As a result, around 1961 the government decreed that half the medical profession's representatives on the Committee on *Nomenclature* should be G.P.'s—previously all were specialists—and subsequent revisions of the *Nomenclature* coefficients and of the monetary fees were more pleasing to the G.P.'s.[20]

Another major decision of the Tripartite Commission is the monetary value for the key letters. These are the monetary ceilings governing collective agreements and, as I have said, tend to be the actual fees in each area. During the late 1960's, three monetary scales existed—for Paris and suburbs; for Marseilles, Lyons, and the commune of Aix-en-Provence; and for the rest of the country. *PC* and *K* were the same everywhere, and the regional differentials applied to home and office visits. Following are the rates issued in 1966:[21]

[20] The successive revaluations of key letters during the 1960's are summarized in "Rapport de la Commission . . ." (note 15), pp. 55–59. The higher rate for general practitioners' work was one of their several victories in French medical politics during the 1950's. A special National Syndicate of French General Practitioners was created in 1951 and later acquired much weight in the once specialist-dominated *Confédération*. Jacqueline Pincemin and Alain Laugier, "Les médecins," *Révue française de science politique*, vol. 9, no. 4 (December 1959), p. 894.

[21] "Arrête du 24 mars 1966 fixant les plafonds des tarifs conventionnels des honoraires des médecins pour les soins dispensés aux assurés sociaux," *Journal officiel* (27 March 1966).

Procedure	Key Letter	Paris	Marseilles, Lyons, Aix	Rest of Country
Office visit for general practitioner	*C*	13	12	11
Daytime home visit for general practitioner	*V*	20	18	17
Office visit for specialist	C_s	24	22	20
Daytime home visit for specialist	V_s	36	32	28
Office visit for neuropsychiatrist	*C.NPSY*	36	33	30
Daytime home visit for a neuropsychiatrist	*V.NPSY*	54	48	20
Sunday home visit	*VD*	18	18	18
Night home visit	*VN*	30	30	30
Simple procedure	*PC*	4.25	4.25	4.25
Complex procedure	*K*	4.25	4.25	4.25
Radiological procedure	*R*	3.15	3.15	3.15

(Free market exchange rate at the time of writing is 1 F = $0.18.)

The patient's payment to the doctor is the franc value of the key letter multiplied by the procedure's coefficients. Let us illustrate by means of procedures mentioned previously:

Appendectomy (*K* 50)	4.25 × 50 = 212.50
Thoracic gastro-esophagectomy (*K* 250)	4.25 × 250 = 1062.50
Intratracheal injection (*PC* 1.5)	4.25 × 1.5 = 6.375
Incision of a deep abscess (*PC* 5)	4.25 × 1.5 = 6.375
Office visit to a general practitioner (*C* 1)	
in Paris	13 × 1 = 13
in the provinces	11 × 1 = 11
Office visit to a professor (*C* 3)	
in Paris	13 × 3 = 39
in the provinces	11 × 1 = 11

If the patient's doctor is covered by a collective or individual agreement, the social security fund reimburses him 70 per cent of the official fee. If the doctor is not covered, the reimbursement is a lower proportion of the official rate, depending on the *tarifs de remboursement* set by the Tripartite Commission for that *département*.[22]

The Tripartite Commission decides the monetary values of the key letters and the regional differentials by a combination of economic research and self-interested bargaining. The Commission's staff reports data on trends in wages and living costs in the country. If wages were known to have risen about 3 per cent during the previous year while living costs rose 2 per cent, medical fees would probably rise in this general zone. The actual figures emerge from bargaining. Sometimes the parties bring their own statisticians and their own economic reports, buttressing their respective cases: the

[22] The lower reimbursement rates set in 1966 are in "Arrête du 9 mars 1966 fixant les tarifs d'honoraires des praticiens et auxiliaires médicaux applicables en l'absence de convention pour les soins dispensés aux assurés sociaux," *Journal officiel* (27 March 1966).

Confédération argues for higher fees, while FNOSS favors no increases or smaller increases. The Ministry of Finance has the final word, since the awards should not threaten the solvency of the insurance system and should not force higher social security taxes.

Before the Tripartite Commission replaced the National Commission on Tariffs in early 1966, the interested parties were weaker and the Ministry of Finance was stronger in the determination of fees. The *Confédération* was represented on the Committee on Nomenclature, which gave advice to the National Commission, but the doctors did not confront their true adversaries in the government in actual bargaining, primarily the Ministry of Finance. The interministerial Commission usually decided from the standpoint of national fiscal policy, tempered by the need to earn the co-operation of all sides in the conduct of social security. The Ministry of Finance has several responsibilities that give it a bias against higher fees. First, it is interested in the financial soundness of social security. If payments to doctors go too high the deficit in social security accounts will rise, and the Ministry of Finance must find more money in the general budget to subsidize what is supposed to be a self-sustaining program. French social security taxes are among the highest in the world—6.50 per cent of the worker's wages plus almost 30 per cent of the employer's payroll—and the Ministry of Finance has always been distressed that they are still insufficient to pay for the deficit-ridden health insurance.[23] Thus demands for yet higher medical fees contradict the Treasury men's attempts to being order into the government's chronically unbalanced social security accounts. Secondly, the Treasury men in France, as in other countries, view wage and price increases as threats to the strength of the franc in international transactions. If they had their way, they would discourage excessive pay increases throughout the economy, but only wages and prices in the nationalized sector are under their influence. Since the Treasury has a voice in setting fees under social security, it is used to implement the Treasury's hard-money aims, particularly when it has been headed by Ministers strongly devoted to stability.[24]

Decisions about the general level of fees have not always been negative, even when the Ministry of Finance was strongest. When necessary to get the co-operation of the doctors increases are granted. Thus, for example, fees were increased in 1960 in order to sugar-coat imposition of a compulsory fee schedule. Until 1960, the charges actually made by French doctors had risen faster than the social security's reimbursements, and a better co-ordination was then sought, since the social security rates would now govern French medicine.

[23] *Social Security Programs throughout the World* (Washington: U.S. Department of Health, Education, and Welfare, revised ed., 1969), comparing France and other countries.

[24] For a complaint by the *Confédération*, see Pierre A. Debuirre, "Rapport du Secrétaire Général pour l'Assemblée Générale de la Confédération," *Médecin de France*, vol. 66, no. 177 (New Series) (November 1960), p. 1054.

Another basic financial decision made by the Commission is the ratio between fees for visits (*C*, *V*, etc.) and technical acts (principally *K*). Professional judgments and medical politics play important roles, and the advice of the Committee on Nomenclature has carried much weight with both the National Commission and the successor Tripartite Commission. As I said before, the Commission in 1962 responded to complaints from the G.P.'s by raising their fees relative to the specialists. The Commission preserved the same value for *K* while raising the rates for *C*, *V*, *VD*, and *VN* one or two francs apiece. Also, the ordinary specialist would no longer earn fees for *C*, *V*, *VD*, and *VN* exactly double those for the general practitioners; he was given a separate fee scale that was now slightly less than double.

Economics and medical politics governed a decision made during the early 1960's to pay radiology according to multiples of its own basic procedure *R* instead of according to multiples of *K*, as it had previously. As a result of medical change, the demand for X-rays and for radiological treatments had greatly increased in postwar France; because of improved personal skills and better equipment, radiologists' productivity steadily mounted; and as a result of France's economic revival and the Common Market, competition among companies lowered the prices of equipment and of film. Consequently, radiologists' profits per procedure and total income rapidly rose, leading the sick funds to suggest lower fees. Meanwhile, the surgeons, internists, and some other clinicians had long believed that a basic radiological procedure should be rated lower than a basic clinical procedure: it is the clinician and not the laboratory man who enjoys the greater glamor and possesses the more confident self-image in French medicine. In order to please the sick funds and keep on good terms with the clinicians, whose referrals are the life blood of their field, the leaders of the radiologists agreed to creation of a special radiological procedure paid at less than the basic clinical procedure (at first, $R = 3$ F while $K = 4$ F). The radiologists' prosperity was assured, their leaders believed, since the Common Market would further reduce costs.[25]

The Tripartite Commission also decides the monetary differentials among fees according to size of community. Like the differentials among procedures in the *Nomenclature*, regional differentials in fees have existed almost since the start of national health insurance, and the National Commission simply perpetuates them with minor modifications. As a rule of thumb, the first differentials in 1934 were supposed to enable the doctor to earn from an office visit the equivalent of half the average daily wage of skilled labor prevailing in that area.[26] Regional differentials in fees customarily existed in French office practice, because of regional differences in wages, living costs, and the

[25] Even after the revision in the rates, radiologists earned far more under social security than any other specialists. *Rapport annuel 1964* (Paris: Inspection Générale de la Sécurité Sociale, 1965), p. 218.

[26] Armstrong, *Health Insurance Doctor* (note 19), p. 176.

eminence of doctors; and social security is supposed only to help finance and not totally alter traditional payment patterns. As wages, living costs, and the professional qualifications of specialists became more uniform in France during the 1960's, the regional differentials in fees were reduced.

Cash Benefits: Sweden

Most fee schedules consist of long lists of advanced specialist procedures customarily performed on inpatients in public or private hospitals. But Sweden's is a list of groups of procedures that a skilled office practitioner can perform upon ambulatory patients—basically tests, advice, and simple treatments. It is assumed that more complex treatments will be performed under national health insurance only to hospital inpatients; the sick fund and the county government will pay the patient's hospital costs, and the doctor will be paid in full by the salary from the county government (if his appointment is nonacademic) or from the national government (if he is a professor). As a result, Sweden's fee schedule is one of the simplest and shortest of any in a national health insurance scheme.

Ambulatory patients come to the doctor at his private office, located either in an office building, in the doctor's own home (a site that is rare in the city but common in the country), or in the hospital outpatient department. A private or insured patient may go to any doctor who will see him. Because of the shortage of physicians and the health consciousness of the population, many office practitioners are booked up long in advance, and some patients go directly to the outpatient clinics of hospitals, where someone will see them sooner or later that day. Home visits to the patient are rare. Unless the patient is a pauper coming to the district medical officer, he pays a fee in cash to the doctor and gets a receipt.

Private inpatient care is possible. Before 1960, one could be treated by a public hospital service chief in the private beds of his service and pay him for his hospital care as well as for his outpatient care. The patient has always been able to pay specialists in this fashion in private clinics. Since 1960 public hospital chiefs no longer can charge their private patients occupying beds in their services, and some service chiefs in Stockholm (and possibly elsewhere) began to hospitalize their private patients in private clinics. Once near extinction in Sweden, because of the high quality of the public hospitals, the private clinics revived.

The entire population is covered by compulsory national health insurance, and therefore the doctor assumes each of his patients may claim reimbursement from the sick fund. His receipt shows his fee and treatments. The patient transmits the receipt to the local branch of the National Insurance Office, which reimburses him 75 per cent of an official fee for that procedure. Under voluntary health insurance before 1955, the reimbursement was about two-thirds. Rural district medical officers, hospital doctors outside Stockholm, junior hospital doctors in Stockholm, and some other doctors must charge no more than the official fee schedule; professors of medicine, chiefs of hospital service in Stockholm, urban district medical officers, and full-time practitioners may charge whatever they like, whether or not the patient will seek reimbursement from the sick fund.

The fee schedule in kronor at the time of writing is as follows:[27]

	Stockholm	*Elsewhere*
Office visits:		
Group 1: visit involving minimum examination and minimum treatment	9	7
Group 2: visit involving simple examination (e.g., taking blood pressure, testing reflexes, etc.) and simple treatments	17	12
Group 3: visit involving more advanced examinations and treatments, graded progressively according to time required, amount of equipment used, and difficulty		
Group 3A	22	17
Group 3B	28	23
Group 3C	35	30
Telephone conversation, renewal of prescription	3	2
Home visits:		
Simple care	20	16
Care including examinations or treatments listed in the Group 3 office visits	25	21

Seventy medical procedures are listed for Groups 3A, 3B, and 3C. Following are some examples:

Group A: heart and lung examinations; suturing and excising wounds; applying plaster casts; gynecological and rectal examinations; posterior rhinoscopy; puncturing and washing maxillary sinus.

Group B: amputation of finger or toe; reducing and setting fractures and dislocations; removing skin tumors; certain optical examinations; operation for adenoids.

Group 3C: pediatric and psychiatric examinations; dilatation and currettage; minor skin grafts; removal of deeply embedded foreign bodies.

If the patient's receipt lists procedures not specified in the fee schedule, the National Insurance Office rates the visit according to the levels of difficulty indicated by the fee schedule, and pays accordingly.

[27] *Taxa för beräkning av ersättning för läkarvård och tandläkarvård enligt lagen om allmän försäkring gällande fr. o.m. den 1 januar: 1965* (Stockholm: Försäkringskasseförbundet, 1964). An English translation and explanation of an earlier edition appears in Hogarth, *Payment of General Practitioner* (note 5), pp. 71–88, 577–85. The free market exchange rate is 1 kr. = $0.19.

Night and Sunday visits, whether in the office or at home, are remunerated at rates 50 per cent higher. Extra payments are possible for the doctor's travel costs on home visits. Separate fee schedules govern reimbursement of radiologists, dentists, and doctors performing tests in the laboratory and tests with certain electrical equipment. Although the reimbursement of the patient follows grouped fees, doctors not governed by the insurance fee schedule can charge more individualized fees, depending on their evaluation of each procedure.

In its general form, the fee schedule has been carried over from the voluntary health insurance system, after many decades of use in the reimbursement of patients. Therefore, as in other countries, the fee schedule is not created anew during negotiations, but it is modified slightly from time to time. The Swedish Medical Association (SMA) long treated the fee schedule gingerly and preferred to avoid taking responsibility for it, lest it become legally or morally binding on the charges of doctors, like the insurance schedule in France. In order to avoid wedges for public control over doctors' fees, the SMA never issued schedules of recommended fees. Formally the SMA considered the insurance fee schedule as a private affair between the National Insurance Office and the public, governing how the Office paid the patient but involving no obligations for the SMA and the medical profession.

But since the fee schedule affected the charges and incomes of doctors in several ways, the SMA became involved in its design. There were no formal bargaining sessions, as in the many countries where the fee schedules represented the sick funds' payments to the doctors, but informal conferences were held involving the SMA, the National Insurance Office, the Royal Medical Board, and sometimes the Ministry of the Interior. The government representatives kept in touch with the Ministry of Finance, which has been the watchdog of the financial solvency of the insurance funds and which must increase its subsidy from general tax funds if the costs of health insurance rise too far.

The absence of formal bargaining sessions and binding contracts was due to the law as well as to the SMA's desire to maintain the freedom of the doctors. Sweden's private economy had long settled its disputes by binding contracts arising out of collective bargaining between employees and employers. The two sides had rights to call strikes and lockouts, but the government exempted itself from such conventional bargaining with its employees. In the public sector, no right to strike existed and wages were fixed by the government, after consultation with the employees' representatives. Most of Sweden's doctors have been full-time or part-time government employees, and the State did not bargain or sign binding contracts with the SMA over salaries or over the fees these doctors could charge during their nonsalaried outpatient work.

By the mid-1960's, this system had serious disadvantages for the staffs of hospitals and for the district medical officers. As a condition for obtaining these appointments, the doctors could charge no more than the official fee schedule. But since no standing mechanism reviewed the fees, they remained almost unchanged during the decade after 1955. The hospital doctors demanded increases in salaries and fees, threatened to strike, and obtained a new system. The *riksdag* in 1965 passed a new law giving the public sector the same procedures as had long prevailed in the private sector: the employees' association would bargain with the government, the employees had the right to strike, and the two sides would fix pay and working conditions in a contract binding on both. Therefore the doctors could strike, but the SMA had to obtain the approval of its parent body, the Swedish Confederation of Professional Associations (SACO). In case of strikes that threaten the national safety, the two sides must submit the dispute to nonbinding arbitration. The contract signed between the hospital doctors and the Association of County Councils in 1965 set both the doctors' inpatient salaries and their outpatient fees in hospitals outside Stockholm. The fees followed the schedule adopted the previous year, after the informal negotiations between the SMA and the sick fund. Therefore the fee schedule acquired an official standing and thereafter has been negotiated more openly between the SMA and the sick fund. Only the full-time private practitioners and some of the prestigious professors and chiefs of service in Stockholm continue to be exempt from the fee schedule.[28]

Before the adoption of open collective bargaining and the extension of the fee schedule's binding effects to the hospital doctors, one consideration in setting the monetary value of medical procedures was the prevailing charges in the country. Since the insurance system had the formal responsibility to reimburse medical costs and since the medical profession was considered free, there was an implied obligation for the sick funds to keep pace with the actual charges. A research division of the National Insurance Office regularly calculates the average charges for all medical procedures, on the basis of the receipts submitted by patients to the sick funds. Reports about average fees for the country as a whole and for individual regions are examined by the conferees and are important influences on the monetary values given to procedures and on the classification of procedures in groups. For example, the empirical finding that doctors' charges are much higher in Stockholm than in the rest of the country is one reason for Stockholm's separate list of fees. A commitment to keep pace with average charges would bankrupt the insurance system if doctors were voracious profiteers and if the

[28] The printed edition of the contract is *Tjänsteförteckning M.M. för heltidsanställda läkare* (Stockholm: Svenska Landstingsförbundet and Sveriges Läkarförbund, LCT 66 nr 4a, 1966). The issues and settlement of the dispute are summarized in the mimeographed annual reports of the Swedish Medical Association to the World Medical Association for 1963 and 1965.

economy experienced rapid growth and price inflation, but neither has been true in Sweden. Possibly no other country has kept its medical fees so stable. The government has used the insurance fee schedule as a brake on actual charges, and these effects will grow as the fee schedule acquires a more contractual status.

According to the surveys of the National Insurance Office, most categories of doctors raised their fees no more than about 5 per cent between 1955 and 1958 and no more than 15 per cent between 1958 and 1963. Throughout this period, the official fee schedule remained almost the same. The increases in charges were slightly higher for the hospital chiefs-of-service and the private practitioners in Stockholm, which persuades some officials to favor controls over them.[29]

Under both the old and new methods of writing the fee schedule, another important consideration for the conferees is the technical character of procedures. The fee schedule classifies work into groups, depending on complexity, difficulty, and time. In their discussions, the conferees try to rank procedures in a common-sense manner according to these dimensions. A group consensus determines the cutting points between, for example, 20-kronor and 30-kronor groups of tasks.

Case Payments in The Netherlands

Fee-for-service is supposed to relate payment and work very closely, by pricing each procedure. But it fits the technical and manual specialties much better than the contemplative and prescribing specialties. Work in the surgical specialties can be itemized, priced, and converted into large incomes under fee-for-service; but the medical specialties sometimes call merely for the periodic examinations, long visits, and therapeutic advice that cannot easily or profitably be itemized on a fee schedule. Salary is the other common method of paying specialists, but often it does not relate income to work level.

Case payment is a flat rate that bases remuneration on the number of patients actually treated. It arose in the Germanic countries during the nineteenth century, primarily in general practice. It has been progressively abandoned, because of doctors' preference for fee-for-service and because medical care increasingly became a series of technical procedures. It survives in general practice in some parts of Austria, but the profession there seems to be pressing successfully for its replacement by fee-for-service.[30]

Holland is the only country where the case method survives without attack. The reasons for this exceptional situation are selective use and an

[29] *Statistisk undersökning rörande de allmänna sjukkassornas utgifter för läkarvård m.m. 1958* (Stockholm: Riksförsäkringsanstalten, 1960), pp. 42–43; and *Statistisk undersökning rörande de allmänna försäkringskassornas utgifter för läkarvard m.m. 1963* (Stockholm: Riksförsäkringsverket, 1962).

[30] Hogarth, *Payment of General Practitioner* (note 5), pp. 350–59 and 377–79.

extremely sophisticated design. Elsewhere, the case method has incurred opposition because it is applied to all medical care, when doctors could earn more by collecting fees for itemized procedures. The Dutch solution is to differentiate payment: the general practitioner receives capitation fees; specialists are paid by fee-for-service for technical, surgical, and comparable procedures; and specialists collect case payments for routine care on ambulatory and hospital inpatients.

Outpatient Care

Table 3 shows the rates in 1966 collected by specialists for ambulatory patients seen in the hospital outpatient clinics and in private offices (Tariff I).[31]

As in referrals to specialists paid by fee-for-service, the patient must present a transfer card. The initial transfer card is issued to a specialist by the patient's general practitioner and is good for one month. During that time, the specialist sees the patient for as many appointments and for whatever care he deems necessary. The specialist himself decides whether to issue renewal cards for a second, third, or additional months. In each specialty, the renewal card is worth less than the transfer card: for example, in ophthalmology, the transfer card is worth f. 9.00 per patient, and each renewal card is worth f. 4.65.

Many Dutch hospitals have salaried medical staffs: they include university-affiliated hospitals and other hospitals in big cities. In other hospitals, doctors have admitting and consultative privileges and earn their entire incomes from fees and case payments. The "all-in" cards are worth more than the "all-out" cards, because they cover both the specialty care and laboratory tests in the hospitals with salaried physicians. Under "all-in" cards, the sick funds pay the hospital and the hospital uses the money to pay the salaries of the specialists and laboratory physicians. The "all-in card A" covers more diagnostic and therapeutic procedures in laboratories than does the "all-in card B." For patients covered by "all-out" cards, the sick fund pays case payments directly to the specialist and pays the laboratory doctors under Tariff VII, described earlier in this chapter.

The loophole for potential overperformance of procedures is the right of the specialist to issue his own renewal cards, according to his own clinical judgment. The renewal factor controls the number of renewal cards for which he shall receive payment. It is computed automatically from the average number of renewal cards issued per transfer card in the health insurance system for that specialty during the previous year, plus an increment of 15 per cent. The statistics are based on the records of the Central Office

[31] *Tarieven* . . . (note 1), pp. 4–11. The exchange rate on the free market at that time was f. 1 = $0.28.

TABLE 3. AMBULATORY CASE PAYMENTS IN THE NETHERLANDS

Specialty	Value of Transfer Card in Guilders	Value of Each Renewal Card in Guilders	Renewal Factor
Ophthalmology	9.00	4.65	0.35
Otorhinolaryngology	9.65	4.85	0.86
Surgery	11.60	5.10	0.65
Plastic surgery	11.60	5.10	1.20
Orthopedics	11.60	5.10	1.15
Urology	18.65	9.65	1.92
Gynecology	12.90	9.00	1.77
Neurosurgery	14.15	9.00	1.82
Psychiatry	18.05	9.65	3.67
Dermatology	12.90	8.35	2.55
Internal medicine			
All-in card A	27.10	13.55	2.28
All-in card B	26.00	13.20	2.28
All-out card	16.75	8.35	2.28
Pediatrics			
All-in card A	21.80	10.80	1.53
All-in card B	21.40	10.80	1.53
All-out card	16.75	8.35	1.53
Gastroenterology			
All-in card	23.65	11.75	4.76
All-out card	16.05	8.35	4.76
Cardiology			
All-in card A	29.80	14.80	2.07
All-in card B	26.40	13.50	2.07
Thoracic medicine			
All-in card A	25.40	13.00	3.52
All-in card B	21.90	11.55	3.52
Rheumatology			
All-in card	22.60	11.80	4.06
All-out card	16.05	8.35	4.06
Allergy			
All-in card	23.25	11.80	5.82
All-out card	16.75	8.35	5.82
Rehabilitation	13.50	6.80	2.42

for the Administration of Specialists' Fees. The extra 15 per cent is designed to give leeway to the urban specialists, whose busy practices include the severely ill requiring long-term care; in the towns and rural areas, the G.P. may take the patient back from the specialist during the late stages of care, but the urban patient is more likely to stay with the specialist until his condition is normal. The renewal factor increases each year, but not by the full 15 per cent; the national renewal rate usually falls short of that year's renewal factor, since not all specialists issue renewal cards at a frequency equal to the factor. The renewal factor is higher for the specialties requiring long courses of treatment (e.g., gastroenterology, rheumatology, psychiatry, allergy) than for specialties whose patients recover quickly (e.g., surgery, ophthalmology, otorhinolaryngology).

If the records of the sick fund show that a specialist has issued renewal cards in excess of the renewal factor in his field, the fund will pay him only for the number within the renewal factor. Since the volume of specialty care is greater and lengthier in the cities than in the smaller towns, some urban specialists get payment for only part of their renewal cards, while nearly all rural specialists receive full payment. The doctor can be paid in full for a patient whom he sees over many months, provided that patient is counterbalanced in his practice by others with many fewer renewals. Presumably most doctors learn to organize their practices according to the renewal norms. The renewal factor does not place an arbitrary ceiling on a doctor's practice and income: if a specialist is so skillful and popular that many G.P.'s send him patients, he will have many transfer cards and many renewal cards, but he cannot build up a large practice at the expense of the sick funds by granting himself many renewals on the basis of few transfer cards.

The size of the case payments is decided by the negotiating sessions between representatives of the specialty associations and the sick funds. The negotiators who first created the fee schedule, capitation fees, and case payment tariff in the late 1940's, postulated a desirable income from insurance practice for each specialty. The negotiators estimated the average amount of time each patient consultation requires in a specialty; they estimated the distribution of each specialty's work day among technical tasks, routine outpatient consultations, and routine inpatient observations. The fees and case payments were set so that the average specialist in the field would earn the target income during the forthcoming year. Various considerations were fitted together in the committee's thinking about the size of the case payment, such as whether the specialty relied primarily on technical procedures or consultations for its effort and income, whether the specialist saw many patients or few, and the amount of time devoted to each patient. Surgeons, ophthalmologists, otorhinolaryngologists, and some others received low fees for each transfer and renewal card, partly because most of their incomes were derived from procedures paid by fee-for-service under Tariff III and partly because their consultations with ambulatory patients of the sort covered by Tariff I were brief. Internists, pediatricians, cardiologists, and some others received high case payments because they must depend on consultations for their incomes and because each patient takes much time. The case payment for an initial transfer card to a dermatologist was fixed low because he sees many patients for brief periods of time.

Having established the case payment schedule in this form, the negotiators try to preserve it by annual increments matching rises in the cost of living. As in the negotiations involving other pay rates for doctors, most statistical evidence and discussion at the sessions concern changes in the cost of living for the population and for doctors since the last round. If the basic structure of Tariff I is challenged—which is very unusual—the negotiators re-examine it by means of the original reasoning about target incomes and the work loads of each specialty.

Inpatient Care

The general practitioner or the specialist himself recommends hospitalization, but, in order to prevent unnecessary and expensive admissions, a control officer of the sick funds must approve and officially is the person making the decision. The specialist collects a payment for each day the patient receives routine inpatient care in his service.[32] The specialist cannot collect one of these payments for a day when the patient's care is covered by a global fee for a technical act performed under the fee-for-service list (i.e., under Tariff III). In order to discourage prolonged and unnecessary hospitalization for mercenary reasons, the daily rate drops sharply after the first five days. For the medical specialties (internal medicine, pediatrics, psychiatry, cardiology, etc.) the daily fees in 1966 were f. 9.90 for each of the first five days and f. 1.65 daily thereafter. For the surgical specialties (surgery, orthopedics, ophthalmology, etc.) the daily fees were f. 8.25 for each of the first five days and f. 1.65 daily thereafter. If a doctor has an "all-in" contract with a hospital, the sick fund sends the case payments to the hospital, as a contribution to his salary; if the specialist has an unsalaried "all-out" contract with a hospital, the sick fund pays him directly. Besides paying doctors or hospitals for routine inpatient care and for special procedures (under the medical Tariffs III and IV), the sick fund also pays the hospitals for the patient's hospitalization costs.

If the control doctor disapproves an application, this simply means that the sick funds will not pay. But the patient can pay the hospital and doctor privately. Disputes between the specialist and the control doctor are resolved by the chief medical officer of the *Ziekenfondsraad*, but such appeals are rare. Nothing could better demonstrate the high prestige of general practice in Dutch medicine than this authority exercised over the specialist by the control doctor, who is usually a former G.P. Such a relationship would be unthinkable in most countries.

Summary

Fee-for-service can be fitted to fundamentally different approaches to public medical care. In many systems, the sick fund or government is a highly visible participant in the doctor-patient relationship, since the public agency pays the bills and may specify conditions that the doctors must meet.

[32] *Tarieven* . . . (note 1), Tariff IV, pp. 68–69.

In other systems, the medical profession tries to keep the procedures of traditional private practice by insisting that the patient pay the doctor, while the public agency does no more than reimburse the patient and has no contact with the profession.

Paying doctors for work performed seems a simple goal, but translating it into practice requires many complex decisions. Not every public medical scheme has the same problems or uses the same criteria, and therefore fee-for-service systems vary considerably. Some schedules cover all procedures in all settings; others cover only the simplest procedures and leave the more difficult work to the salaried doctors in hospitals and polyclinics. The fee schedules result in part from rational planning by experts and by committees; but they are also the result of internal maneuvering among specialties within the medical profession. The precise combination of rational calculation and medical politics varies among countries. Elaborate formulae sometimes are included to discourage repeated performance of the same procedure without clinical justification. Fee schedules usually are written by doctors, with some representing the interests of the profession while others speak for the sick funds or government.

IV

TYPES OF PAYMENT: SALARY

In salaried systems of payment, the doctor receives a lump sum from an organization for medical services during a specific period of time. The payment system ties the doctor to the organization; payment does not depend on a variable personal relationship between doctor and patient, as do capitation and fee-for-service payments. The type of doctor-patient relationship varies according to conditions specified by the organizations retaining the doctors' services.

Salaried systems are very common in the world: nearly every country has many doctors who receive a salary from some unit of government; numerous doctors in each country have salaried relationships with private organizations; and some younger doctors are virtually salaried assistants to older private practitioners. Entire medical specialties, such as public health, usually have consisted of officers of some organization and usually have been paid by salary. Until recently, most clinical specialties in each country were on a composite basis: some specialists were paid salaries for some or all of their time, other specialists earned fees. Since the spread of public hospitals and national health insurance in the late nineteenth century, increasing proportions of the doctors in many countries have been paid by salary; since the Bolshevik Revolution, several countries have adopted national health services retaining nearly all their doctors on salary. The trend in the world is toward increased salary practice, since organized medical care often involves salaried arrangements and since the world trend is toward greater organization of medical care. In nearly all countries, the trends are for organized medical care to be governmental and therefore for doctors increasingly to have a salaried relationship with governments. Even in America, with its nearly unique mixture of private and public medical care, increasing organization is causing a steady rise in salaried practice.[1]

[1] "Will the Hospital Soon Be Your Boss?" *Medical Economics*, vol. 40, no. 12 (17 June 1963), pp. 75–156; and Herman M. Somers and Anne R. Somers, *Doctors, Patients, and Health Insurance* (Washington: The Brookings Institution, 1961), p. 52.

Salaried systems are quite varied because of cross-national differences in medical organization, in national prosperity, and in the demands and power of the medical association. In most countries, the hospital and polyclinic specialists are paid by salary, while specialists and general practitioners working outside these establishments earn their incomes by some other method; in some countries both general practitioners and specialists are salaried. In some countries, only a portion of the doctors in a category (e.g., only some of the specialists) are salaried; elsewhere nearly all the members of the category (e.g., all the specialists or the entire medical profession) are so paid. Most salaried doctors are allowed to practice under different conditions outside their salaried working hours, but in some countries one or several salaried arrangements cover their full work schedule. The amount of salaried time varies: in some countries, it is short; elsewhere it occupies a full work day. Relationships between doctor and the paying organization vary: some countries define the doctor and the organization as equal contracting parties; elsewhere the doctor is defined as the organization's employee. Sometimes the doctor is allowed to make extra charges for medical work during his salaried hours, but the trend in the world is to make the salary full payment for all medical procedures performed in accordance with the contractual or employment conditions. The methods of determining salaries and the amounts differ greatly among countries.

The fixing of doctors' salaries often becomes involved in governments' larger economic plans, since salaried medical work usually is part of organized systems involving other facets of the economy. In contrast, capitation and fee-for-service rates are set more autonomously; if dependent on any organized system or subject to any higher external constraints, these are part of a separate medical sector, such as national health insurance.

This chapter will concentrate on the salaried arrangements for clinicians in public medical systems. For the sake of brevity and simplicity, I will not discuss the payment of public health doctors, medical administrators, or clinical research scientists, unless they are covered by the salary scales for clinicians. Most such doctors in the world are paid by salary.

The Soviet Union

Like all other employed persons, doctors are paid by salaries drawn from the general revenue of the government. Each economic sector has its own wage scale, and Soviet doctors are paid according to the scale for all employees in health.

Wages in health follow procedures introduced in 1931. Positions on all Soviet pay scales are distinguished according to the characteristics of the job and of the individual: arduousness; education, skill, and other personal qualifications; managerial or other responsibilities; the incumbents' length of service; importance of the industry in the entire economy; and geographical location of the installation. The categories of the pay scale of each occupation are drafted by the Ministry employing it; in health, the first draft is prepared by the Ministry of Health. The categories and wage rates then are written in detail during conferences between the Ministry and the trade union representing that occupation—in health, the Ministry of Health and the Medical Workers Union. Since the economy is centrally planned and directed, and since someone must designate priorities in spending, higher levels make the final decision. The State Commission on Staffs—now located in the Ministry of Finance—writes the final draft, which is issued as a decree of the Council of Ministers of the government. The wage decrees bind all government agencies, trade unions, and employing organizations. The salary schedule of each enterprise is filed with the local office of the Ministry of Finance, which supplies the money and is guardian over the payment system.[2] Once salary scales remained unchanged for several years, but the 1964 reforms prescribed annual review.

Following are the basic pay scales in rubles per month for doctors, after the reforms announced in 1964:[3]

Work Site	Number of Years of Experience: Less than 5	5–10	10–25	25–30	More than 30
Hospitals and polyclinics in small towns	105	115	125	140	170
Regional and rural medical centers in villages and small towns	100	110	120	130	170
Other medical installations in villages and small towns; urban public health and first aid centers	95	105	115	125	170
Urban hospitals and polyclinics	90	100	110	125	165
Other medical installations in cities	85	95	105	120	165

Directors of hospitals and of other medical installations receive higher rates on the average. But there is considerable overlap: practitioners with

[2] The Soviet wage determination system is described in, Abram Bergson, *The Structure of Soviet Wages* (Cambridge: Harvard University Press, 1944), pp. 155–56, 172–76; Solomon P. Schwarz, *Labor in the Soviet Union* (New York: Frederick A. Praeger, 1952); Emily Clark Brown, *Soviet Trade Union and Labor Relations* (Cambridge, Mass.: Harvard University Press, 1966); and Murray Yanowitch, "Trends in Soviet Occupational Wage Differentials" (New York: dissertation for Ph.D., Columbia University, 1960).

[3] N. K. Pitilimov, *Oplata truda medetsinskich i farmaceutitseskich rabotnikov* (Moscow: PROFIZDAT, 1966); A. V. Rott and K. M. Pavlenko, *Novaya oplata truda rabotnikov zdravookhraneniya* (Kiev: Zdorov'ya, 1965); and U. Danilov, "Chtoby kachestva meditsinskogo obsluzhivaniya bylo vyshe," *Sotsialisticheskii trud*, no. 1 (1965), pp. 7–13. 1 ruble = \$1.10 at the official exchange rate. Earlier salary scales can be found in, Grigory N. Kaminsky, *Okhrana zdorov'ya v sovetskom soyuze* (Moscow: Narodny Kommissariat Zdravookhraneniya, 1935), pp. 114–19; Henry E. Sigerist, *Medicine and Health in the Soviet Union* (New York: Citadel Press, 1947), pp. 313–14; and B. F. Konnov, *Pravovoe regulirovanie truda meditsinskikh rabotnikov* (Moscow: GOSIURIZDAT, 1960), pp. 19–20.

seniority can earn more money than directors of small establishments. Following are the rubles per month earned by directors:

Hospitals by size (number of doctors)	Other medical installations by size (number of doctors)	Years in Practice	
		Less than 30	More than 30
Less than 10	Less than 10	145 rubles	180 rubles
11–35	10–25	155	195
36–60	26–40	165	215
61–85	41–55	175	215
86–110	56–70	185	221
111–135	71–85	195	230
136–160	86–100	205	230
161–185	101–115	215	230
186–210	116–130	225	230
211–250	131–165	235	235
Over 250	Over 160	250	250

Chiefs-of-services in hospitals and in polyclinics receive supplements to their basic pay rates according to the sizes of their departments. Size is measured by the number of doctors working under them.

Chiefs-of-Service in Hospitals (number of subordinates)	Chiefs-of-Service in Polyclinics (number of subordinates)	Additional Rubles per Month
Less than 3	Less than 6	10 rubles
3 to 6	6 to 12	17
Over 6	Over 12	22

In return for his salary, the doctor is expected to work six or six and one-half hours a day and six days a week in his hospital or polyclinic. This has always been the work day for the Russian urban professional; there is no interruption for lunch, which is taken after the working period. Some urban doctors and probably all rural doctors must be available for emergencies, but most polyclinics and hospitals have separate emergency staffs. In other economic sectors, workers sometimes have been pressed to work overtime without extra pay; but this was always less common in medicine, and it is now avoided throughout the economy.

One group of doctors, the professors in the Medical Institutes and the clinical scientists, have long been paid according to separate salary scales. Professors and scientists have always been highly respected in Russia, and the salary scales during and after Stalin have placed them among the richest people in the country. According to pay scales announced in 1942, instructors in Medical Institutes were paid as much as chiefs of service in hospitals; docents (the next higher rank) were in the same bracket as hospital directors; and many professors had salaries double those of hospital directors.[4] Some

[4] Compare the salaries in, Sigerist, *Medicine and Health* (note 3), pp. 313–14; and Alexander Korol, *Soviet Education for Science and Technology* (New York: John Wiley & Sons, 1957), p. 304.

professors received even higher "personal salaries" outside the educational pay scale. Directors and scientists in clinical research laboratories were paid by another scale that placed them on a par with professors and docents.[5] In addition to their base salaries, professors and scientists could earn extra pay enabling them to surpass most industrial managers and engineers. Eminent professors and scientists could be elected to various categories of membership in the Academy of Medical Sciences, paying them increments up to half their base salaries. Many leading men held several jobs, such as professor in a Medical Institute, director in one or two laboratories, editor of journals, memberships on committees, and so on.[6] The result was enormous incomes, excessive concentration of power in the hands of *grands patrons* in some fields of medicine, discontent among many lower-ranking doctors, and frequent misgivings in the Ministry of Health. Excessive multiple job-holding has been discouraged by the Ministry since the 1950's, but has not completely disappeared.

Multiple jobs have been common throughout the sciences. For example, in 1962 the 103 members of the Academy of Sciences held 1,037 jobs. Enormous incomes resulted until 1959, when the government forbade one man to collect more than one full-time salary and when the size and number of part-time salaries were regulated.[7]

The advantageous position of the academicians and scientists in medicine diminished but was not eliminated as a result of reforms of the wage structure recommended by the State Committee on Labor and Wages during the 1950's. The gap between high and low classes in many salary scales was reduced. High pay grades were reduced; for example, professors in medicine and in other fields had a pay cut. Bonuses and other extra payments were reduced, so that base salary became a larger proportion of the employee's income. Limits were placed on the number and size of "personal salaries."[8]

According to the pay rates announced in 1964, the professor of medicine receives one and one-half times the salary he would have earned in the basic salary scale for physicians. The docent is paid according to the rates for all physicians, depending on his seniority and the location of the teaching hos-

[5] Galina V. Zarechnak, *Academy of Medical Sciences of the U.S.S.R.* (Washington: Public Health Monograph No. 63, U.S. Department of Health, Education, and Welfare, 1960), p. 21.

[6] Ibid., pp. 21–22. Russians get numerous fringe benefits in addition to pay, and the professors, scientists, and directors in the medical services have always gotten the most generous rewards, such as good apartments, free transportation, comfortable vacations, etc.

[7] Subcommittee on National Security Staffing and Operations, *Staffing Procedures and Problems in the Soviet Union* (Washington: U.S. Government Printing Office, 1963), p. 44.

[8] Walter Galenson, "The Soviet Wage Reform," *Proceedings of Thirteenth Annual Meeting of the Industrial Relations Research Association* (1961), pp. 250–65; Nicholas DeWitt, *Education and Professional Employment in the U.S.S.R.* (Washington: National Science Foundation, 1961), pp. 539–42; Yanowitch, "Wage Differentials" (note 2), pp. 32–38; and Brown, *Union and Labor Relations* (note 2), chap. 10.

pital. The medical faculties can still earn supplements for clinical practice or for writing. For example, for clinical work, the professor receives an additional 3 to 5 rubles an hour, or 15 rubles a day. The docent can collect an additional 1.5 to 2 rubles an hour, or 7.5 rubles a day. Lower faculty ranks receive lower rates.[9]

Nearly all Soviet doctors are paid by a salary scale that applies to all employees in health; scales differ in other economic sectors, but they are governed by the same principles and are determined by the same procedure. From this Soviet baseline, countries vary in two directions. Some have special salary scales and procedures for doctors alone. Others have a standard salary scale for all government employees, including doctors.

Great Britain

Britain, like most European countries with salaried medical sectors, has a special scale and procedure for doctors. Salary has been associated with a rank hierarchy in the hospitals, and a set of standard ranks was established after 1948. The group of doctors in a specialty in a hospital is called a "firm" and is headed by a "consultant." A firm is assigned a fixed number of beds; patients are admitted to those beds if they suffer from the conditions in which the firm specializes. A "consultant" is not synonymous with a fully qualified "specialist": the former holds a hospital appointment and is in charge of a "firm"; since there are more licensed specialists than consultantships, some must await openings and meanwhile may help consultants run their firms. The grades, ranked by experience and responsibility are called "consultant," "senior hospital medical officer," "senior registrar," "registrar," "junior hospital medical officer," "senior house officer," and "house officer." Smaller firms may have only some of these ranks. The rank of "senior hospital medical officer" was created at the start of the hospital service for mature doctors who were neither trainees nor fully qualified specialists, but who had always done miscellaneous tasks in the hospital without official status in specialty work; the rank was gradually abolished during the 1960's, as it became customary for the senior hospital doctors to have credentials in a specialty. As postgraduate clinical experience in hospitals became routine for young English doctors, whether planning to specialize or enter general practice, the lower ranks (registrar, junior registrar, and house officer) were redefined so that their incumbents no longer were considered specialty trainees.[10]

[9] Rott and Pavlenko, *Novaya oplata truda* (note 3), pp. 102–4, 131–33, 166–67, 173.

[10] The hospital service is described in, Rosemary Stevens, *Medical Practice in Modern England* (New Haven: Yale University Press, 1966); and Almont Lindsey, *Socialized Medicine in England and Wales* (Chapel Hill: The University of North Carolina Press, 1962), chaps. 10 and 11. The staff structure is described and evaluated in the Platt Report, known more formally as *Report of the Joint Working Party on the Medical Staffing Structure in the Hospital Service* (London: H. M. Stationery Office, 1961).

Since 1948, the pay of hospital staffs has been affected in two ways: periodically the salary rates for all ranks have been examined and increased;[11] and the functions and size of some ranks have been examined and altered. The first salary scale was written by an impartial committee of experts and nonpartisan public figures, headed by Sir Will Spens and assisted by a staff drawn from the Ministry of Health and from the British Medical Association. The Committee relied upon a questionnaire survey of doctors, sponsored by the medical societies, to learn the actual economic position of hospital doctors. The Spens Committee specified various standards that the salaries should meet. The lower hospital ranks, who had been underpaid before the war, should be compensated sufficiently to alleviate hardships, free them from dependence on private means, and relieve them of the need for outside jobs. Pay would be commensurate with responsibility and skill: the Committee crystallized the formerly amorphous rank structure of hospitals, suggested a series of pay grades, and recommended a salary scale with automatic annual increments. In the past, consultants had concentrated near London, where lived the wealthiest private patients. Since the National Health Service needed a wide geographical distribution of specialists of all ranks, rates would be the same throughout the country. Prewar incomes had varied greatly among specialties, causing unbalanced recruitment. The Spens Committee recommended the same pay scales for all specialties, in order to ensure sufficient recruitment into necessary but less popular fields like ophthalmology, radiology, and anesthesiology.[12]

The Spens Committee's mission was to help set the first pay rates. Thereafter, the pay of hospital doctors, like that of all other National Health Service employees, was supposed to be settled by one of the "Whitley Councils." Each Council includes representatives of Health Service employees and management. Deadlocks within Councils are settled by arbitration. The mechanism later was used to settle some disputes, but was inadequate to cope with major controversies involving the consultants; the latter preferred to negotiate directly with the Government, and the Medical Council merely approved the result.[13] A new procedure was necessary that would keep doctors' pay under regular review and that would settle disputes at the highest level of the government, befitting a profession that deemed itself especially important. A Royal Commission investigated the problems of doctors' pay after the bitter controversies of the 1950's—particularly those involving the

[11] The changing rates from 1948 through 1959 are summarized in *Royal Commission on Doctors' and Dentists' Remuneration 1957–1960: Report* (London: H. M. Stationery Office, Cmnd. 939, 1960), pp. 300–2.

[12] *Report of the Inter-Departmental Committee on Remuneration of Consultants and Specialists* (London: H. M. Stationery Office, Cmnd. 7420, 1948), esp. pp. 6–13.

[13] H. A. Clegg and T. E. Chester, *Wage Policy and the Health Service* (Oxford: Basil Blackwell, 1957), esp. pp. 60–63.

general practitioners—and it proposed a new procedure as well as new pay rates.

The consultants' spokesmen before the Royal Commission recommended transfer of their pay questions from the Whitley Council on the grounds that the government side in the bargaining represented only low-level civil servants acting on instructions from the Treasury; the consultants' negotiators never confronted the real decision-makers; and only a high-ranking Review Body responsible to the Prime Minister could make an authoritative decision.[14]

The Commission recommended and the government created a "Standing Review Body of eminent persons of experience in various fields of national life to keep medical and dental remuneration under review and to make recommendations about that remuneration to the Prime Minister."[15] A division of functions then evolved: the Ministry of Health negotiates with the medical profession about the structure of the payment system; the Review Body gives a monetary interpretation to the agreed payment system. The Review Body in theory does not arbitrate; officially it is a consultant to the Prime Minister, and the actual payment decisions are made on the government's responsibility. But of course the Review Body's recommendations carry great weight with the Treasury and Cabinet, and it is overruled only under unusual circumstances. The membership of the Review Body is picked after conversations involving the Prime Minister's office, the Ministry of Health, and the medical and dental associations; since its task is defined as calculating fair incomes, its membership is drawn from economic and actuarial backgrounds rather than from health. Like a Royal Commission, the Review Body includes distinguished members whose decisions command respect. The Review Body considers all medical and dental compensation, but the perennially embattled general practitioners have attracted its attention most often.

The Review Body decides two dimensions of the size of payment, namely the actual amount and the length of each award. The Review Body has functioned much like the Royal Commission that preceded it: other government agencies, private economists, and the professional associations submit facts about the income levels of doctors, dentists, and the other professions used as reference groups. Since the Royal Commission recommended that the pay of professionals should be stable, the adjustments are not made automatically every year, as they are in some other national medical care schemes. A fair income is calculated for the period from the date of announcement to

[14] "Witnesses for the Joint Consultants' Committee," *Minutes of Evidence Taken before the Royal Commission on Doctors' and Dentists' Remuneration* (London: H. M. Stationery Office, 1959), pp. 1099–1100, 1148–52.

[15] Royal Commission . . . (note 11), p. 145.

the date of the next review. At first the Review Body planned to re-examine pay about once every three years; when the first two predictions proved inaccurate, the duration of each award was reduced to two years or less. A basic problem is to calculate a sum that is not merely fair at the moment of the award but will remain fair on the average throughout the three-year or two-year period.

Usually the Royal Commission and the Review Body are pressed by the medical profession to maintain its economic position relative to other professions. Thus movements in the wage and price structure of the country were the decisive influences on the Commission's and Review Body's thinking. Both the Commission report and the Review Body's first report estimated the probable trend in incomes among the other professions used for comparison during the next three years, and then they fixed doctors' and dentists' incomes so these sums would be relatively high at first but relatively low at the end of the period.[16] Thus price inflation and rising incomes were assumed; if incomes were declining, the logic would call for another way of calculating doctors' pay for the three-year period. If the estimates of national trends were too conservative, then doctors' pay would average lower than the desired relation over the three-year period; if the estimates of trends were too high, doctors would gain relative to the professions used for comparison. The Review Body's first report said that the Royal Commission had underestimated the rise in prices and other incomes between 1960 and 1963, and thus doctors earned an average income lower than expected. By awarding a pay increase of 14 per cent, the Review Body hoped to make up for lost ground and achieve parity with the comparison professions during the subsequent period.

But wages and prices in Great Britain during the 1960's rose faster than productivity, and the government ordered a freeze and then a period of restraint. Wage increases would be justified only if they fostered increases in productivity or prevented serious malfunctions in the economy. Therefore the seventh report of the Review Body used criteria other than parity with the incomes of other professions. Rather, it emphasized recruitment into medicine and the necessary distribution of doctors in various ranks: concluding that not enough doctors were entering and remaining in the junior hospital ranks and in general practice, the Review Body recommended changes in the pay structure to improve their positions relative to other doctors and other professions. Since the Review Body's seventh report antedated ministerial directives banning pay awards to preserve or attain parity among occupations, it used as secondary criteria in its reasoning the movement of wages and prices elsewhere in the economy.[17] After 1968, the Review Body

[16] Ibid., p. 437; "Doctors' and Dentists' Remuneration (Review Body's Report)," *Weekly Hansard: House of Commons, Parliamentary Debates*, no. 586 (25 March 1963), cols. 124–31.

[17] *Review Body on Doctors' and Dentists' Remuneration: Seventh Report* (London: H. M.

resumed fixing pay primarily in the light of the levels of other occupations.

Following is the full-time structure in the hospital service recommended by the Review Body in 1969.[18] In addition, specialists can earn fees for home visits and lectures to nurses. The figures are in sterling, which on the present free market is £1 = 20s = $2.40.

MAIN GRADES:	
Consultant	£3,470 + 9—5,275
Medical assistant	2,100 + 14—3,810
Senior registrar	2,120 + 5—2,760
Registrar	1,790 + 4—2,200
Senior house officer	1,570 + 2—1,790
House officer	1,250 + 2—1,450
OTHER GRADES:	
Senior hospital medical officer	2,700 + 8—3,640
Junior hospital medical officer	1,680 + 8—2,200

"3,470 + 9—5,275" means that the starting full-time salary is £3,470, the consultant can receive 9 seniority increments, and his final pay in this grade is £5,275. If a specialist has already received several seniority increments under previous national pay awards, a new salary award to the hospital service results in assigning him to his place in the seniority scale with a higher basic pay rate than before. Few consultants are full-time, and therefore most receive less than the full-time salaries. But private practice yields them considerably higher total incomes.

Besides the basic salaries, the superior doctors receive "distinction awards." They are higher salary rates designed to motivate better performance and induce the leading consultants to practice within the hospital service. The procedure for bestowing the distinction awards will be described in chapter IX.

SPECIAL SCALES FOR HOSPITAL STAFFS

Special salary scales are common for hospital doctors in much of Europe and in many other countries. In many societies, the staffs of public hospitals are employees of or contractors with the national Ministry of Health, in

Stationery Office, Cmnd. 2992, 1966). The ministerial white papers on incomes are *Prices and Incomes Standstill* (London: H. M. Stationery Office, Cmnd. 3073, July 1966) and *Prices and Incomes Standstill: Period of Severe Restraint* (London: H. M. Stationery Office, Cmnd. 3150, November 1966). The second white paper stated that "pay increases will not in general be regarded as justified during the period of severe restraint on the grounds of comparison with the level of remuneration for similar work or on the grounds of narrowing of differentials" (*Prices and Incomes* [Cmnd. 3150], p. 7).

[18] *Review Body on Doctors' and Dentists' Remuneration: Tenth Report* (London: H. M. Stationery Office, Cmnd. 3884, 1969), pp. 16–17.

others they are employees of or contractors with the municipality or province. Physicians in teaching hospitals receive their salaries from either the Ministry of Education, the Ministry of Health, or the local government, according to the administrative location of the teaching hospitals in that country.

In most countries, salaries of all hospital doctors are low. This is particularly true where per capita national incomes are low: tax resources are insufficient to pay more than nominal salaries. Under such conditions, the hospitals are also underfinanced in many other ways: nurses' pay is low; not many graduate nurses are employed; and few modern hospital buildings can be constructed.

Pay within the medical staff varies by rank. Although grumbling about pay is common, pressures to raise it have been weak in the past, since the higher ranks did not depend on their salaries entirely and since the lower ranks lack political influence. Usually the higher ranking doctors, particularly the chiefs-of-service, have had lucrative outside private practices. The younger doctors have been postgraduate medical students getting their specialty credentials and awaiting senior posts. The younger men have been in no position to revolt for higher pay, since usually their principal concern was to please their chiefs-of-service and gain the latter's patronage. In most countries, hospital medical staffs are broad-based pyramids: each service has few senior doctors and many young ones. Instead of needing to raise pay to recruit enough doctors, most governments have found they have more candidates than positions: to become a service chief in a public hospital is usually a stepping-stone to the largest private practice, since the job is public certification of professional leadership. In return for his salary, the doctor must work at the hospital most of the morning and until mid-afternoon—8 A.M. to 2 P.M. in some countries, more or less in others.

The foregoing has been true in the public general hospitals of many of the countries I visited, notably France, Switzerland, Spain, Italy, and Greece. For example, following are the medical staff structure, salaries, and hours governing the 1,360 doctors in the 120 hospitals of the Ministry of Social Welfare of Greece in 1963:

Rank of Doctor	Drachmas per Month: Athens, Piraeus, Salonika	Drachmas per Month: Rest of Country	Daily Hours: Winter	Daily Hours: Summer
Chief-of-service	4,200–5,000	6,000	9:30–1:00	9:00–12:30
Chief resident	3,100–3,500	4,500	9:00–2:00	8:30–1:30
Assistant doctor	2,300–2,600	3,000	8:30–2:00	8:00–1:30

(Present free market exchange rate is 1 drachma = $0.033)

In the Athenian and provincial hospitals that I visited, about half the doctors were service chiefs, one-quarter chief residents, and one-quarter assistant doctors. The junior ranks are considerably smaller in Greece than in many other countries, since young Greek doctors usually prefer to enter general practice. But in Italy, where the salary scale was much like that in Greece in the early 1960's, the junior ranks were much larger than the senior: for example, in one 1,700-bed Rome hospital, there were at the time of my visit in 1962, 22 service chiefs, about 50 chief residents, 118 assistant doctors, and several dozen volunteers—a staff structure duplicated in many other urban hospitals throughout Italy.

The salary scale for Greek hospital doctors is fixed by a law of the National Chamber of Deputies or by a decree of the executive, and thus it tends to remain the same for many years. Such statutory scales with their consequent inflexibility typify hospital doctors' salaries in many countries; only negotiating machinery or a standing review body can bring about frequent changes. The Greek salary scales are unusual in providing a large differential in favor of jobs in the provinces. The differentials are designed to attract doctors away from the largest cities, where they find the best opportunities for private practice and the more sophisticated life. But monetary advantages alone have proved insufficient—chapter IX will show this is true in other countries—and the Greek government now forbids any doctor to practice in the larger cities until he has worked for three years in the provinces.

Low pay carries dangers. In particular, the chiefs-of-service may neglect their official duties in favor of their more lucrative private practices, conducted elsewhere in the city. Therefore many countries during the 1960's tried to raise the salary rates for their hospital staffs.[19]

Standard Salary Scales

Several countries have basic salary scales for all government employees, including doctors.[20] Therefore, if the country has a national health service, a substantial proportion of its doctors are paid like any other civil servants and may even be subject to all civil service regulations. If different scales exist, the doctors are not treated separately from laymen as in Western countries,

[19] See, for example, the higher rates for Italian hospital doctors in, Carlo Palenzona, "Période de réforme sanitaire, disputes entre médecins, disputes entre ministères," *Concours médical*, vol. 89, no. 7 (18 February 1967), p. 1328.

[20] Specialists in wage administration disagree whether separate or universal salary scales should apply to all professionals. Collett believes that separate scales should be avoided, since every profession then presses for special treatment and higher pay, and no rational total structure can develop. Doctors have recently become particularly successful in these maneuvers. Merrill J. Collett, "Building the Framework of the Pay Plan," in, Kenneth O. Warner and J. J. Donovan (editors), *Practical Guidelines to Public Pay Administration* (Chicago: Public Personnel Administration, 1963), p. 39. But Belcher believes that the labor market and incentive profiles in the professions are so different from those of management that the professions should be paid by independent procedures. His reasoning implies a separate scale for each profession. David W. Belcher, *Wage and Salary Administration* (Englewood Cliffs, N.J.: Prentice-Hall, 2d ed., 1962), pp. 539, 541.

but the scales for administrators and employees (including doctors) are different from the scales for the Ministry of Education (including its professors of medicine). Most of these countries are less developed societies that attempt to maintain simple and standardized administrative structures. But one example of this salary system is found in Sweden.

Sweden

Although the Swedish public services are highly decentralized in finance and in management, personnel policy is centralized and standardized. Although many activities are administered by local governments, many categories of national and local employees are regulated according to common civil service rules and pay scales. Although most of the country's medical services are managed and financed by provincial, city, and communal governments, the doctors are paid according to nationwide salary scales applying also to nonmedical employees.[21]

Labor conflicts were once common in Sweden, but for several decades working conditions and wages have been settled by nationwide collective bargaining between employers and employees. The Confederation of Swedish Trade Unions (LO) has functioned since 1898. Two similar national organizations have existed since the 1930's to protect the interests of salaried workers of all types, the Central Organization of Graduate Workers (SACO) and the Central Organization of Salaried Employees (TCO). For purposes of negotiating wages and working conditions, the Swedish Medical Association is affiliated with SACO and the Swedish Nurses Association with TCO. Basic pay scales for salaried government employees are negotiated from time to time (often annually) by conferences between the labor representatives (SACO and TCO) and government representatives from the section on salaries of the Department of Civil Affairs, from the Ministry of Finance, from the Council of Local Governments, and sometimes from other agencies. In theory, the two sides are not bargaining and the Cabinet and *riksdag* are free to enact as law whatever salary scales they wish, but in practice the government representatives agree to recommend to the *riksdag* whatever scales the conferences write.

In practice, preparing the basic salary scales is not so difficult. The more complicated problem is the second stage, when each occupation's jobs are fitted to the scales. In general form, the scales remain the same year after year, with minor revisions; each new scale has a slightly higher monetary value than the previous one, but usually only moderate raises are possible because of limited rises in tax revenue and competing demands from other

[21] The structure and weaknesses of the government salaried system are described by Gunnar Heckscher, *Svensk statsförvaltning i arbete* (Stockholm: Studieförbundet Näringsliv och Samhälle, 1952), pp. 319–21, 333–40.

government agencies. SACO, TCO, and the government favor salary scales that differentiate employees by responsibilities, work, and education. SACO argues that the university-trained should get the highest pay, to recoup the time and money invested in training, an argument that strengthens the doctors' position in wage demands and that ensures support by the SACO leadership. A desire to avoid levelling is one reason why the college-educated (including doctors) have their own labor confederation and do not approach the government through the larger TCO. The conferences try to devise salary scales that will fit many occupations and that will provide geographical differentials, the latter primarily to compensate for differences in living costs.

The basic salary scales for salaried government employees in 1966 appear in Table 4.[22]

A particular job is assigned to a salary class, and most of the salary negotiations concern these assignments. Some jobs are rated C5, B4, B1; others are KB6, A15, KA9, and so on. Slightly different jobs in the same occupation with similar responsibilities and qualifications—such as a professorship in medicine and the direction of a hospital—may be given the same pay class. (In the cited case, often the former is U27 and the latter is C1 or B7.) Comparable jobs in different occupations may be in the same pay class, if the budgets of their respective services allow, if the collective bargaining sessions produce the same results, and if the occupations enjoy the same priority in public policy. Thus doctors in various pay grades have counterparts in other occupations; some of the latter jobs resemble the medical ones, but, as I shall show later, many medical jobs have higher pay than comparable jobs in other occupations. One of the common complaints about the Swedish salary structure is that rates are tied to jobs and not to individuals, and that seniority cannot be rewarded by increments.[23] The same is true for doctors—they get salary raises only by job promotions—but the rigidity is less irritating to them than to other government employees, because they have large supplementary incomes from private practice.

The principal groups of salaried doctors covered by these general civil service salary scales are hospital physicians, district medical officers, and the faculties of medical schools. In theory SACO should negotiate with the Department of Civil Affairs, but in practice each side delegates this technical work of job rating to the medical administrators best qualified: the Swedish Medical Association represents the medical profession and speaks for SACO; the Royal Medical Board, the medical officials of the Council of Local Governments, and someone from the section on salaries of the Department of Civil Affairs speak for the public employers. SACO and the SMA keep in

[22] *Löne- och anställningsvillkor m.m.* (Stockholm: Sveriges Akademikers Centralorganisation, 1966). The free market exchange rate is 1 kr. = $0.19. The basic rates are increased by cost-of-living allowances of 10 per cent or 11 per cent.

[23] Heckscher, *Svensk statsförvaltning* (note 21), pp. 334–38.

TABLE 4. SALARY SCALE FOR SWEDISH GOVERNMENT EMPLOYEES

Employees of National Government	All Teachers	Employees of Municipalities and County Councils	Kronor per Year in Regions with Various Costs of Living		
			Region 3	Region 4	Region 5
A1		KA1	10,392	11,052	11,700
A2		KA2	10,932	11,604	12,300
.		.	.	.	.
.		.	.	.	.
.		.	.	.	.
A9	U1	KA9	15,672	16,656	17,640
A10	U2	KA10	16,536	17,480	18,600
.	.	.	.	.	.
.	.	.	.	.	.
.	.	.	.	.	.
A21	U13	KA21	30,708	31,752	32,796
A22	U14	KA22	32,508	33,516	34,524
A23	U15	KA23	34,404	35,388	36,348
A24	U16	KA24	36,348	37,320	38,292
A25	U17	KA25	38,472	39,384	40,320
A26	U18	KA26	40,692	41,592	42,456
A27	U19	KA27	43,092	43,896	44,700
A28	U20	KA28	45,600	46,308	47,076
A29	U21	KA29	48,204	48,876	49,572
A30	U22	KA30	51,000	51,588	52,200
A31	U23	KA31	53,916	54,408	54,960
A32	U24	KA32	57,000	57,408	57,864
A33	U25	KA33	60,024	60,564	60,936
			All Regions		
		KB1	60,936		
	U26	KB2	64,176		
C1	U27	KB3	67,392		
C2	U28	KB4	70,764		
C3	U29	KB5	75,012		
C4	U30	KB6	80,268		
C5	U31	KB7	86,688		
C6		KB8	94,476		
C7		KB9	103,932		
C8		KB10	115,356		
B1			48,480		
B2			51,060		
B3			53,760		
B4			56,604		
B5			59,604		
B6			62,760		
B7			66,096		

touch, but SACO invariably accepts the SMA's decisions. The SMA delegation includes representatives from the medical group whose jobs are being discussed, such as professors or hospital specialists. Fitting the jobs of hospital doctors to the salary scale is negotiated separately for each county, but usually the agreements are the same throughout the country, in accordance with guidelines emerging from the larger bargaining sessions in Stockholm. Resulting from the negotiations are very specific lists of job descriptions in particular organizations in particular cities, with pay grades and hours of work.[24]

Like management-employment relations throughout the Swedish economy, the annual negotiations are calm, painstaking, and lengthy: many memoranda are exchanged and many meetings are held. Lately, deadlocks have become unusual. When they occur, the Ministry of Interior is empowered to impose new salary scales by decree and does so occasionally. During less harmonious periods in the past, the doctors sometimes called strikes (euphemistically called "blockades") against county governments that wished to pay less than the national norms. For example, during the late 1950's the SMA struck against the public hospitals of Göteborg, which did not wish to pay high enough wages to its hospital residents. During the strike, the SMA urged doctors not to take jobs in these hospitals. During the 1930's and 1940's, the Association of Young Doctors won higher rates for residents by threatening or calling strikes against many public hospitals.

Doctors occupy very high positions on the salary scales: professors, hospital directors, and the leading hospital chiefs of service are U27 and B5 through B7; other hospital chiefs of service and senior specialists are B5, or range between KB1 and KB5; other specialists may vary between A27 and A30 and between KA28 and KA31; junior hospital doctors are paid between A23 and A26 or between KA24 and KA29; some doctors working in municipal polyclinics come under the foregoing salary scales and may be paid between KA27 and KB4. (All these are approximations, and publicly employed doctors in smaller hospitals, smaller polyclinics, or less important jobs may have lower pay classes.) District medical officers are KA21–KA24; assistant district medical officers are KA19–KA22; and temporary appointees to these posts also are KA19–KA22. Some physicians earn second salaries. For example, professors in the clinical specialties may be paid 36,000 kr. to 48,000 kr. annually as chiefs of service in the teaching hospitals. Some chiefs of service in nonteaching hospitals may earn up to 36,000 kr. in addition for outpatient work, for administration, or for other duties.

Other occupations have lower positions on the basic salary scales and do not earn second salaries. For example, only recently did the other university professors rise into the same bracket as the professors in medical schools. Compared to other occupations, medicine has larger proportions of its members on the B and KB scales. About two-thirds of the public employees paid according to Plan A are in the lower half of the scale, but virtually no doctors are included. Nearly all the civil government employees paid according to

[24] E.g., *Specialbestämmelser till 1947 ars allmänna tjänstereglemente för Stockholms kommunalstyrelse* (*T 47*) *och till bestämmelser om arvodesanställning* (*Arv 48*) (Stockholm: Stockholms Stads Lönenämnd, 1961).

Plans B and KB are in salary classes 1 through 4, but many doctors are in classes 4 through 6.

Invidious comparisons can easily be made, since the salary ratings of all government jobs are highly public. For example, the rates for all the employees of Stockholm are published in the city's annual yearbook, *Särtryck ur Stockholms Kommanalkalender*. The extreme visibility of salary grades doubtless puts pressure on the negotiators to develop a complete wage structure that they can justify and that will minimize discontent. Probably for this reason, the differentials between medicine and other occupations narrowed during the 1960's.

The prospective rewards of private practice influence the salary decisions of negotiating committees. Doctors without rights of private practice earn more than those with such rights; for example, in several hospitals that I visited in 1962, the director was B6 and the service chiefs B1—according to the salary ratings then used. Doctors whose specialties afford less opportunity for private practice also get more than others; for example, in some of these hospitals, in 1962, the head anesthesiologist was B4. (Since the full-time house staff in anesthesiology was no more deprived than the full-time house staffs in other fields, they were paid alike, namely A26 for the chief resident and A23 or A22 for the other residents.)

United Arab Republic

The government plans a nationwide medical system that will fill the over-all deficit and urban-rural imbalance in facilities: all hospitals will become part of a national system organized regionally; rural health centers, begun during the 1940's, will be multiplied. It is hoped that national health insurance will be feasible; perhaps eventually it will be replaced by a national health service supported by general tax funds. To meet the needs of the future, the classes of medical schools have been expanded, and new schools have been established.[25]

Like many underdeveloped countries, pre-revolutionary Egypt paid all its government employees according to simply constructed salary scales, classified government-employed doctors as civil servants, and therefore paid doctors according to regular civil service rates. Thus the expansion of public medical services under Nasser has increased the number of salaried doctors and has increased the proportion of the medical profession who are salaried employees of the government. Following is the salary scale for salaried government employees, including doctors, at the time of my visit in late 1961:[26]

[25] Egypt's current problems and future plans are described in, Ahmed Kamel Mazen, "Development of the Medical Care Program of the Egyptian Region of the United Arab Republic" (Stanford: dissertation for Ph.D., Stanford University, 1961) and *The United Arab Republic Yearbook* (Cairo: Information Department, 1959), pp. 370–88.

[26] Mazen, "Medical Care Program" (note 25), p. 29. The tourist exchange rate in the late 1960's was 1 EL = 100 piastres = $1.30, the official rate was 1 EL = $2.30.

Grade	Average Annual Pay in Egyptian Pounds
1	1,050
2	870
3	660
4	480
5	360
6	240
7	174
8	138

For each salary grade, the beginning pay is slightly lower than the average, and the maximum pay for the grade is slightly higher. The doctor receives regular seniority increments from the lower to the higher rates within each grade. Job promotions bring the doctor higher pay grades. At times "war allowances" are added, to compensate for price inflation. The highest ranking government employees have salaries above Grade 1, between EL 1,200 and EL 6,000 annually. Wage workers are paid rates below that of Grade 8.

Egyptian college professors—including the faculties of medical schools—are paid outside the general government scales:[27]

	Part-Time Salary	Full-Time Salary	Full-Time Salary with No Other Job	Seniority Increments
Dean	—	EL 1,260–1,800	EL 1,620–2,160	EL 100 every 2 years
Professor	EL 300–600	960–1,500	1,320–1,860	100 every 2 years
Assistant professor	300–600	780–1,080	1,020–1,320	75 every 2 years
Instructor	300–600	480–780	660–960	50 every 2 years
Demonstrator:				
With M.D.	—	360–480	360–480	40 every 2 years
With M.B., Ch.B.	—	180–240	180–240	30 per year

The basic salary scales are administrative decisions of the government. Rates are low because national income and tax revenues are low, and because civil servants always have been numerous. As in many other underdeveloped countries, government employment is one of the few job opportunities for the educated and many civil service posts are created. Insulated from outside political pressures by the executive authority of the government and by the

[27] John L. Wilson and Joseph J. McDonald, "Medical Education in the Arab Middle East," *Journal of Medical Education*, vol. 36, no. 9 (September 1961), p. 1196. Wilson publishes the rates in U.S. dollars in 1961, when 1 EL = $2.38, but I have converted them back to Egyptian pounds.

weakness of pressure groups, the Ministry of Finance and the Civil Service Commission have been able to maintain approximately the same salary scale and have modified it by purely financial considerations. At times, Egypt's per capita national income and tax revenues have declined, and meanwhile heavy claims on the budget have come from economic development, military preparedness, and international political adventures. In order to economize, pay scales of the civil service sometimes have been slightly reduced and the automatic seniority increments occasionally have been suspended; cost-of-living bonuses have risen and fallen from time to time, according to budgetary stringencies. In other countries, the combination of economic growth, price inflation, and private pressure group activity usually have produced a steady rise in the government salary scales, but Egypt has been unable to maintain the necessary economic base. Like many underdeveloped countries, it has depended excessively on foreign sales of one agricultural product (cotton), and poor crops or downturns in world demand have sometimes caused domestic depressions; like many underdeveloped countries, the population's growth has outpaced economic expansion.

Medical jobs have occupied certain positions on the civil service and educational salary scales for many years. These customary ratings persist, so no periodic negotiations occur, like those common in Europe. The Medical Syndicate's leaders sometimes confer informally with the Ministry of Health officials about salaries, particularly when new services and jobs are being created. As yet professional associations and trade unions have had only limited strength and limited functions, but they may expand in the future, and professional associations like the Syndicate may perform an integral consultative role in the public medical services.

Chiefs of service in nonteaching public hospitals fall into the better-paying grades of the civil service salary scale. The junior hospital doctors are in the medium grades. The rural health officer, who does general practice and runs a small hospital in a rural area, usually has been assigned Grade 6; usually he gets a free house and some small fees, such as twenty piastres per home visit.[28] Most hospital doctors are paid from the budget of the Ministry of Public Health; so are the rural health officers now, although once they were paid by the Ministry of Social Affairs when it was responsible for all rural development programs. Over half of Egypt's 11,000 doctors hold some sort of salaried government job, primarily with a hospital, polyclinic, or rural health center controlled by the Ministry of Health.

The chiefs of service in urban hospitals are expected to work half-days and are free to conduct private practices after about 2 P.M. Many younger hospital doctors conduct private practice or hold private jobs during after-

[28] Sadek Antonios Bouktou, "Organisation of Medical Care in the Rural Districts of Egypt," *Bulletin of the International Social Security Association*, vol. 7, nos. 1–2 (January–February 1954), p. 23.

noons or evenings. Once younger doctors could hold a second government job, but the régime has sought to spread the work in recent years by forbidding multiple public jobs. The medical faculty usually chooses part-time appointments to be free for private practice, and many professors own private clinics. Once rural health officers could be employed part-time, but recently the government has tried to make these appointments full-time. The régime hopes the medical service some day will become entirely full-time, but this requires adequate salaries that the government cannot yet support and a loyalty to the public service that has been developed in Egypt only since the Revolution of 1952.

Turkey

The most highly standardized pay scale for all government employees, including doctors, has existed in Turkey. Several Ministries of the national government run medical services. The Ministry of Health and Social Assistance manages hospitals (totalling two-thirds of the country's beds), local polyclinics dispensing specialized and general care, and public health services. The hospitals and polyclinics may be used by all classes of the population but, as in much of the eastern Mediterranean, persons are screened according to ability to pay: poor people are exempt from payment if they bring letters from their mayors ("*muhtars*' certificates"); in theory others should pay fees, but in practice many get *muhtars*' certificates too. Thus, as in many underdeveloped countries, the Ministry of Health's services are the nucleus of what will become a free national health service when investment in medical care increases.

A compulsory health insurance law is administered by the Workers Insurance Institute of the Ministry of Labor. For many years it covered only workers—but not their dependents—in major urban industries, a group constituting only 2 per cent of the population. In 1965, national health insurance was extended to all employed persons. To treat its subscribers, the Workers Insurance Institute owns and operates hospitals and polyclinics. Turkey's large and influential Army has medical services for its personnel, as do some of the state-owned economic enterprises. Some municipalities own and manage hospitals and polyclinics for their citizens. Besides the numerous publicly owned installations, hospitals and clinics are run by some charitable associations, factories, and other private organizations.[29]

[29] Overviews of the country's medical services appear in *The Organization and Legislation Concerning Health and Social Assistance in Turkey* (Ankara: Ministry of Health and Social Assistance, 1956); André Prims, "Problemen van Gezondheidszorg in Turkije," *Sint-Lucastijdschrift*, no. 1 (1963); and Robert J. Myers, *Report on Social Security Systems in Turkey* (Washington: Social Security Administration, 1961). An explanation of the Social Insurance Law of 1965 can be found in *Bu Genelge, 506 Sayili Sosyal Sigortalar Kanununun . . .* (Ankara: T. C. Calisma Bakanligi Isci Sagligi Genel Md., Sayi 915–1–22/1232, 1965).

The Turkish government service has always been highly centralized, and many doctors hold their appointments directly from the Ministry of Health or the Workers Insurance Institute. All doctors employed by any Turkish government agency—whether by a national Ministry or by a local government—are paid according to one pay scale. Called the Barem scale, it applied in the past to all salaried employees of all Turkish government agencies. The fact that all, whether doctors or civil servants, were compensated according to the same salary scale follows from the traditional Turkish belief that all public employees are alike servants of the state.

Following are the Barem scale and the salary grades for Turkish physicians at the time of my visit in early 1962.[30]

Salary Grade	Barem Scale	Salaries of Doctors in Turkish Lira per Month
1	150	2,400
2	125	2,100
3	100	1,500
4	90	1,250
5	80	1,100
6	70	950
7	60	800
8	50	700
9	40	600
10	35	500
11	30	450
12	25	
13	20	
14	15	

The Barem scale resulted from attempts to rationalize the Ottoman state administration during the nineteenth century. To correct the previous lack of organization, budgetary unpredictability, and corruption in the Ottoman civil service, an extremely standardized and rigid salary system was created for all public employees. The system was extended by Ataturk in 1929 and persists today because of administrative convenience, the ever-present danger of favoritism to one group, and the difficulty of inventing a flexible and generally acceptable set of inter-occupational differentials. The Barem scale's numbers originally referred to units of gold. Now it is a set of ratios that is translated into Turkish lira by the government's statutory and budgetary actions. As can be seen in the table, increments are larger among the higher rather than among the lower salary brackets. Among employees covered by

[30] Sabahattin Payzin, "Medical Manpower in Turkey," *Conference on Teaching of Preventive Medicine* (Shiraz, Iran: Central Treaty Organization, 1961), p. 259. The table shows the basic salary grades that are used for fixing the salaries of particular jobs. It omits the intermediate five-point intervals where many doctors fall because of the automatic triennial pay increases. At the time of writing, the official exchange rate is 1 TL = $0.09.

the Barem scale, the highest salaries are ten times the lowest. Not all Turkish government employees are paid according to the Barem scale: wage workers, such as laborers, are paid by other procedures, and classifying someone as a weekly wage worker is one of the few ways that a government agency can pay an individual a special rate.

Its name comes from Bertrand François Barrême, a seventeenth-century arithmetician and accountant, who suggested a basic numeral scale to guide the international exchange of money. Barrême-type scales have been unfashionable in Europe for many years, but the Turkish government sought some way of tying its salary payments (expressed in the dubious Turkish currency) to gold.[31]

As in much of Turkish public life, the monetary values of the Barem scale are fixed by government action, with much less of the pressure group lobbying than would surround such crucial economic decisions in any Western legislature. Government regulations fix many of the wages and working conditions throughout the Turkish economy. The population has long been accustomed to central direction by the government, and trade unions, professional associations, and other private pressure groups are little developed.[32] The customary Turkish practice of passing legislation applying standard procedures to a great variety of public and private activities gives narrow-interest groups little opportunity to demand special treatment and little leverage in the political structure.

Although salary decisions are made centrally, they are not made secretively or undemocratically. The form and monetary value of the Barem scale are contained in a law adopted by the democratically elected Grand National Assembly, and there is considerable debate in both the legislature and the press. For example, during the last major revision of the Barem scale in 1954 and 1955, the popular press, professional journals in economics and public administration, and other media carried complete news and many articles with expert advice.

If there is enough money in the budget, all Barem scale monetary values are increased by the same percentage. But since Turkey is a poor country with steadily mounting defense expenditures, general pay increases occur only infrequently. As a result of the budget deficits and price inflation during the 1950's, the cost of living rose faster than government salaries, and public employees as a class suffered a decline in real income.

[31] The history and recent structure of the Barem scales can be found in, Feyzi Magat et al., *Barem* (Ankara: Titas Basimevi, 1941), and Joseph B. Kingsbury and Tahir Aktan, *The Public Service in Turkey* (Brussels: International Institute of Administrative Sciences, 1955), chap. 4.

[32] *Labour Problems in Turkey* (Geneva: International Labour Office, 1950). So too, the population has long been accustomed to the national government taking the initiative in many sectors of economic development. Zvi Hershlag, *Turkey: An Economy in Transition* (The Hague: Uitgeverij van Keulen N.V., 1958).

Since the same pay scale applies to all Turkish salaried occupations in the public service, the problem for an individual occupation cannot be to secure a very high money value or a particularly advantageous scale for itself alone, as is the goal in many other countries. Rather, an occupation seeks to have its jobs placed in the higher salary grades. In addition, an occupation seeks supplements that are not part of the official Barem scale, such as cash bonuses for high performance or fringe benefits, like free housing or expense accounts.

There is only limited scope for these inter-occupational variations. Each occupation has low positions on the scale for its neophytes; each has some of the highest Barem scale points for its leading executives and professors; moving up the scale depends on seniority and the job promotions that come with seniority. Some occupations start at a higher grade than others whose neophytes begin with less education—for example, young doctors begin at point 30 on the Barem scale, while occupations with less educational preparation start slightly lower—but the differences among occupations in starting points and spread are small.

In the early 1960's, the youngest and lowest ranking doctors, such as hospital residents, started at point 30 (450 TL). Hospital specialists, assistant professors of medicine, and local public health officers fell in the range of 50 to 80 points (700 through 1,100 TL). Some general practitioners in polyclinics reached this level, because of pay increases due to seniority. Chiefs-of-service in hospitals fell in the range of 70 through 100 points. The highest Barem scale positions are held by only a small number of Turks, but doctors are included. There are less than one hundred jobs rated at scale value 150 but some professors of medicine are included, because of the prestige of the universities in Turkish life.[33] Officials in the Ministry of Health and some hospital directors may be paid according to scale positions 100 and 125 (1,500 through 2,100 TL).

The fact that the individual rises on the Barem scale both by seniority and by promotion creates a need to match the two. When an individual's seniority gives him a salary rating much higher than his current job and equivalent to a higher job, the Ministry tries to promote him. This creates persistent administrative problems: the number of jobs at higher ranks are too few, particularly in Western Turkey; often the only available higher jobs are in the underdeveloped areas of Eastern Turkey, which most doctors avoid. As a result anomalies sometimes occur: a doctor with seniority may have attained a higher or equal salary to his superior, who obtained the same Barem scale position through promotion; doctors in equivalent jobs in the same organization often receive different pay because of seniority differences. In order to

[33] The salary is "high," of course, by Turkish standards. But 2,400 TL equals $284. This sum is reduced by income taxes, according to the rates published in Payzin, "Medical Manpower" (note 30), p. 259.

avoid these problems, personnel policy in the medical services—as in the rest of the government—is fitted to the rules of the salary system. Since pay increases must be conferred by seniority and since pay differentials are supposed to match rank, promotions tend to be given by seniority rather than by merit. Consequently, personnel policy serves the payment system instead of the latter serving the former.

Another complication is budget ceilings: sometimes the Ministries of Health and Labor (like other ministries) fail to get enough money for all their functions and wages, and thus cannot pay the entire increase in salary costs due to higher Barem scale positions. Since the higher Barem scale payments due to seniority must be met under civil service regulations, often the Ministries must give them priority over pay increases due to job promotions. The situation gives the Ministries one of their few areas of discretion in determining pay: executives may ask doctors to fill higher jobs without formal appointments, but the appointments and the higher Barem scale positions are assured once the budget increases sufficiently.

In return for their salaries, full-time hospital doctors work from 8 A.M. to 2 P.M., five days a week, and 9 A.M. to 12 noon on Saturdays. Many general practitioners employed by polyclinics and other installations work from 9 A.M. to 5 P.M. every day, as do doctors in public health and preventive medicine. Part-time physicians work a fraction of these hours, according to their contracts, and are paid proportionately. Since salaries are low, the doctor is left free for additional jobs or private practice during the rest of the day.

If the Turkish experience can be generalized, it appears impossible to maintain a single pay scale indefinitely for all government employees. New agencies arise and claim they have special staffing needs requiring extra payments. New occupations arise with rank structures and skills that cannot easily be fitted to the standardized scale and its incremental structure. In the late 1950's and 1960's several new government agencies were created and were given the right to pay at higher rates and by principles different from those of the Barem scale.[34] The drawback was that recipients of these special and "temporary" pay rates did not gain the social security benefits associated with the Barem scale. As we shall see in chapter IX, it became obvious that nearly all doctors preferred working in the cities to working in the less developed parts of the country, as long as they were paid only on the basis of rank and seniority. Therefore, after 1963 they too obtained special treatment in the form of large supplements for practice in the less developed areas.

[34] The mixture of pay rates within and beyond the Barem scale can be found in the personnel survey of the government, reported in, Devlet Istatistik Enstitusu, *Devlet Personel Sayimi* (Ankara: I Genel ve Katma Butceli Kurumlar, Publication No. 473, 1965), esp. p. 41.

SUMMARY

Salaried systems are very common in the world. Every country has some salaried doctors working in polyclinics or offices. In a few countries, a large proportion of the medical profession has a salaried relationship with government agencies, and they administer most of the medical care.

Probably salaried practice is destined to spread. Its principal alternative, fee-for-service, is maintained throughout general and specialty practice only in countries with a long tradition of private office practice, where the medical association is strong, and where the economic base of the country is sufficient for either private payments or an insurance mechanism. Salaried national health services supported by tax revenues and occasionally by foreign subsidies may grow in underdeveloped countries: the average citizen is not covered by health insurance and welcomes free care, and many doctors require salaried jobs to make a living. In developed countries, salaried practice may spread too, unless national health insurance schemes are constructed to protect the office practitioner working on a fee-for-service basis: in all countries, the part-time salaried doctor with a supplementary private practice is a formidable competitor for the full-time office practitioner. Even in America, the rise of medical research, medical education, specialized hospital care, and other forms of organized practice have greatly increased the minority of salaried doctors.

While salaried medical practice may create anxieties among competing private practitioners, it may not disturb the incumbents, particularly if salaries are high and if opportunities exist for supplementary private practice. Often part-time salaried jobs are important bases for building private practice, and doctors may compete to get them.[35]

Salary systems are quite varied. Some are generous, others are meager because of either national economic policy or a low national income. Some encompass a wide range and produce conflicts of interest within the medical profession, others treat doctors much alike regardless of status. Many apply to specialists alone, some cover all practitioners. Some are carefully designed to allocate doctors among jobs and regions and to reward performance; other systems are simple and inflexible. Some are constructed especially for doctors, other salary systems apply to nonmedical occupations as well.

The over-all structure and individual rates of a salary system can be de-

[35] Instead of full-time private practice, most Turkish doctors favor full-time or part-time salaried employment by government medical installations, according to the survey reported in, Carl E. Taylor et al., *Health Manpower Planning in Turkey* (Baltimore: The Johns Hopkins Press, 1968), p. 56. But, said the Turkish doctors, the pay should be adequate. Most of the Finnish doctors in full-time private practice would prefer to have salaried appointments as hospital specialists, according to the poll conducted by Elina Haavio-Mannila, "Tietoja Suomen lääkärikunnan rakenteesta ja osallistumisesta avosairaanhoitoon," *Suomen Lääkärilehti*, no. 25 (1965), pp. 1712–13.

signed carefully in order to achieve goals in public policy and in the allocation of personnel. Recruitment can be encouraged by high rates or discouraged by low ones. Administrators can try to attract persons into certain regions, specialties, or jobs by the offer of high rates. Persons can be discouraged from staying in certain positions too long by pay offers that are not commensurate with age and stage of career. Excellence and stable service can be rewarded with special supplements. The potential influence of salary upon the career choices of individuals and upon the structure of medical practice arouses the anxiety of medical associations in many countries and induces them to seek a voice in the administration of payment.

V

TYPES OF PAYMENT: CAPITATION

In capitation systems the doctor receives a single fee for each person for an extended period. During this time, the doctor provides all necessary care for that person without additional charges, and the person is expected to take all his medical problems to that doctor. Since the capitation fee covers only the one doctor-patient pair, referrals to other physicians and facilities must be financed separately. In most countries using capitation systems widely, they are employed only in the remuneration of general practitioners, and specialists are covered by a different system. Capitation systems are very rare; doctors in nearly all countries—whether general practitioners or specialists—are paid by fee-for-service or salary.

Great Britain

The most extensive use of capitation in the world is in general practice in the National Health Service. Medical associations usually avoid capitation arrangements and abandon existing ones if they believe fee-for-service will be more remunerative. The British Medical Association (BMA) preferred capitation during 1946 for several reasons that might not govern such a decision today. As I shall discuss in more detail in chapter VI, the BMA was most anxious to avoid a bureaucratized salaried system that it believed was being planned by a Labor government hostile to doctors. Thus capitation was considered the best possible compromise. Its long usage before and during National Insurance gave capitation a certain sanction. The poverty of the whole nation during the war years and the poverty of working class districts long before were still salient in 1946; the postwar economic boom was not foreseen, and few believed the country could afford an expensive and unpredictable fee-for-service system.

Like any payment system, capitation fees can be designed to achieve various planning goals. The payment of general practitioners has been bitterly disputed throughout the history of the National Health Service because of disagreements over the aims, over the best methods of accomplishing the goals, and over the adequacy of the fees.[1] On the eve of the passage of the Act, the task of recommending policy guidelines was given to an impartial committee of experts and nonpartisan public figures, under the chairmanship of Sir Will Spens. The Spens Committee recommended and the Ministry of Health agreed that capitation fees should be set in order to achieve target incomes. The Committee reasoned from two premises: capitation fees plus all other remuneration should be sufficient to place the total average annual income of general practitioners in a just relationship to the incomes of other occupations; capitation fees and other remuneration should be fixed at a level ensuring recruitment of the optimum number of able young doctors into general practice.[2] Since then, relativities, recruitment considerations, or some mixture of the two criteria have guided compensation decisions.

Subsequently the Ministry tried to maintain parity between the general practitioners and other professionals. But at the start, the Committee had recommended two basic changes from the past: the status of general practice should be raised relative to other occupations, and incomes should be distributed more equally among general practitioners. Survey data had shown that nearly half the country's general practitioners between the ages of forty and forty-nine was earning less than £1,000 in 1939; some were earning incomes only slightly higher than those of their working-class patients. The Spens Committee decided that fewer general practitioners should earn low incomes, on the grounds that their training was long, their skill great, the work arduous and responsible. Unless more G.P.'s could earn better incomes, said the Committee, all the able doctors would become specialists and only the least competent would enter general practice. Financial anxiety was said to have affected adversely the quality of general practice during the 1930's. The Committee believed it necessary not to raise the entire income scale for G.P.'s, but only to reduce the proportion earning very low incomes. The following table presents the central theme in the committee's reasoning: it compares the actual and recommended distribution of incomes in 1936–39 currency among general practitioners aged forty to forty-nine. The actual sums to be paid would exceed the 1936–39 figures, because of the changing value of money, but the table shows the planned distribution.[3]

[1] The troubled story of general practice in the Service is presented in Almont Lindsey, *Socialized Medicine in England and Wales* (Chapel Hill: The University of North Carolina Press, 1962), chaps. 6–9.

[2] *Report of the Inter-Departmental Committee on Remuneration of General Practitioners* (London: H. M. Stationery Office, Cmnd. 6810, 1946).

[3] Ibid., p. 5. At present the free market exchange is £1 = 20s. = $2.40.

Income Levels	Actual	Recommended
Under £700	20%	7%
£700–£1,000	22.5	20
£1,000–£1,300	21	24
£1,300–£1,600	17.5	24
£1,600–£2,000	10	16
Over £2,000	9	9
	100%	100%

Other aims were also mentioned by the Spens Committee. General practitioners should receive similar incomes throughout their careers, with a peak in the forty to forty-nine group. If high incomes were achieved early in life, able people would be attracted into general practice. Consequently, the Committee recommended a flattening of the extreme differences in incomes that doctors in many countries have long experienced over their life cycles. If possible, the Committee added, remuneration should vary according to individual ability.

The Treasury and the Ministry of Health needed to plan expenditures. Therefore they did not fix a capitation fee for each patient on a doctor's list and pay the resultant costs. Rather, they allotted a Central Pool of money, in the light of the approved income goals for general practice. From the Pool, each general practitioner would draw various payments, including capitation fees for all persons on his list. The reasoning behind the first Pool illustrates how the calculations were made as long as the Pool system was used. The first Pool was set at a size so that all payments would result in a net real income for the hypothetical average G.P. 20 per cent higher than before the war. First the Pool was built up: the average annual net income of a prewar G.P. was estimated, increased by 20 per cent to fulfill the Spens recommendation of higher status, and increased by 20 per cent more to correct for price inflation since 1939; the result was multiplied by the number of G.P.'s working in 1939; the average practice expenses of the prewar G.P. were multiplied by the number of doctors and increased by 20 per cent for price changes; the total was further increased by 3 per cent to account for the expansion of the population. Then the Pool was reduced by 5 per cent, on the assumption that this proportion of the population would pay general practitioners as private patients. The Pool was distributed among the Executive Councils, which paid the doctors. After other charges against the Pool—transportation costs for rural doctors, fees for treating temporary residents, etc.—the remaining money gave general practitioners capitation fees of between 16s. 6d. and 17s. per patient, depending upon the area in which they practiced. Since the Central Pool was designed to pay doctors an average income and not to guarantee a minimum capitation fee, if the portions of income earned from these other charges had been very high throughout the country, capitation fees would have been lower—as the G.P.'s finally discovered to their distress in 1964. The system aimed only at bringing about a desired *average* income; some doctors earned more than others, since they had longer lists of patients and earned more capitation fees. During the first eighteen years of the National Health Service, the formulae for calculating the inputs and outputs of the Pool were occasionally revised.[4]

The aim of giving doctors a certain average income meant that England did not have a completely consistent capitation system. Capitation was merely the administrative mechanism for producing the desired income. It was adopted because other methods were resisted by the profession (i.e., salary) or were uncontrollable and were resisted by the government (i.e., fee-for-service). The Central Pool was calculated as if a salary were paid to each doctor. Thus what went in were salaries; these allowed the Treasury to plan spending and pleased the government. What came out were capitation fees and other payments, and they pleased the doctors. But the actual workings of the system ultimately displeased everyone. The general practitioners and the government disagreed about the interpretation of the Spens Committee guidelines and about the length of time the guidelines were supposed to bind the government: the general practitioners complained that their pay had never reached the levels recommended by the Spens Committee, largely because the 20 per cent increase to compensate for wartime price inflation was not enough. The absence of an automatic review procedure led to recriminations and strike threats. The accounting of the Central Pool was difficult to understand. Because so many charges other than capitation fees were deducted from the fund and tended to reduce capitation fees, and because the incomes of doctors depended on these special charges and length of lists of patients, the distribution of income among G.P.'s departed from the Spens Committee's intentions. Disputes over the Pool system increased during the 1960's, thereby nullifying the anticipated pacifying effects from creation of a standing Review Body.

In 1965 the Ministry of Health and the British Medical Association agreed to abolish the Central Pool and to use a more straightforward system.[5]

[4] Methods used at various times are described in, James Stirling Ross, *The National Health Service in Great Britain* (London: Oxford University Press, 1952), pp. 226–27; James Hogarth, *The Payment of the General Practitioner* (Oxford: Pergamon Press, 1963), pp. 34–37; and *Review Body on Doctors' and Dentists' Remuneration: Third, Fourth and Fifth Reports* (London: H. M. Stationery Office, Cmnd. 2585, 1965), pp. 9–13.

[5] "Second Report of Joint Discussions between General-Practitioner Representatives and the Minister of Health," *British Medical Journal Supplement* (16 October 1965), pp. 153–59; and *Review Body on Doctors' and Dentists' Remuneration: Seventh Report* (London: H. M. Stationery Office, Cmnd. 2992, 1966), esp. chap. 6 and appendix 3. The profession's case against the Pool was stated in "Revised Memorandum of Evidence to the Review Body on Doctors' and Dentists' Remuneration," *British Medical Journal Supplement* (6 June 1964), pp. 219–26. The profession's proposal for a new payment system and new Terms of Service appear in "A Charter for the Family Doctor Service," ibid. (13 March 1965), pp. 89–91. The disputes over general practitioners' pay during the 1960's are sum-

The Review Body in 1969 recommended for a fifteen-month period the following schedule of capitation fees, basic payments to doctors regardless of length of list, and fees on an item-for-service basis.[6]

1) Basic practice allowance: full rate	£1,150	0s.	0d. a year
2) Standard capitation fees:			
a) for each patient aged under 65	£1	1s.	6d. a year
b) for each patient aged 65 or over	£1	10s.	0d. a year
3) Payments for "out-of-hours" responsibilities			
a) Supplementary practice allowance: full rate	£230	0s.	0d. a year
b) Supplementary capitation fee for each patient in excess of 1,000 on the list (1,000 per doctor on the combined lists of doctors in partnership)		2s.	9d. a year
c) Fee for visit requested and made between midnight and 7 A.M.	£1	0s.	0d. a visit
4) Additions to the basic practice allowance (full rates):			
a) To a doctor whose main surgery is situated in an area that has been "designated" as underdoctored for a continuous period of three years up to the date of payment	£400	0s.	0d. a year
b) To a doctor practicing with others in a central surgery in such a way as to satisfy the agreed definition of group practice	£200	0s.	0d. a year
c) Seniority payments (subject after 1969 to attendance at a prescribed number of sessions of postgraduate training):			
i) To a doctor whose name has been continuously included in the Medical Register for fifteen years and who has been a principal providing unrestricted general medical services under the National Health Service for at least the last five years	£210	0s.	0d. a year
ii) To such a principal, after ten more years of practice in the general medical services, an additional	£210	0s.	0d. a year
iii) To such a principal, after a further ten years of practice in the general medical services, an additional	£260	0s.	0d. a year
d) Allowance for pre-entry vocational training (not payable to a doctor who qualifies for any of the seniority payments)	£175	0s.	0d. a year
5) Postgraduate training allowance	£20	0s.	0d. a year for five years
6) Standard fee for item or course of service carried out in pursuance of public policy		15s.	0d.
7) Fee for doctor included in obstetric list providing complete maternity medical services	£15	17s.	6d.

---

marized in, Rosemary Stevens, *Medical Practice in Modern England* (New Haven: Yale University Press, 1966), chaps. 20 and 21.

[6] *Review Body on Doctors' and Dentists' Remuneration: Tenth Report* (London: H. M. Stationery Office, Cmnd. 3884, 1969), pp. 14–15. Some items were recommended in *Review Body on Doctors' and Dentists' Remuneration: Ninth Report* (London: H. M. Stationery Office, Cmnd. 3600, 1968), chap. 4.

Other maternity medical service fees to be increased *pro rata*

8)	Temporary resident fee, as defined at present: full rate	£1 3s. 6d.
9)	Rural practice funds to be increased by	6 per cent

The basic capitation fee was modified in two ways. First, elderly patients were thought to cause doctors more work, and each elderly inhabitant on a list therefore would bring the G.P. a higher fee. Second, the supplement for each patient beyond the first 1,000 on a doctor's list was designed to motivate the G.P. to acquire medium-sized lists, thereby discouraging short lists and equalizing the distribution of inhabitants among doctors. Once the British payment system eliminated the loading beyond a certain number of persons on a G.P.'s list in order to discourage lists that were undesirably long but still permissible under the rules, but by 1966 the lists had become less unequal in length than before.

Every capitation system has rules limiting the length of lists, and England's remained in effect under the revised payment procedures. Since the early 1950's, the maxima have been 3,500 for a single practitioner, 4,500 for a member of a partnership (provided the average list in the partnership is for no more than 3,500 persons), and 2,000 for each permanent assistant. Exceptions to these ceilings are permissible in severely underdoctored areas.[7]

Before 1966, three-quarters of the incomes of general practitioners came from capitation fees and loadings. The system initiated in 1966 contained so many other payments that less than half the average doctor's income was derived from capitation fees. Since the fee was lower than it would have been under a straight capitation system, the changes were another mode of discouraging long lists. Certain flat payments were recommended without regard to the length of the doctor's list. Each G.P. received a basic practice allowance to cover expenses: anyone with a list of at least 1,000 persons would receive £1,150 annually—according to the award in 1969—while doctors with shorter lists (fewer patients) received proportionately less. Every doctor would receive a basic payment for availability at night or on weekends, either to subscribe to a stand-by emergency service or to compensate himself. Incentive payments were available for those entering underdoctored areas or group practice. Seniority payments were given.

Special payments were provided for particular procedures. Fees could be collected from the Service for night visits, immunizations, the taking of cervical smears, maternity care, and some other procedures. Rents and actual expenditures for the wages of nurses and technicians were reimbursed.

[7] The distribution of British G.P.'s by length of list appears in *Annual Report of the Ministry of Health for the Year 1965* (London: H. M. Stationery Office, Cmnd. 3039, 1966), p. 77.

The Ministry of Health agreed to this elaborate payment structure to satisfy the general practitioners' complaints about the complexities of the Central Pool and the excessive simplicity of straight capitation. Thereafter the G.P. would receive the exact fees announced by the government; he would not live in suspense until the calculations from the Central Pool were announced. The doctor would earn additional income from the more time-consuming patients and from some extra work. His practice expenses would be paid for, either by a flat rate or in keeping with his own expenditures: they would not be paid at the discretion of the National Health Service, thereby requiring him to meet its standards. Increases in practice expenses would not cause decreases in the profession's income for services rendered.

The Netherlands

Every licensed physician in Holland has the right to participate in national health insurance, and nearly every general practitioner has some insured patients. In industrial towns where nearly everyone is covered by insurance, most patients will see general practitioners under the system; thus most of the patients coming to the average G.P. will be on his list, and most of his income will come from capitation fees. In big cities and wealthy suburbs like The Hague, Amsterdam, Wassenaar, and the Haarlem region, many people are not covered by the official scheme, private patients (some covered by private commercial insurance) constitute a larger share of general practice, and more of the G.P.'s income comes from private fee-for-service payments. Since coverage is by health insurance, usually all members of a family go to the insured person's doctor; under some circumstances, other family members may ask for another doctor, but this is unusual. (In a National Health Service covering the entire population by statute, as in England, it is easier for members of the same family to select different doctors.)

The maximum limit on length of lists varies by locality: it is 3,000 persons in many places, 3,500 in Amsterdam, 3,600 in Rotterdam, and 4,000 or more in a few growing and temporarily underdoctored communities. Because the geographical distribution of general practitioners is fairly even in Holland, long lists are unusual. In 1959 the average list had 1,878 persons, two-thirds of the subscribers were on lists smaller than 3,000, and only 4 per cent were on lists longer than 4,500.[8] The official ceilings may be exceeded temporarily to include new children and new spouses of members already on a doctor's list. (If a doctor's list is closed, any other patient may still see him privately.) For the first 2,000 persons registered with him, the G.P. receives f. 24.86

[8] Hogarth, *Payment of General Practitioner* (note 4), p. 454. The distribution of doctors by length of list in 1950 and 1951 in Amsterdam—where general practitioners were fewer in number relative to the population—appears in, Arie Querido, *The Efficiency of Medical Care* (Leiden: H. E. Stenfert Kroese N.V., 1963), p. 37.

each; for each additional person, he receives f. 18.83. (All figures are those for 1968, when the free market rate for one guilder was $0.28.) As in England before 1966, the loading is designed to discourage long lists. Unlike England, short lists are not discouraged by lower capitation fees. One of the problems of the English system is the equalization of lists, in part by motivating doctors with small practices to take additional patients. But in Holland a small national health insurance practice is not considered a policy problem, since many doctors have large private practices and since there are few long insurance lists needing to be redistributed.[9]

Straight capitation is modified or supplemented in certain ways in Holland, but not as extensively as in Great Britain. In order to guarantee them satisfactory incomes, doctors on some islands and in some sparsely populated areas are given special payments and higher capitation fees. Some G.P.'s are paid transportation allowances. If a G.P. needs to treat a person who is not his regular patient, he collects f. 6.25 for an office visit, f. 7.25 for a home visit, and double these fees for night and Sunday care. All are eligible to receive obstetrical fees if called by midwives, who normally perform deliveries and collect insurance fees. If the area lacks a druggist, a G.P. is authorized to run his own dispensary and receives an extra small capitation fee of f. 10.28 for each patient, and this becomes an important part of his income. Until 1956, small extra capitation fees were paid for each patient older than sixty-five in order to compensate for the extra work, but these were abandoned on the grounds that the customary capitation fee was sufficient; a special voluntary sick fund for the elderly was begun in 1957, with public subsidies supplementing the subscribers' small fees, and the medical profession's leaders agreed that doctors should donate any extra work, without special compensation, as their contribution to the scheme.[10]

Since payment is basically a multiplication of the capitation fee by length of list, the G.P.'s income from insurance practice can be calculated very easily and at minimum administrative costs. The Dutch G.P. receives a quarterly pay check from the sick fund.[11]

Decisions about length of lists and the size of the capitation fee are made by a committee responsible to the *Ziekenfondsraad* and the Cabinet, on the basis of recommendations from negotiating sessions between officials of the sick funds on the one hand and, on the other, representatives from the Royal Dutch Medical Association and from the Union of General Practitioners. Because specialists are paid according to a long fee schedule, their compensa-

[9] This is not to say that no one questions the official ceilings. As in England, some Dutch observers believe the best care can be given only to lists shorter than the present maxima, and they favor reductions.

[10] Details about all extra payments appear in, Hogarth, *Payment of General Practitioner* (note 4), pp. 459–62.

[11] Ibid., pp. 462–63.

tion is reviewed annually. The round of negotiations always includes general practice; the capitation fee is re-examined annually, and often slight increases result.

Two considerations dominate the negotiations concerning the size of the capitation fee. First, the fee must be set within the financial limits of the insurance system. The available money is fixed by the size of the payroll tax and by the number of taxpayers, both beyond the control of the negotiators. Maximum social security rates are specified by Parliament, and the annual rates are set by the Ministry of Social Affairs, after consultation with the sick funds and with the government's Social and Economic Council. The social security rates change very little, in contrast to general tax revenues; the latter are more flexible but cannot be used to finance the costs of the insurance system. In most countries with national health insurance, the sick funds are supposed to be self-supporting, but in practice the costs of hospitalization, drugs, and medical care outrun the yield of the payroll taxes and require heavy subsidies from the Treasury. Under such conditions, the doctors feel free to press for higher fees, since the only result will be to increase an existing Treasury subsidy. But the Dutch have always attempted to run health insurance on true insurance principles, with the funds paying full hospitalization costs and covering all their expenses out of the payroll taxes. Consequently, although the representatives of general practitioners ask for higher capitation fees each year, everyone knows that the arithmetic of the system can at best produce only a small increase, and the financial realities dominate the conversations.

Treasury subsidies were given when rapid increases in costs created large deficits during the late 1940's and early 1950's. But they have since been reduced, and the government would prefer that most of the program be self-sustaining. Some subsidies are earmarked for specific purposes: for example, one helps finance medical care for the aged, since they pay low voluntary rates and have no employers to contribute payroll taxes.[12]

The second consideration prominently discussed in negotiating sessions is the desirable annual income for a general practitioner. The two sides try to fix a capitation fee that will produce a reasonable living for a G.P. with a list of reasonable length. The logic and mood of the decisionmaking sessions are illustrated by Dekker's description of the events during 1954–55, when the insurance system was revised and when the capitation fees were altered.[13] The sick funds and the Royal Dutch Medical Association decided that the

[12] The financial accounting of the sick funds is summarized in, L. V. Ledeboer, *De Ziekenfondsverzekering in Nederland* (Amsterdam: Ziekenfondsraad, 1965), pp. 27–31; and *Verslag van de Ziekenfondsraad over het Jaar 1964* (Amsterdam: Ziekenfondsraad, 1965), pp. 60–91.

[13] Gerard Dekker, "Social Security and the Fees of General Practitioners in the Netherlands," *World Medical Journal*, vol. 3, no. 4 (July 1956), pp. 237, 248.

fee should be set by an objective formula and not by collective bargaining between interested parties. It was decided that a list of 3,000 patients was a reasonable number for good care. It was judged that a successful doctor should earn enough from 3,000 patients to cover practice expenses, cost of living, four weeks of vacation annually, and insurance against illness, accidents, invalidism, old age, and widow's and orphan's pensions. A sufficient number of doctors with well-arranged practices agreed to open their normally confidential books to accountants from the sick funds and the Royal Dutch Medical Association. From these data, the negotiators agreed upon a capitation fee.

The principal pressure for change in rates arises from increases in the cost of living, but higher practice expenses are also cited by the medical associations during the annual conferences. Periodic surveys of doctors' books are made by accountants, just as in 1954–55, in order to identify rises in practice expenses. The cost of living is known from national economic statistics. If the cost of living has risen within the past year or if the incomes of other groups have increased, the capitation fee will be raised, provided the insurance system has the money. To some extent the system has an inherent capacity to keep doctors' incomes at parity with the rest of the economy: if other occupations have been getting pay raises, the social security taxes on payrolls should be yielding more revenue, and thus more money is available for doctors. If living costs rise faster than the incomes of the sick funds—as they did during the mid-1960's—the G.P.'s demand larger increases in fees than the sick funds are able or willing to grant, and the normally harmonious Dutch health insurance system becomes embroiled in unaccustomed conflicts.

Spain

In the few countries where capitation is used throughout a national medical system, usually it is applied only to general practitioners. Since capitation implies a lasting relationship between a citizen and a doctor, it is assumed that capitation is inappropriate for specialists: specialists see patients only on the intermittent occasions of serious illness and have no permanent responsibilities to the individual patient; since a specialist performs different services for different patients, and since specialties are unlike in work, nothing so standardized as capitation seems to fit them. Therefore nearly all specialists in the world are paid by fee-for-service or by salary. But the tradition of capitation fees has been so strong in Spain that the national health insurance fund has attempted to pay its polyclinic specialists and some of its senior hospital specialists by capitation fees. All general practitioners under national health insurance are also paid by capitation fees.

During the twentieth century, many Spanish government agencies and private organizations developed health insurance funds and clinical services for their employees or clientele. The *Instituto Nacional de Previsión* (National Welfare Institute) was created in 1908 and housed in the Ministry of Labor, with the task of developing social insurance for workers. At various times under the monarchy and republic, it initiated and expanded voluntary insurance schemes, including one for sickness. The new government of Generalissimo Francisco Franco in 1942 made social security compulsory. The health insurance program of the *Instituto Nacional de Previsión* was renamed the *Seguro Obligatorio de Enfermedad* (Compulsory Health Insurance—SOE) and, like the rest of social security, it has been financed by a payroll tax on both employees and employers. At first, social insurance extended only to industrial and urban employees and—since the country was predominantly rural and had high unemployment—only a minority of the population was covered. But during the 1950's and early 1960's, the program has been extended to small farmers, farm workers, housemaids, and others, and now over half the population is covered. Inclusion of one taxpaying worker under the health insurance program extends coverage to his spouse, children, father, mother, and grandparents (if any). A law adopted in 1963 extended the various social security programs and began the task of unifying the administration and benefits of the numerous public and private funds into a single system, probably emulating that of France.[14]

The various insurance schemes initiated by the *Instituto Nacional de Previsión* and other Spanish organizations have had closed medical panels (i.e., subscribers could not use insurance funds to pay any doctor, but had to choose among those under contract to the sick fund). Many sick funds in the world begin on closed panel principles, but usually the medical associations secure legislative endorsement of free choice, as national health insurance becomes compulsory and expands. The same pressures are evident in Spain—the reforms begun in 1963 will extend treatment of subscribers to any physicians who have been admitted to any social security practice—but as yet insurance practice is not open automatically to any licensed physician.

Each general practitioner is supposed to have a list of 650 insured persons. He treats them and their dependents. If 650 new people become covered by health insurance in the community, a new general practitioner is hired by

[14] The Spanish social security system is described in, Manuel Alonso Olea, *Instituciones de Seguridad Social* (Madrid: Instituto de Estudios Politicos, 2d ed., 1967). National health insurance and SOE are described in, Enrique Serrano Guirado, *El Seguro de Enfermedad y sus problemas* (Madrid: Instituto de Estudios Politicos, 1950); and Enrique Martin Lopez et al., *Estudio sociologico sobre el Seguro de Enfermedad* (Madrid: Ministerio de Trabajo, Secretaría General Técnica, 1964). The reforms begun in 1963 and the future directions of social security are described in the special issue of *Revista de Politica Social*, no. 61 (January–March 1964); Manuel Alonso Olea, *Sobre los principios cardinales del proyecto de Ley de Bases de la Seguridad Social* (Madrid: Ministerio de Trabajo, Servicio de Publicaciones, 1964); and Jesús Romeo Gorría, *Ley de Bases de la Seguridad Social* (Madrid: Ministerio de Trabajo, Instituto Nacional de Previsión, 1963).

the local office of social security. Insured persons may not go to any outside doctor under the scheme, but they can see him for private fee-for-service payments. An insured person may choose any enrolled local general practitioner whose list has not yet reached 650. All dependents must use the insured person's doctor.

This is the ideal procedure for determining the length of general practitioners' lists. In practice, G.P.'s have shorter lists if SOE subscribers are too few in their areas, and longer lists if the area has many SOE subscribers and not enough doctors who meet the standards for admission to SOE practice. Because of the rapid expansion of SOE coverage in recent years and because of the considerable movement of the population from rural areas to cities, most urban G.P.'s have more than 650 names on their lists, and most rural G.P.'s have less.[15]

Since insurance appointments are desirable and doctors are too numerous, there is much competition for posts. Formal procedures ensure that the best applicants are hired: according to an automatic formula prescribed by law, each applicant receives points for his grades in medical school, number of years in practice, number of postgraduate examinations passed and certificates required, and other objective facts. There is little administrative opinion or favoritism, and the new appointments are given to a waiting list ranked by number of points. Half of all new jobs are filled from the waiting list entirely by this automatic process; to prevent talented persons from being shut out by an excessively mechanical system, the other half of the G.P. and specialist posts are filled by doctors receiving supplemental points through a special examination in an open competition announced each year. (Such nearly automatic selection methods, designed to eliminate the once rampant favoritism, exist in many organizations throughout Spanish society.) The closed panel system has the advantage of restricting insurance care to the best general practitioners. Because of the large number of medical school graduates, many lacking sufficient clinical experience, the quality of general practice would otherwise be a great problem for Spanish national health insurance. Some other European countries have the same problem of deficient training among general practitioners, but free choice of doctors means that the sick funds must pay whomever the patient selects.

According to his appointment, the general practitioner must devote several hours a day, six days a week, to office hours and home visits for insured patients.[16] In most cities and towns, he holds his office hours in a polyclinic

[15] Statistics on length of list appear in, Martin Lopez, *Estudio sociologico* (note 14), vols. 2 and 3 passim, and vol. 5, pp. 20–25.

[16] The work loads vary considerably. Among G.P.'s, according to a survey in the early 1960's, about one-third work between five and fifteen hours a week, about one-third between sixteen and twenty-five hours, and about one-third more than twenty-five hours. Most specialists and pediatricians under contract devote between five and fifteen hours a week to SOE practice. Martin Lopez, *Estudio sociologico* (note 14), vol. 4, p. 146.

owned by social security. The rural G.P. sees these patients in his regular office, usually located in his own home. For his basic fee the G.P. is not obligated to see his insured patients outside these office hours, although he may do so voluntarily. In Madrid and Barcelona, the social security polyclinics maintain emergency services for those patients who require care outside their general practitioners' office hours, and G.P.'s can earn extra salaries by participating. It is assumed that the G.P. has several other medical jobs and possibly a little private practice outside his insurance hours. Since a social security appointment is public proof of superior professional standing, the doctor can readily get such additional jobs.

During the late 1960's the G.P. received 15.505 pesetas a month for each family unit on his list. (The free market exchange rate for one peseta was $0.017.) He obtained more than one fee for the same family only if these individuals were separately insured under the payroll tax and had registered with him separately. The Spanish capitation system thus differs from that in other countries, where the doctor receives a separate fee for each *person* on his list. Beginning in March 1966, each general practitioner obtained in addition to his capitation fees a basic practice allowance of 1,250 ptas. a month. This grant was designed to alleviate the financial plight of the rural G.P.'s: when SOE was expanded to cover many agricultural workers, during the early 1960's, the rural doctors earned lower fees than they had received from these workers' private sick funds; later, during the 1960's, the movement of the Spanish population from the countryside to the city reduced the number of patients covered by any insurance and curtailed the lists of rural G.P.'s under SOE. (The rural G.P. can earn fees from social security for each delivery, if the community lacks an obstetrician.)

Besides general practitioners, SOE appoints pediatricians to treat the children of insured persons on an ambulatory basis. The general practitioner sees the adults, and the local pediatrician sees the children. A pediatrician is appointed for every area with 1,950 insured persons, and additional pediatricians are appointed for larger populations. The capitation fee during the late 1960's was 5.16886 ptas. a month for each insured person. Not all these insured persons have children, and some have several. Therefore the pediatrician's work is created by only part of the people on his list. It is estimated that the 1,950 insured persons will give the average pediatrician 809 children, but in practice considerable difference in work load results from lists of similar length, because of class and regional differences in birth rates. Like the general practitioner, the pediatrician receives a basic practice allowance of 1,250 ptas. monthly at the time of writing.

The specialist is expected to work several hours daily in the polyclinic, with the rest of his time free for other jobs and for private practice. He is responsible for all work in his field in a district containing a certain number of families covered by social security; at least a dozen general practitioners work in the specialist's district, and they refer to him all patients requiring his skills. The payment system is designed to give the specialist an income appropriate for his field. At one time the sick funds tried to pay all specialists the same total, in an amount equal to that earned by a general practitioner with the maximum list. This reasoning encountered a dilemma: all general practitioners might be considered alike, but different specialties are given different amounts of work by the same population. For example, in a country like Spain, possessing a high birth rate and great solicitude for maternal and child health, an obstetrician can be kept fully employed by a smaller number of families than a radiologist. Therefore, different list sizes and different capitation fees for various specialties were necessary to achieve similar pay rates. For example, during the early 1950's, the desired income was 3,250 ptas. monthly for all specialists, and therefore surgeons and pediatricians were made responsible for areas with 13,000 insured persons with a fee of 0.25 ptas. for each person; radiologists and dentists were assigned 15,600 people with a fee of 0.20 ptas.; urologists and psychiatrists had 19,600 people, each with a fee of 0.165 ptas.; and obstetricians had 9,500 people for a fee of 0.33 ptas.[17]

The calculations have become more flexible, because an identical income no longer is sought for all specialists. But the procedure is still to postulate a desirable income for each specialty from social security work, estimate the population size that will produce a reasonable work load for that specialty, and then calculate the capitation fee. At the time of writing, 17,000 ptas. monthly is the target income for surgeons and gynecologists, about 11,000 ptas. is sought for gastroenterologists, and other totals are proposed for each remaining specialty.[18] For the total capitation fee, the specialist is expected to provide any medical or surgical or combined care needed by a number of insured persons in a district. On page 96 are some capitation fees and the sizes of specialists' lists that are expected to produce a reasonable amount of work.[19]

If a specialist's list includes substantially more than his numerical quota, his district boundaries are reduced or an additional specialist is appointed. Many specialists have less than the optimum number of insured persons, and they are guaranteed a minimum monthly income: 3,360 ptas. for the senior

[17] The complete fee schedule from that period appears in, Serrano Guirado, *Seguro de Enfermedad* (note 14), p. 361; and *Relations between Social Security Institutions and the Medical Profession* (Geneva: International Social Security Association, 1953), p. 500.

[18] The target incomes resemble the salaries paid to specialists at clinical centers and hospitals owned by SOE: during the late 1960's, 12,418.56 ptas. monthly for all chiefs of service in the surgical specialties; 8,064.00 ptas. for senior internists and some others; 5,967.36 ptas. for most assisting physicians.

[19] The complete schedule of capitation fees and of salaries for work in hospitals and other organizations under social security appears in *Boletin Oficial del Estado*, no. 53 (3 March 1967), pp. 2927–28.

	Capitation Fee in Pesetas per Month			Number of Insured
	Medical Care	Surgical Intervention	Total	
Surgery	0.91636	0.21953	1.13589	12,000
Assistant surgeons	0.45817	0.21953	0.67770	12,000
Anesthetists	—	0.30545	0.30545	12,000
Obstetrics	1.00750	0.20125	1.20875	10,000
Assistant obstetricians	0.50375	0.04875	0.55250	10,000
Internal medicine	0.91636	—	0.91636	12,000
Gastroenterology	0.91636	—	0.91636	12,000
Dermatology	0.45818	—	0.45818	20,946
Pediatric consultants	0.22885	—	0.22885	41,140
Urology, complete care	0.45818	0.12020	0.57838	20,946
Gynecology, complete care	0.45818	0.19160	0.64973	20,946

specialists, 1,680 ptas. for the assisting surgeons, and 840 ptas. for the other assisting physicians.

All doctors receive certain supplements, whether they are in general or specialty practice. For every three years of service under social security, the doctor's pay check is raised 10 per cent. Every July and December, a bonus is paid equal to one month's income. Like the G.P.'s, all specialists receive the basic practice allowance of 1,250 ptas. monthly.

Summary

Capitation systems are rare in the world. Without a prior history of voluntary capitation arrangements between doctors and patients, organized medicine may resist the establishment of one as the standard payment system in a large public medical system. Capitation fees are usually part of a set of close and permanent bonds between a doctor and individual persons—not merely temporarily ill patients—and therefore they are usually used for general practitioners rather than for specialists. Under such circumstances, general practitioners and specialists usually have different payment systems and there are great differences in the size and flexibility of their incomes. Capitation can survive only if there are clear-cut differences in the work and ambitions of G.P.'s and specialists, so that the G.P.'s do not compare themselves with specialists and are not tempted to enter the specialists' payment system. The essence of capitation is its stability and predictability: the fee remains nearly the same for several years; the length of the doctor's list changes slowly and the list system may discourage patients from changing doctors too often; the doctor's work load, his income, and the costs of the health service remain nearly the same over long periods. Consequently, capitation pleases medical administrators and budget officers. Probably it arouses the least discontent among doctors when its own stability is matched by a stability in the economy; the incomes of other professionals do not rise ahead of those of doctors;

sick funds' tax resources remain stable; doctors and their patients lead stable and predictable economic lives. A standing mechanism is particularly necessary to review capitation fees, since the rigidity of fees and lists may cause the doctor's lead over the rest of the economy to diminish during periods of unusual prosperity.

Capitation can be designed in several ways. The rates can differ by types of patient, in order to compensate for the more time-consuming patient. The capitation fees can vary in order to discourage lists of lengths contrary to public policy. Supplementary payments can guarantee minimum incomes and offer incentives not adequately furnished by simple capitation. The basic practice allowances that have been added in several countries move the payment system in a direction closer to salary.

VI

DEVELOPMENT OF PAYMENT SYSTEMS

The adoption of national health insurance or a national health service makes inevitable certain changes in the working conditions and economic positions of doctors. Money becomes available to pay for patients who otherwise might have been treated free or not at all. For the remaining patients, the source of the payments changes from the individual to an organization. As a condition for collecting payments, the doctor must accept the financial procedures of the third party; sometimes the third party may announce rules protecting the clinical and financial interests of the patients. Besides changing the payment procedures, the third party may transfer care from traditional sites into polyclinics or hospitals, or it may acquire and reorganize the establishments where the doctors already work.

Governments usually avoid trouble from the doctors and sick funds by continuing familiar practices. But these procedures may break down, necessitating completely new ones. One example is the history of the capitation system in Great Britain, as we shall see later in this chapter. English general practitioners in the mid-1940's fought salary and favored universal extension of the familiar capitation system throughout the National Health Service. But when their pay lagged and did not relate closely enough to the work created by different patients, the general practitioners attacked the capitation system in the 1960's as strongly as they had opposed alternative payment systems two decades earlier. Another example of a situation calling for change is the unremitting strike waves of general practitioners and specialists against the sick funds and hospitals of Italy during the 1960's. As national health insurance expanded and as the number of public hospitals grew, the sick funds and governments had tried to preserve the familiar mix of capitation, salary, and fee-for-service. But when pay lagged and the remuneration system did not seem to differentiate fairly according to doctors' work and responsibility the profession demanded something new.[1]

[1] Convenient summaries of these events appear in Carlo Palenzona's articles for the French medical journal *Concours médical*. See the issues of 30 June 1963, 3 August 1963,

Whether a completely new set of medical institutions is proposed or whether a major change is suggested in institutions that have evolved for years and are patently unworkable, basic innovations usually arouse the ire of the medical profession, unless the government is simply enacting the doctors' proposals. In the West, and in countries with a Western-oriented medical tradition, the medical profession has several apprehensions about medical reforms enacted by laymen. The profession wishes full responsibility for providing medical care to patients. It wishes freedom to make any diagnoses and to prescribe any treatments according to its judgment, and it demands continuous improvements in facilities. It wishes a recognized position in society commensurate with its conception of its own importance, so that it will gain necessary recruits, co-operation, facilities, and rewards. In some countries, good treatment is thought to presuppose completely free mutual choice between doctor and patient and complete privacy between them. These attitudes toward national health insurance and national health services were distilled in the "Twelve Principles of Social Security and Medical Care" adopted in 1948 by the Second General Assembly of the World Medical Association (WMA):

Whenever medical care is provided as part of Social Security, the following principles should govern its provisions:

I. Freedom of choice of physician by the patient. Liberty of physician to choose patient except in cases of urgency or humanitarianism.

II. No intervention of third party between physician and patient.

III. Where medical service is to be submitted to control, this control should be exercised by physicians.

IV. Freedom of choice of hospital by patient.

V. Freedom of the physician to choose the location and type of his practice.

VI. No restriction of medication or mode of treatment by physician except in case of abuse.

VII. Appropriate representation of medical profession in every official body dealing with medical care.

VIII. It is not in the public interest that physicians should be full-time salaried servants of the government or Social Security bodies.

IX. Remuneration of medical services ought not to depend directly on the financial condition of the insurance organization.

X. Any Social Security or insurance plan must be open to the participation of any licensed physician, and no physician should be compelled to participate if he does not wish to do so.

XI. Compulsory health insurance plans should cover only those persons who are unable to make their own arrangements for medical care.

XII. There shall be no exploitation of the physician, the physician's services or the public by any person or organization.

---

27 February 1965, 18 September 1965, and 1 January 1966. The agreement that was supposed to settle the disputes is summarized in Palenzona's article "Période de réforme sanitaire, disputes entre médecins, disputes entre ministères," *Concours médical*, vol. 89, no. 7 (18 February 1967), pp. 1325–31.

Written when the WMA was dominated by national medical associations who opposed any alternatives to private medical care except for the indigent, Principle XI was an attack on any form of national health insurance or national health service. Most medical associations have since adjusted to national medical care systems, and their recent resolutions insist instead upon substantial representation on all governing and administrative bodies.[2]

Despite the unusual publicity surrounding disputes between doctors and governments, the doctors are motivated no differently from any other profession: they contend that the solution of the social problems in which they specialize is urgent and requires the highest social priorities; they believe that their training gives them alone the knowledge and skills to solve these problems; and they conclude that society must give them the facilities and freedom to solve these problems at their discretion. Changes in established relations are usually opposed by doctors out of fear of reduction in their status, autonomy, and performance. When remuneration is at issue, doctors usually demand more money and more authority over the management of the payment system as part of their pressure to gain the most means and the greatest autonomy. Confronted by a group claiming to have a monopoly of knowledge and skill in matters of life and death, laymen usually give the doctors what they ask, short of repealing all changes or completely abdicating power. The medical market represents an important exception to the simple rule that monopsonists use their bargaining power to obtain advantageous procedures and minimum prices: the doctors' political influence enables them to influence the terms of the market, and the monopsonist is most interested in buying peace.

The Persistence of Traditional Methods

A country's current payment system under its public medical services is usually the arrangement it had before the services were created by government: traditional payment systems generally spread when the enactment of national health insurance or a national health service creates a need for standard nationwide administrative institutions. If the decision is made by a democratic legislature, organized medicine usually makes advantageous alliances with the conservative political parties; if the decision is made by executive decree, the administrators usually make concessions to the doctors in order to motivate their voluntary co-operation. Any change in traditional payment systems makes them even more profitable, as a result of the profession's demands or the laymen's gesture of conciliation.

[2] The W.M.A. principles appear in *First Decade Report of the World Medical Association 1947–1957* (New York: The World Medical Association, 1957), chap. 12, p. 2. An example of the more recent views of national medical associations is the statement of policy on health insurance adopted by the Canadian Medical Association in 1960 in, Edwin A. Tollefson, *Bitter Medicine: The Saskatchewan Medicare Feud* (Saskatoon: Modern Press, 1964), pp. 67–68.

All the present payment systems have a long history.[3] Often in eighteenth- or nineteenth-century Europe, all the payment systems existed simultaneously in a country. Flat rate systems—capitation, case payments, and salary—always have been common, because the first organized purchasers of medical services preferred them. Fee-for-service was used for those members of the public who paid privately.

Flat rate methods were associated with a stable relationship between a closed medical panel and an organization. The citizen as insurance subscriber or as taxpayer paid the sick fund or government regularly, and this third party paid a doctor regularly. Salaried systems are very ancient: early physicians were often paid fixed sums by kings or armies to render specified services for particular periods or for unlimited calls. In a few countries, such as Scandinavia and Russia, substantial proportions of the country's doctors were offered salaried jobs by the government to give ambulatory treatment to the general public. When hospitals acquired regular medical staffs, small salaries were paid to the doctors by the governments, Churches, or private associations that owned the hospitals.

Capitation fees were paid by many of the guilds that retained doctors and by many of the social welfare associations formed by urban and town workers after the Renaissance. Often founded initially to pay members' burial expenses and provide other welfare services, during the nineteenth century these clubs began to help pay members' medical expenses. Since members paid regular fees to the club, the financing of care was most predictable and remained within the limited resources of the club if the doctors accepted some regular payment for each member, bearing some relation to the member's annual subscription payment but having no relation to the volume of services rendered. Many clubs made agreements with doctors to care for their members in return for an annual fee per member.

The participating doctors were willing to accept capitation systems, since the alternatives were far less profitable. General practitioners in nineteenth-century working class areas shared the economic risks of their frequently unemployed and impoverished clients. Annual capitation fees from the treasury of a medical club were preferable to unpaid bills rendered to individuals on a fee-for-service basis. Often workers had a sufficient real income from part-time farming or personal handicrafts, but they might not have had enough cash to pay medical bills, and the capitation system ensured that the doctor would get his share of the worker's limited and easily spent cash. Thus the clubs usually solved the doctor's collection problem; any impending bankruptcy of the club was known in advance. During the late nineteenth century,

[3] Not much has been published about the past history of medical pay, and evidence is sparse. See René Sand, *The Advance to Social Medicine* (London: Staples Press, 1952), part 1 passim; George Rosen, *Fees and Fee Bills: Some Economic Aspects of Medical Practice in Nineteenth Century America* (Baltimore: The Johns Hopkins Press, 1946); and Brian Abel-Smith, "Paying the Family Doctor," *Medical Care*, vol. 1, no. 1 (January–March 1963), pp. 30–32.

general practice in many Northwest European cities was highly competitive—as it remains in much of the world—and the system of clubs and capitation fees meant that each participating doctor had a predictable minimum income. Probably nearly every participating doctor had an extra and variable income from private patients who were not club members. To an urban specialist of this period, a capitation system would be a financial comedown; but to the general practitioners who were tied to the economic plight of workers, the system provided security. The clubs favored the capitation system because of predictability, economy, and administrative simplicity. Fee-for-service systems require a large clerical staff to receive and pay the many separate bills, and the clubs lacked the necessary funds and personnel. Some general practitioners earning fixed capitation fees were able to relate income more closely to work by selling the drugs they prescribed, a combination surviving today in Holland and parts of England.

Fee-for-service existed, but the rate structure was simple until modern times, when the rise of modern surgery and modern clinical science generated a large number of differentiated procedures requiring various amounts of work. At earlier periods when doctors merely diagnosed illnesses, prescribed treatments, and performed a few standard therapies themselves (such as bleeding, cupping, and blistering), the fee schedule itemized the visit and only a few other procedures.[4] In countries where the doctor sold the medicines that he prescribed, these medicines were responsible for a more detailed price list and often brought the doctor most of his income.

Negotiated Settlements

When national health insurance is enacted, the existing sick funds usually survive as administrative agencies within the official system. National health insurance is merely designed to strengthen the financing of medical care by spreading the risks to more people, by converting subscribers' voluntary contributions into taxes enforceable under law, and by requiring that administrative procedures meet certain minimum standards.

The statutes or decrees creating national health insurance or a national health service usually specify the coverage, taxes, and benefits. The instruments creating national health insurance usually state the criteria that the pre-existing private sick funds must meet in order to participate in the official system. Almost never is the procedure for paying doctors specified in the statute or decree. One reason—but not the only one—for this omission is to postpone the decision: the doctors would accept a legislative statement only of the payment system that is most favorable to them; the sick funds and the

[4] A few countries have preserved and extended into national health insurance the simple fee schedules that were based on the visit. See the discussions of Sweden in chapter III, supra, and Italy in chapter VII, infra.

government would prefer a legislative statement of whatever payment procedure can keep costs low; and, since the enactment of national health insurance or a national health service is embroiled in many other controversies, the legislators usually decide to avoid an additional source of trouble that might block adoption of the entire scheme. Another reason for omitting the specific payment system from the original statute is to avoid future as well as current trouble: if it were frozen into the statute, opponents of modernization could block legislative amendments. After creation of health insurance or the health service, the government might then try to negotiate an amicable arrangement with the doctors. Or the government might say that its responsibility is only to ensure money for the sick funds and care for the public, and that the funds have the responsibility to negotiate their own procedures with the doctors. If the decision is left to the sick funds, the doctors induce them to continue the familiar payment system. If the sick funds must adopt a common method, it is the one previously used by most.

Great Britain

The erratic course of general practitioners' pay illustrates the willingness of governments to woo the doctors with concessions, even when the result is to change important administrative structures when the doctors change their minds. The constant factor has been the doctors' concern with their prosperity and independence. At first, their anxiety about potential dangers to their traditional position led them to favor capitation as a standard procedure in general practice throughout the National Health Service. They continued to favor capitation while doctors in other countries fought it. But ultimately the British G.P.'s became disillusioned with capitation and obtained fundamental modifications.

Before the enactment of the National Insurance Act of 1911, many Friendly Societies sponsored closed medical panels and paid their doctors by capitation. The Friendly Societies, insurance firms, and comparable private associations were allowed to participate in National Insurance if they met certain administrative standards. The British Medical Association (BMA) insisted on freedom of choice between doctor and patient; thus any general practitioner could join the scheme, and any insured patient could ask to be included on the list of any participating general practitioner. Two-thirds of Great Britain's doctors joined, including nearly all the general practitioners in working class neighborhoods. Since the BMA wished to avoid making the doctor subordinate to the Approved Societies, the statute created a series of regional Insurance Committees that would represent the Approved Societies, the doctors, and other interested groups. The doctor would be paid by the public Insurance Committee and not by a private Approved Society. Each Insurance Committee could adopt whatever payment system it wished:

most selected capitation, since the Friendly Societies and doctors in working class districts were accustomed to it. The capitation system brought the doctor a predictable income and would not strain the funds. No doctor depended on capitation for his total income, and its limiting effects on income did not seem serious. Since most people were not covered by National Health Insurance, every general practitioner earned some or most of his income from private practice, conducted by fee-for-service. A few Insurance Committees changed from fee-for-service to capitation after controversies over the administrative restrictions designed to discourage physicians from billing their Insurance Committee for more procedures than were medically necessary.[5]

The capitation system therefore spread as a result of the National Insurance Act. The National Health Service made it universal. During the public debate between 1944 and 1946, it was clear that general practice would be included in the service, but the system of payment was not yet certain and was not spelled out in the drafts of the National Health Service Bill. The only precedents for a comprehensive medical service offering general practitioner care to the entire population—the U.S.S.R., European rural medical officers, and the colonial medical services of England and of other colonial powers—all paid doctors by salary. Some policy proposals, such as the Ministry of Health's White Paper of 1944, suggested creation of local health centers administered by local governments and employing salaried general practitioners. Gradually it became clear during 1945 and 1946 that specialists, public health officers, and other special groups of doctors would be paid by salary. Early drafts of the health service bill gave to every G.P. a "basic salary" of £300 a year, designed to give young doctors a cushion while they were building a practice. Although this basic salary was intended to be no more than a fraction of total income, many medical leaders interpreted it as the first step in making all income consist of salary. After issuance of the White Paper, the BMA repeatedly announced it would oppose any administrative arrangement that would make general practitioners salaried employees of either the national or local governments. The BMA insisted that the doctor remain an independent practitioner and free professional. Meanwhile specialists' representatives were issuing similar but less public warnings.

During late April 1946, the Ministry of Health inserted into the Bill certain administrative changes enabling the general practitioner to work within the National Health Service while retaining the status of independent contractor. As often happens during controversies about medical reform, the

[5] Hermann Levy, *National Health Insurance* (Cambridge: University Press, 1944); R. W. Harris, *National Health Insurance in Great Britain 1911–1946* (London: George Allen & Unwin, 1946); and James Hogarth, *The Payment of the General Practitioner* (Oxford: Pergamon Press, 1963), pp. 13–30.

safest and most widely acceptable solution was to perpetuate the earlier situation. The general practitioners would deal neither with national or local governments but with regional Executive Councils representing the public and the medical profession. The Councils would admit doctors to practice under the scheme and would pay them. The £300 "basic salary" for everyone became a £300 "fixed annual payment" only for new entrants into general practice; in later years it was transformed into a graduated "initial practice allowance." As before, each general practitioner would have a list of regular patients, and the Executive Council would pay a fixed sum for each patient. Asking a private fee from any patient on one's own list would be a violation of one's contract with the Executive Council, but the G.P. was left free to seek private patients among people not on his list. Originally a way for the Friendly Society to prepay the costs of a worker-member, capitation now was becoming the accepted method for paying for every citizen's general practitioner care.[6]

But there are several ways to arrive at capitation fees, and the method of calculation and the size of the fee have been almost constantly at issue between the general practitioners and the National Health Service. The payment of the G.P.'s has been the most severe area of controversy in the Health Service. A series of special investigating committees has examined the doctors' complaints, and the profession's representatives have frequently conferred with officials from the Ministry of Health. Each dispute results in important concessions to the doctors over procedure and money; at best, the government has merely delayed and limited these concessions. Nothing could better demonstrate the power of the medical profession in public medical care than the recurring concessions by the National Health Service, despite the fact that it is virtually a monopoly buyer of general practitioner services.

The simplest capitation system would pay each doctor for each person on his list from the revenue of the Treasury or sick fund, according to an agreed rate. But the third party needs to predict and limit its expenditures during the forthcoming year. One problem of administering a capitation system is that unexpected increases in population can increase costs beyond previous plans and can create deficits. Another problem is that a person sometimes changes doctors and joins a new list without being removed from the original doctor's list; the third party may pay a considerable sum unnecessarily because of this "inflation" of lists. The British government's solution was to

[6] The creation of the National Health Service and the early negotiations with the general practitioners are reported in, James Stirling Ross, *The National Health Service in Great Britain* (London: Oxford University Press, 1952), pp. 90–93; Harry Eckstein, *The English Health Service* (Cambridge: Harvard University Press, 1958), pp. 144–46, 156, 196–99; Harry Eckstein, *Pressure Group Politics* (London: George Allen & Unwin, 1960), pp. 98–100.

continue and elaborate the "Pool" method that had been used in a simpler form under National Health Insurance. Its characteristics and the doctors' complaints were summarized in chapter V.[7]

At first the general practitioners insisted on retention of the Pool, to the gratification of the Ministry of Health, which favored its budgetary predictability.[8] But when the profession discovered that the complex calculations of the Pool made the payment outcomes unpredictable for individual doctors and deprived the negotiators of effective control over the results, the Ministry readily dropped it in favor of a more direct payment system that would enable the physician to foresee his earnings, even though it reduced the Ministry's ability to forecast its costs.

Before the Pool was abandoned altogether, the government shifted its methods of calculation in order to please the profession. When the doctors reversed themselves, the government usually followed. For example, one issue was whether the size of the Pool should be calculated as a multiple of the number of citizens or the number of doctors. They do not increase together: after World War II, the number of general practitioners at first rose faster than the British population, and the doctors' average income would have declined if the Pool had continued to grow with the population. One might expect logically that the amount of money for capitation fees should vary with the population covered—as it did until 1952—but the government thereafter readily agreed to the profession's demands that the Pool should grow with the number of doctors.[9] The statistics showed fundamentally different trends during the 1960's: the population began to grow faster than the number of doctors. The profession reversed itself and asked that the Pool—or a substitute payment procedure—again be based on the size of the population. The straight capitation system adopted in 1965 met this demand.

So long as the general practitioners insisted on retaining capitation, it was the mechanism for distributing the Pool. It was an inefficient method for achieving the income targets envisioned by the Spens Committee, and it did not guarantee adequate profits after practice expenses. Much of the discon-

[7] Full details about the complaints, the work of the investigating committees, the negotiations, and the outcomes have been published elsewhere: Almont Lindsey, *Socialized Medicine in England and Wales* (Chapel Hill: The University of North Carolina Press, 1962), chaps. 6–8; Eckstein, *Pressure Group Politics* (note 6), chap. 6; and Hogarth, *Payment of General Practitioner* (note 5), pp. 30–49.

[8] ". . . the Council wishes to record its firm conviction that any departure from the Pool method of payment would be a breach of the undertaking given by the Government to the profession when it entered the Service." From the "Preliminary Memorandum of Evidence presented by the British Medical Association," *Royal Commission on Doctors' and Dentists' Remuneration: Minutes of Evidence* (London: H. M. Stationery Office, 1958), p. 238.

[9] The award by Justice Harold Danckwerts is quoted in, Ross, *National Health Service* (note 6), pp. 387–88. It was elaborated on in the report of the Working Party of Representatives, *Distribution of Remuneration among General Practitioners* (London: H. M. Stationery Office, 1952).

tent of the profession was due to the persistent failure of its preferred method to achieve goals that could be attained more efficiently by the payment technique that it wished to avoid, namely salary supplemented by practice allowances or aided by State-owned facilities. By the mid-1960's the frustrated doctors asked for numerous supplements that would reward extra effort, guarantee minimum incomes, defray operating costs, and alter capitation in many fundamental ways.[10]

The Ministry agreed to nearly every proposal. Extra capitation fees were offered for all persons over sixty-five, on the grounds that they created more work. Payments were available for night visits, immunizations, and weekend duty. Every doctor would receive a practice allowance for overhead expenses, and some specific expenses like rent and staff salaries would be reimbursed. G.P.'s would obtain extra payments for seniority. The National Health Service Act was amended to allow doctors to elect payment by salary, and the Ministry agreed to experiment with fee-for-service. Parliament created a public corporation to give capital grants or loans to doctors, for the improvement of their facilities. At a time when wages and prices were curbed throughout the economy, the general practitioners received a large pay increase.[11]

Sweden

Fear of salaried employment led British general practitioners to press the National Health Service to perpetuate the capitation system. Anxiety about the creation of a salaried service also led Swedish office practitioners to insist on the use of a traditional payment method, but in their case it was fee-for-

[10] The profession's demands appeared in "A Charter for the Family Doctor Service," *British Medical Journal Supplement* (13 March 1965), pp. 89–91; and "Revised Memorandum of Evidence to the Review Body on Doctors' and Dentists' Remuneration," ibid. (6 June 1964), pp. 219–26. Events during the 1960's are summarized in, Rosemary Stevens, *Medical Practice in Modern England* (New Haven: Yale University Press, 1966), chaps. 20–21; Stanley S. B. Gilder, "Crises in British General Practice," *World Medical Journal*, vol. 13, no. 2 (March–April 1966), pp. 48–49; and *General Practice and the National Health Service* (London: Young Fabian Pamphlet Number 9, 1965). The anger of the rank-and-file G.P. is documented in the survey reported by David Mechanic and Ronald G. Faich, "Doctors in Revolt: The Crisis in the British Nationalized Health Service," in, Ian Weinberg (editor), *English Society* (New York: Atherton Press, forthcoming). The demands and tactics of the general practitioners were criticized by supporters of the National Health Service, such as Brian Abel-Smith, "The Cure that Failed," *Manchester Guardian Weekly*, 25 February 1965, p. 13.

[11] The new payment system is summarized in chapter V, *supra*. The new contract between the government and the general practitioners and the new remuneration arrangements are reported in detail in "Second Report of Joint Discussions between General Practitioner Representatives and the Minister of Health," *British Medical Journal Supplement* (16 October 1965), pp. 153–59; "Third Report of Negotiations on Family Doctor Service," ibid. (7 May 1966), pp. 135–45; and *Review Body on Doctors' and Dentists' Remuneration: Seventh Report* (London: H. M. Stationery Office, Cmnd. 2992, 1966), chaps. 6 and 8.

service on a reimbursement rather than a service basis. Sweden has had a long tradition of sick clubs, like those of northwestern Europe. Many arrangements were medical and burial benefit provisions sponsored by medieval guilds. Some were village benefit associations dating even earlier. Declining during and after the Reformation, sick clubs revived during the nineteenth century, when associations of diverse types multiplied. Some medical benefit clubs had no other function; other people were covered by insurance schemes and benefits sponsored by temperance societies, fraternal orders, trade unions, and other associations. The State approved and regularized these sick clubs and health insurance schemes by legislation passed in 1891 and in subsequent years. By 1955, 70 per cent of the population was covered by some kind of voluntary health insurance.

In much of northwestern Europe, as I have said, sick clubs formed alliances with particular doctors and paid them by capitation. This was unusual in Sweden; the sick clubs customarily helped the patient pay his fees and thus offered no more than cash benefits insurance. So many of the country's limited number of doctors already had regular commitments to other organizations—primarily their part-time salaried relationships with the local or national governments—that they could not enter into the kind of exclusive contract with sick clubs that creates a capitation tradition throughout a country. A distinction developed between salaried care for the poor and private fee-for-service for anyone capable of paying. The State offered some office practitioners salaries to make themselves available, particularly in underdoctored areas, but the salaries were not supposed to cover all their work: the salaried district medical officer was supposed to charge any other patients. Many people used the district medical officer as their general practitioner, and the sick clubs helped them pay their fees by reimbursement.

Made compulsory and virtually universal in 1955 by national statute, Swedish health insurance continues to be a cash benefits rather than a service benefits system. The system has been preserved at the insistence of the Swedish Medical Association (SMA) and withstood a test of strength between it and the Social Democratic Cabinet during the late 1940's.

Since 1932, the Social Democrats have had majorities or pluralities in the *riksdag* and have led all Cabinets. The Social Democrats were originally dedicated to nationalization of industry and social services, but the pragmatic responsibilities of government and the need to compromise with coalition partners have attenuated their Marxist ardor. In 1938 the Social Democrats won one of the few absolute majorities in Swedish electoral history. World War II prevented the Social Democrats from carrying out their pledges to introduce nationalization into an economy previously dominated by private enterprise and co-operatives. When the postwar elections deprived the Social Democrats of their majority and gave strategic *riksdag* seats to the Communists, the public appeared to be demanding action impatiently.

In 1946 the *riksdag* enacted a bill for compulsory national health insurance. Implementation was delayed for several years in order to settle questions of finance and the organization of health services. To devise a medical plan, the government appointed a commission headed by Dr. Axel Höjer, a left-wing Social Democrat and director-general of the Royal Medical Board. In 1947, shortly before initiation of the National Health Service, the Höjer Commission issued a report influenced by discussions of a possible salaried service in Britain. The report proposed a gradual evolution toward a Swedish national health service consisting entirely of full-time salaried doctors without rights of private practice. The Höjer Report took as its model Sweden's salaried district medical officer. But he had never been full-time; and another model in Swedish medical tradition had a stronger hold on the doctors, namely the private office practitioner who collected fees.[12]

The Höjer Report was greeted by an uproar from the SMA, from the conservative political parties, and from business groups—an uproar of the kind that the Swedish political and social system attempts to avoid. In settling problems, Swedes take pride in being calm and reasonable (*lagom*). The entire social and political structure is criss-crossed by lines of communication and negotiation, enabling groups to compromise their diverse interests, avoid a public fuss, and announce unanimously agreed solutions. Visionary goals are viewed skeptically. Dogmatic attacks on one's opponents and intransigent demands are bad form.[13]

The Höjer Commission had violated the unwritten code by issuing an official report that expressed the ideal aspirations of one ideological faction instead of presenting an agreed solution cleared with all interested groups. The SMA retaliated against Höjer by refusing to deal with him in his capacity as director-general of the Royal Medical Board, an unusual sanction in Swedish public life. When Höjer's periodic reappointment was due in 1952, the Cabinet had to replace him with someone acceptable to the SMA, and Höjer spent the next eight years abroad. Meanwhile, political trends weakened the left wing of the Social Democratic party: the Communists lost popular votes and *riksdag* seats, the Liberals gained, and Social Democratic reliance upon the Agrarian party increased. The Agrarians favored an insurance mechanism and subsidies in health and other sectors of the economy,

[12] The Höjer Report is described in, Gunnar Biörck, *Medicin för politiker och några andra uppsatser* (Malmö: Allhem, 1953); and Wilfrid Fleisher, *Sweden: The Welfare State* (New York: John Day Co., 1956), pp. 139–41. The arguments of the doctors and of the Report's supporters are presented in many issues of *Svenska Läkartidningen* during late 1947 and 1948, e.g., Albert Grönberg, "Mammon och medicinmannen: Ett inlägg i debatten om läkarkårens socialisering," ibid., vol. 45, no. 15 (9 April 1948), pp. 711–14.

[13] François-Régis Bastide, *Sweden* (London: Vista Books, 1962), passim, esp. pp. 74–79; Dankwart A. Rustow, *The Politics of Compromise: A Study of Parties and Cabinet Government in Sweden* (Princeton: Princeton University Press, 1955), esp. chap. 8; and Hans L. Zetterberg, "National Pastime: Pursuit of Power," *Industria International 1960–61* (1960), pp. 160, 162.

but not socialization. So, in 1953 national health insurance was enacted in a form that made it available to most of the population but disturbed the working conditions of doctors as little as possible. The SMA participated in the negotiations leading to the 1953 law and the settlement was worked out in a manner typical of Swedish public life: the Cabinet agreed that the compulsory system would be a cash benefits scheme as it had been under voluntary insurance, and therefore the doctor would see and charge insured patients exactly as if they were private patients coming to his own office; the SMA reluctantly accepted compulsory health insurance, while retaining misgivings about possible future controls over fees and work; the *riksdag* approved the law almost unanimously. Compulsory national health insurance went into effect in January 1955.

Harmonious Acceptance of Salary

Since medical professions in some countries have fought the actual or imagined prospects of salaried employment, one might think it universally opposed by doctors. But people will accept any payment system if all the alternatives seem worse. Therefore, in many circumstances medical professions have welcomed salaried methods.

Great Britain

While the general practitioners during the late 1940's were fighting salary, the specialists were welcoming it. Consultants and general practitioners underwent different economic histories long before the National Health Service. Many English general practitioners had regular relationships with groups of patients, and the capitation system evolved. But since a consultant performs advanced medical procedures and is used occasionally and unpredictably, groups of patients cannot easily prepay him by subscription. National Health Insurance covered only general practice, and consultants were not affected by its payment decisions.

The prewar consultant divided his time between private office and hospital, but the key to his status has been his relationship to the hospital. Traditionally in English medicine the specialist is thought to be the hospital doctor, while the G.P. is supposedly strictly an office practitioner and refers to the consultant any patient requiring hospitalization. (Of course, there have always been G.P.'s with hospital privileges and specialists without them, but in principle English medicine has always assumed a clear organizational discontinuity between the two classes of doctor.) In his private office or in patients' homes, the consultant treated private patients and collected cash fees for individual procedures; he hospitalized his patients in the private beds of voluntary hospitals or in a private clinic (called a "special hospital" or "nursing home"). Many consultants donated considerable time to treating the poor and teaching undergraduate and graduate medical students in urban voluntary hospitals. To be asked to donate much time was a mark of professional eminence and served the charitable traditions of the English hospital. Usually consultants enjoyed high income and high class status. To earn such incomes despite the sometimes considerable donation of time, consultants charged high fees. This so-called "Robin Hood policy" was feasible when English class inequalities were great and when the rich had a greal deal of money.[14]

The system had disadvantages. Consultants had collection problems. Some may have felt uncomfortable when overcharging their private patients. Fees varied with the individual doctor's judgment of the patient's pocketbook and did not necessarily relate to work done or professional skill; the same patient would be charged differently by various doctors, according to the doctors' economic needs and their perceptions of the patient's wealth. Since the consultant donated his time to charitable care and student teaching, he was not strictly obligated to the hospital. Finances might induce him to give to his private patients more time and attention than to other patients.

The compensation system was disadvantageous for younger hospital doctors. Unable to earn private fees, the trainee spent at least a decade in hospital posts for only a nominal salary. The large rewards did not begin until the consultant was in his forties.[15]

One disadvantage for the consultant was his dependence on his professional and class inferior, the general practitioner, for private patients and therefore for his livelihood. The consultant could recruit few patients directly but depended on the G.P. for referrals. Therefore consultants had to woo general practitioners by various tactics, ranging from flattery to split fees. During the Depression, severe competition developed among some consultants for patients and for the favor of G.P.'s.[16]

Not all specialists depended on referrals and fees. Some doctors worked at hospitals owned by local authorities and received salaries.[17] Therefore a

[14] *The British Health Services* (London: Political and Economic Planning, 1937), pp. 240–41; and Brian Abel-Smith, *The Hospitals 1800–1948* (London: William Heinemann, 1964), passim.

[15] Ffrangcon Roberts, *The Cost of Health* (London: Turnstile Press, 1952), pp. 171–72; and Stevens, *Medical Practice* (note 10), p. 58. The poverty and struggles until middle age and the rapid increase in wealth and power thereafter are recalled by Sir James Paget, *Memoirs and Letters* (London: Longmans, Green and Co., 3d ed., 1903), pp. 86, 103, 105, 188–97.

[16] Competition for patients occurred in both general practice and specialty practice, and at times the struggle for money was particularly severe among G.P.'s. The unethical work that sometimes resulted was criticized and satirized in George Bernard Shaw's writings, such as *The Doctor's Dilemma; The Intelligent Woman's Guide to Socialism and Capitalism* (London: Constable and Co. Ltd., 1928), p. 461; and *Everybody's Political What's What?* (New York: Dodd, Mead, and Co., 1944), chap. 24.

[17] Stevens, *Medical Practice* (note 10), p. 60.

precedent existed for salaried employment, although unattractive facilities and arbitrary management placed it in low repute.

During the planning and early debates on the National Health Service, no-one doubted that hospitals would be reorganized and that the working conditions and compensation of consultants would be changed in some way. But the early planning statements, such as the White Paper of 1944, were vague and made negotiated settlement possible. Most of the early controversies about the proposed service centered on the BMA's fears that its principal constituency, the general practitioners, would become salaried employees of local governments. Since their future status had not yet been specifically defined, the consultants and their spokesmen, the Royal Colleges, remained quiet. Some early opinion polls of the medical profession showed that consultants were slightly more favorable than general practitioners toward an organized and salaried health service. Many consultants, particularly the underpaid trainees, welcomed salaries for time they had previously donated. Because of their experience in hospitals, the consultants did not find an organized system as distasteful as did an individualistic G.P. A salaried and contractual relationship with a hospital seemed better than total dependence on referrals by general practitioners.[18]

Opinion polls and conferences between the Ministry of Health and the medical societies revealed the doctors' specific apprehensions. At least as strongly as the G.P.'s, the consultants wished to avoid an employment relationship with local authorities, since the latter had sometimes treated their medical officers of health arbitrarily, had managed many of their hospitals bureaucratically, were perceived by doctors as excessively leftist and demagogic, and were usually under obligation to officials of much lower class than the consultants.

During 1945 and 1946, the Ministry revised the draft with concessions designed to mollify the doctors, and the consultants' principal objections were removed. The hospitals were to be run not by the local authorities but by a special hospital service responsible to the Ministry of Health. Consultants would sign contracts not with the lowest units but with Regional Hospital Boards, only one level below the Ministry. The teaching hospitals of London and other cities, where the leading consultants practiced, would retain their own governing boards. Consultants would be allowed considerable scope for private practice, including provision for private beds in the National Health Service hospitals. Besides salaries, consultants would receive fees for home visits. Some private hospitals would be left outside the service. While many general practitioners were apprehensive about their status in the service, the Bill and subsequent regulations incorporated many concessions to the con-

[18] Harry Eckstein, *The English Health Service* (Cambridge: Harvard University Press, 1958), pp. 148–54.

sultants and to other hospital doctors. While the BMA denounced the Ministry of Health and refused to meet its representatives, the Royal Colleges and the Ministry were negotiating amicably. Ultimately the BMA Council was compelled to recommend that the medical profession join the National Health Service upon the latter's initiation in 1948, in large part because the consultants and the Royal Colleges were certain to co-operate. Instead of having fought salaried payment under national ownership, the consultants had been largely responsible for their creation.[19]

Soviet Union

In many underdeveloped countries, a large proportion of the doctors must rely on salaries from public agencies for much of their income. Since few citizens earn adequate incomes, neither individuals nor sick funds can pay enough fees to support extensive private office practice. As the government expands medical services, the proportion of doctors in salaried work rises. The doctors eagerly seek these jobs, since full-time private practice is too insecure.

The leading example of a large medical profession conditioned to accept salaried work is in the U.S.S.R. Many doctors depended on salaries from the start of medical care in Russia. Compulsory health insurance was never enacted, but several government agencies provided medical services for various clienteles and employed part-time or full-time salaried doctors. Some doctors worked for the Army. Some were employed in the polyclinics and small hospitals that factories were required by law to provide for their workers. About one-sixth of the doctors at the start of World War I were salaried employees of local governments (*zemstvos*) and performed work much like that of the salaried rural health officers of contemporary Scandinavia. Each *zemstvo* doctor was assigned to give all medical care to all residents of a district: most worked in a house or small hospital provided by the *zemstvo*; some devoted most of their time to house calls, conducted by horseback or sleigh. Many of the more famous doctors were salaried professors on the faculties of medical schools or on the staffs of research laboratories.

The physicians of St. Petersburg and Moscow could earn much or most of their incomes from private fee-for-service payments from the aristocracy and middle class. Probably *zemstvo* doctors collected some private fees from residents of their districts. Private fee-for-service was not unknown in the countryside, since the numerous midwives and folk practitioners were paid in this way, but it was the aim of the *zemstvo* system to provide all necessary care to rural areas through salaried physicians and *feldshers*, if the necessary

[19] Stevens, *Medical Practice* (note 10), pp. 76–94; Abel-Smith, *The Hospitals* (note 14), chap. 29; and Arthur J. Willcocks, *The Creation of the National Health Service* (London: Routledge and Kegan Paul, 1967), pp. 69–72, 106.

money and personnel became available.[20] (*Feldshers* were medical personnel who learned to do some medical work, often after apprenticeship to a doctor. The Soviet government has retained *feldshers*, since they are indispensable to the rural medical services. Now they are trained in special schools.)

Strong traditions of private practice and fee-for-service never developed in Russia. In most countries, dedication to such entrepreneurial values and skill in keeping one's own accounts develop only if the medical profession is part of a large urban business class. But capitalism and urbanization had barely begun in Russia before World War I intervened. Some doctors came from the commercial classes and shared their pecuniary, autonomous, and aggrandizing tendencies, but there were not enough to shape the character of the entire profession. Many doctors came from the traditional intelligentsia and could neither assimilate nor admire the commercial spirit. The small market for private practice and the necessary conditions for any publicly supported fee-for-service system were destroyed by World War I, by the Revolution, and by the military destruction and epidemics during the Civil War. By the beginning of the 1920's, the number of doctors had diminished, fewer people could afford to pay private fees, the medical problems of the country had increased, and the economy was disorganized. Even when the New Economic Policy of the 1920's authorized private business—including the doctor's freedom to practice privately—most doctors depended on governmental salaried jobs in order to earn their living, and few earned much from private practice.[21]

In many countries the reorganization of medicine is hard fought, but no such struggle stood out in Russia. Many doctors were anti-Communist and disliked the new trends, but their disagreements with the Commissariat of Health were overshadowed by the Civil War. By defeating far more powerful domestic enemies, the Soviet government was left in a position to dictate its terms to the doctors, as have few other governments. The doctors were further weakened by the reorganization of their professional associations under State direction. Another reason for the doctors' weakness was the destruction of private practice by the country's economic collapse; instead of exacting concessions from the government by threats to withdraw into private practice, the doctors needed salaried government jobs in order to live.[22]

[20] Pre-revolutionary Russian medical organization is described in, Henry E. Sigerist, *Socialized Medicine in the Soviet Union* (New York: W. W. Norton & Co., 1937), pp. 64–82; and C. E. A. Winslow, "Public Health Administration in Russia in 1917," *Public Health Reports*, vol. 32, no. 52 (28 December 1917), pp. 2191–2219. The economic problems of the often underemployed private practitioner and the underpaid *zemstvo* doctor are described in Vikenty Veressayev, *The Memoirs of a Physician* (New York: Alfred A. Knopf, 1916), esp. chaps. 18–21. The desperate competition for salaried jobs in Czarist Russia is described in ibid., pp. 58, 78–80, 302. Like all underdeveloped countries, Russia had too few doctors for the population's medical needs, but too many for those able to pay privately.

[21] Sigerist, *Socialized Medicine* (note 20), p. 122.

[22] The widespread poverty of doctors in Russia just after the Civil War and their dependence on salaried jobs are reported in, W. Horsley Gantt, "A Review of Medical

Yet another reason why the new system was created so easily was that war and civil war left the government with few doctors and installations to reorganize and therefore with few vested interests to overcome. Thereafter a virtually new medical profession and a new set of facilities were created by the Soviet government in its own image. In 1917 there were fewer than 20,000 doctors and possibly as few as 11,000; at the end of the First Five Year Plan in 1932 there were over 76,027, and the number has continued to grow rapidly.[23] The many young doctors included members of social groups whose members had never before entered the liberal professions or business and thus lacked any entrepreneurial preconceptions about medicine. Children of workers and peasants were given preference in medical school admissions during the 1920's; not only did salaried medical practice represent a welcome rise in social status, but many felt deep gratitude to the new régime for this opportunity and thus were disposed to accept the system. For the first time many women attended medical school; they found a medical system with fixed hours, a work site provided by the State, and a guaranteed salary far preferable to the uncertainties of fee-for-service or private practice. For a short period during the 1920's, and again after Stalin's death, the organized representatives of the doctors acquired a role sought by professionals everywhere, namely a voice in the procedures and levels of their remuneration.

Decolonization: Cyprus

Many countries are now acquiring salaried medical professions because of their colonial heritages. The trend usually—but not always—is accepted by the local doctors, because the salaried medical service always was an integral part of modern medical facilities from their creation. During the colonial period in each instance, organized medical services are provided by the colonial country and are staffed by doctors sent by the mother country and paid according to the salary schedules of the mother country's civil service. Gradually citizens of the colony are trained in medicine and enter the colonial medical service. After the departure of the colonial power, the organized medical service and its salaried medical staff become a department of the new independent government. As the government expands its medical services, an increasing amount of the country's medical care is carried out by salaried doctors, and salaried government employment becomes increas-

Education in Soviet Russia," *British Medical Journal* (14 June 1924), pp. 1055, 1058; and Nikolai Semashko, "Das Gesundheitswesen in Sowjet-Russland," *Deutsche Medizinische Wochenschrift*, vol. 50, no. 22 (30 May 1924), p. 722. During the short-lived March Republic, the medical profession itself proposed a governmentally owned and financed national health service under professional control. Mark G. Field, *Doctor and Patient in Soviet Russia* (Cambridge: Harvard University Press, 1957), pp. 48, 51.

[23] G. F. Konstantinov, *Zdravookhranenie v SSSR: Statisticheskii Spravochnik* (Moscow: MEDGIZ, 1957), chap. 2.

ingly important to the medical profession. Since the colonial medical service is part of the larger colonial civil service, its doctors are paid according to a scale covering nonmedical officials, and medical salaries may remain part of the regular civil service pay scales long after independence. Such an orderly transition to an indigenous salaried medical service can be seen in many former British colonies.

English doctors have worked in her colonies for many decades. At first the employment conditions were heterogeneous: some went on contracts with business firms or other organizations; many were military officers; many were missionaries; many were under contract to individual colonial governments. Since so many colonies were tropical and disease-ridden, the Colonial Office in London encouraged the development of courses in tropical medicine in English schools of medicine and schools of public health, and it actively recruited doctors. The posts were usually full-time and salaried. A unified West African Medical Staff was created by the Colonial Office in 1902, with common working conditions and pay scales. Eventually in 1934, the unified Colonial Medical Service was created for all the colonies, as one of the unified occupational structures in a reorganized colonial service.[24]

Each British colony has had its own public service, staffed by its own citizens and supported by its own tax funds. In practice the Colonial Service based in London interlocked with the local public service: some or many of the posts would be filled by Englishmen assigned by London, while other posts were filled by local citizens. Members of the Colonial Service would enjoy benefits prescribed by Parliament and by regulations of the Colonial Office, such as paid home leave, free transportation from the colony to England for home leave, free housing or housing allowances in the colony, pensions, etc. Depending on its affluence and policies, the colonial legislature might provide some fringe benefits to locally recruited employees. In his responsibilities, the member of the Colonial Service assigned to a local post was a member of the public service of that colony, like any local citizen. All branches of the Colonial Service had the same salary scale, although one occupation might have more members in high pay grades than another. Some differentials in basic salary existed among colonies, but they were small. Since members of the Colonial Service tended to occupy the higher posts in the public service of each colony and since Colonial Service members throughout the world had similar basic pay, similar pay scales resulted for the public services of different colonies.[25]

The Colonial Medical Service was part of the unified Colonial Service. In each colony, its members performed administrative, public health, and therapeutic tasks. They managed and staffed hospitals and clinics for the

[24] Charles Jeffries, *The Colonial Empire and Its Civil Service* (Cambridge: University Press, 1938), pp. 10, 16–17, 26, 42–45, 76–77.

[25] Ibid., chaps. 7–9 passim.

population, did sanitary and other preventive work, cared for government employees, and (in some of the larger colonies) trained nurses and medical assistants. Usually English doctors in the Colonial Medical Service gave all the organized medical care in the colony at first, gradually local doctors acquired medical training in England (and later in other countries), these local doctors entered the local medical service at the lower ranks, and eventually only a few Colonial Medical Service officers remained. Members of the Colonial Medical Service were paid according to the same salary scales applied to other members of the Colonial Service in that colony, but their starting point usually was slightly higher. Usually (but not always) members of the Colonial Medical Service had full-time contracts forbidding private practice.[26]

Cyprus passed through the stages typical of many former English colonies. For several decades its colonial government had a medical service. At first staffed entirely by members of the English Colonial Service, gradually it was converted to a Cypriote organization. Some Cypriotes began to go to England for medical education, and some returned to join the island's medical service. Then other Cypriotes began to get medical training in Greece and Turkey. As more Cypriotes entered the island's medical service at the junior ranks, the members of the Colonial Medical Service became a shrinking minority at the higher ranks. On the eve of independence, only the Director of Medical Services and one hospital doctor remained from the Colonial Medical Service; the hospital doctor's departure and the Director's replacement by two Cypriotes (a Minister of Health from the Turkish community and a Chief Medical Officer from the Greek community) completed the changeover.

The medical services continued to function as before, with the same facilities and personnel. At the time of my visit during early 1962, there were 86 doctors in the government service and 312 in private practice. The government then ran one large general hospital, six district hospitals, fifteen local health centers, and several public health programs. The local health center doctor is primarily concerned with patient care, but he and his superior, the district medical officer, also perform sanitary inspection. As in most countries, Cyprus has private clinics owned by doctors; by hospitalizing the patient in his private clinic rather than in the public hospital, the private practitioner continues to treat the patient and continues to collect fees. Any Cypriote is entitled to use a doctor or hospital in the public medical service, but he must pay fees unless he presents a *muktar's* certificate.

Before independence the salaries of the Cypriote medical service were set, as in other British colonies. General standards were laid down by the Colonial Office and by Parliament. A set of salary scales for all occupations in the Cypriote government—including the doctors—was worked out by a Selection

[26] Ibid., chap. 12.

Committee consisting of representatives from some of the government departments. The Committee was responsible to the governor. Its pay scales had to be approved by the Governor; they also had to be approved by the Secretary of State for the Colonies in London before becoming official, but this step nearly always was no more than a formality. This administrative machinery was adapted during decolonization. A new Civil Service Commission replaced the Selection Committee as the body that wrote pay scales. The Ministerial Council (i.e., the Cabinet) and the House of Representatives replaced the Governor and the Colonial Office as the bodies ultimately deciding the pay scales and the Ministry budgets. Doctors continued to be paid according to a salary scale governing other professionals and civil servants.

During the last revision of the salary scale for doctors and all other occupations, in 1954, the Selection Committee deliberately streamlined the payment system in preparation for independence, when all employees would be native Cypriotes. Cost-of-living allowances, rent allowances, and certain other supplements designed particularly for members of the Colonial Service were abolished.[27] This pay scale was used during the first months after independence. Thereafter the Civil Service Commission added several grades to the scale and raised the rates, primarily for the doctors in hospitals. The need to motivate doctors to stay in Cyprus and to accept full-time salaried jobs gradually resulted in a pay scale different from that of other professionals and civil servants in the government.

Israel

Instead of pressing for abandonment of salaried methods, the medical profession may fight to preserve them, if the alternative is less advantageous. An example is the unsuccessful attempt by the principal sick fund of Israel to shift to the capitation system.

For many years most Israelis have received their general practitioner care in polyclinics owned by the sick fund of the General Confederation of Jewish Labor (the *Kupat Holim* of *Ha'histadrut Ha'klalit*). A group of salaried general practitioners works in each polyclinic. Until the 1960's, patients belonging to *Kupat Holim* were assigned to a polyclinic but not to an individual general practitioner: a lay clerk at the reception desk would give the patient a ticket to see one of the doctors. To earn his salary, each doctor was supposed to see a certain number of patients during fixed working hours each day. The doctors did not like their work depending upon the authority and judgment of a layman using statistical work norms. Many patients complained that the

[27] *Revision of Salaries 1954* (Nicosia: Cyprus Government Printing Office, 1954). The organization of the colony's health services at that time is described in, G. F. Neild, "The Health and Social Services of Cyprus," *Journal of the Royal Army Medical Corps*, vol. 104, no. 2 (April 1958), pp. 51–62.

assignment system was too impersonal, that they would rarely see the same doctor on successive visits, and that they might not be able to see a doctor if all had completed their day's quotas.[28]

The controversy became a political issue during elections in the late 1950's. When the political parties controlling the Parliament and the *Histadrut* lost votes, the leadership of *Histadrut* and *Kupat Holim* decided to change the patient assignment system in the polyclinic and create family doctors on the English pattern. Every patient would be permanently assigned to one doctor, each general practitioner would have a list, the doctor would be responsible for his patients at all times, and the G.P. would be paid by capitation rather than by salary.

The Association of *Kupat Holim* Doctors rejected this proposal for several reasons. For the first time doctors would be obligated to make night calls, and these would interfere with the private practices many conduct outside their fixed polyclinic hours. A salaried system has made the *Kupat Holim* doctors equal, but capitation would suddenly introduce inequalities of pay, status, and power according to length of list. Thus the capitation system was opposed by doctors with shorter lists, such as the elderly, those in rural areas, and those in overdoctored areas. It is risky for a medical association to agree to sudden changes in the payment system, since its internal balance of power will change suddenly and unpredictably, and therefore the Association's leaders were skeptical.

A compromise was devised that eliminated the assignment clerk but changed little else. Doctors continue working fixed hours for a salary. Each doctor has a list of patients that see him during his office hours, but the polyclinic maintains an emergency service for visits outside these hours.[29] If they had had a free choice, the doctors might have selected fee-for-service, but capitation was plainly a last resort, particularly since it implies unlimited responsibility for the patient.

Introducing Novel Changes

It is very unusual for a democratic legislature to enact any fundamental reorganization in the medical services or in doctors' pay. The medical association usually gains enough allies from the political parties of the Center or Right to block unacceptable legislation. Legislators who do not support doctors because of economic ideology may be reluctant to antagonize the physicians or to disrupt medical services.

[28] Joseph Ben-David, "The Professional Role of the Physician in Bureaucratized Medicine," *Human Relations*, vol. 11, no. 3 (1958), pp. 255–56 and 259–60; Marver H. Bernstein, *The Politics of Israel* (Princeton: Princeton University Press, 1957), pp. 323–24.

[29] Itzhak Kanev, *Summary of the Report and Statistical Abstract 1955–1958* (Tel Aviv: Central Kupat Holim, 1960), pp. 17–18.

Cutright may be correct that democratic governments are more likely to adopt social security programs than are authoritarian governments.[30] But most social security schemes merely offer monetary benefits and differ from health insurance, which affects the working conditions of a powerful profession. Authoritarian governments may be more successful in enacting legislation opposed by the doctors.

An example that is far from unique is the long delay in the enactment of Medicare in the United States, because of the American Medical Association's effective alliance with the Center-Right coalition and with strategic committee chairmen in Congress. Medicare was enacted in 1965 only because the least offensive bill was offered in an unusually favorable political climate: the Democratic landslide victory of 1964 sent an overwhelming majority of supporters to Congress and suggested strong public approval; one of the ablest legislative tacticians in American history sat in the White House; the bill confined national health insurance to the single category of people over sixty-five; the bill was liberally amended to please the doctors and to disturb very little their customary methods of practice and payment.[31]

Even when a determined Cabinet enacts a bill in a legislature that customarily operates by clear-cut majority rule, the medical profession often forces the government to amend the law. For example, the medical profession of Saskatchewan in 1962 struck against an official insurance scheme little different from those already commonplace throughout the world. One different—and disturbing—feature was a clause that could be interpreted as giving the government a monopoly in the purchase and evaluation of medical services: "With respect to a beneficiary or a dependent of a beneficiary, the commission is the agent of the beneficiary for all purposes." The doctors responded with unusual fury: instead of suspending administrative relations with the sick funds in the manner of protest customary in Europe, they halted care to patients. The government's subsequent concessions to the doctors included allowing the private sick funds to act as carriers in the official scheme, giving the doctor freedom in his insurance participation and in his billing methods, allowing doctors to choose either service benefits or cash benefits arrangements, and abandoning a new program of care in polyclinics. The individual physician could elect any method of remuneration. The doctors failed to accomplish their unrealistic goal of forcing the government to repeal compulsory health insurance—its creation was the government's only

[30] Phillips Cutright, "Political Structure, Economic Development, and National Social Security Programs," *American Journal of Sociology*, vol. 70, no. 5 (March 1965), pp. 537–50.

[31] The enactment of Medicare is described in, Richard Harris, *A Sacred Trust* (New York: New American Library, 1966) and Theodore R. Marmor, "The Politics of Medicare, 1965" (Boston: Harvard Interfaculty Program on Health and Medical Care, Harvard School of Public Health, 1966). The fate of earlier bills for national health insurance is described in, Stanley Kelley, Jr., *Professional Public Relations and Political Power* (Baltimore: The Johns Hopkins Press, 1956), chap. 3.

victory in the affair—but, like the medical professions in most countries, they succeeded in moulding it to their interests.[32] Scarred from its pyrrhic victory, the government hesitated to introduce the usual controls against possible venal multiplication of procedures by doctors until the medical association came to its rescue.[33]

Germany

When a medical system violates many of the central watchwords of professionalism, it will encounter ceaseless trouble, as the turbulent history of German health insurance shows. The German experience also illustrates the difficulty of finding a completely new arrangement when existing institutions prove unsatisfactory to the doctors.

The German national health insurance law of 1883 was the first of its kind. It antedated the professional organization and collective self-consciousness of modern medicine, and therefore the government did not have to bargain with the doctors over the draft. It contained numerous features that the medical professions of other countries subsequently learned to dread, largely in the light of the German precedent. The law gave the sick funds themselves the responsibility for providing medical care to beneficiaries.[34] It contained none of the safeguards for professional responsibility and autonomy that medical associations have since demanded in legislation, such as recognizing the pre-eminent position of licensed doctors in the provision of care, guaranteeing the right of any doctor to treat any subscriber, recognizing freedom of choice between doctor and patient, and so on.

The sick funds were strengthened in their customary relations with the doctors, since they (and not the medical profession) were responsible for giving care under the law, their incomes were higher because of tax collections, more people were covered by insurance, and therefore the doctors depended on the funds more than ever for their livelihoods. Sick funds continued their previous methods of hiring closed panels of physicians, paying them by low flat rates wherever possible, and sometimes regulating their prescriptions and their granting of sick leaves. The procedures and levels of pay usually

[32] Robin F. Badgley and Samuel Wolfe, *Doctor's Strike: Medical Care and Conflict in Saskatchewan* (New York: Atherton Press, 1967); Edwin A. Tollefson, *Bitter Medicine* (Saskatoon: Modern Press, 1964); Eugene Feingold and Marjorie Taubenhaus, "Physician Response to a Governmental Health Plan: The Saskatchewan Experience," in, Roy Penchansky (editor), *Health Service Administration* (Cambridge: Harvard University Press, 1968); and James A. Schnur and Robert D. Hollenberg, "The Saskatchewan Medical Care Crisis in Retrospect," *Medical Care*, vol. 4, no. 2 (April–June 1966), pp. 111–19.

[33] Gordon Forsyth, *Doctors and State Medicine* (London: Pitman Medical Publishing Co., 1966), p. 146.

[34] "Gesetz, betreffend die Krankenversicherung der Arbeiter," *Reichs-Gesetzblatt*, no. 9 (21 June 1883), part B.

were not negotiated with the doctors' representatives but were proclaimed unilaterally by the funds; doctors who did not like a fund's payment system were not hired or faced discharge.

In response, medical societies soon arose as pressure groups to represent doctors in disputes with local sick funds, and the national association of these regional societies became the spokesman for legislative reform. Fee-for-service gradually spread; but the doctors were still dissatisfied and strikes were common, because fees were low, particularly during the Great Depression. Service benefits continued to be used. Closed panels for individual funds were abandoned, but limits remained on the number of doctors eligible for all insurance practice. Funds still sometimes regulated doctors' clinical decisions in the name of economy. No regular consultative machinery existed for negotiation over fees and working conditions.[35]

A chronic problem has been the limited money available for doctors' fees. Generously financed national medical care schemes require heavy taxes on employers and large State subsidies. But the political parties representing business in 1881 rejected Bismarck's bill proposing higher taxes on employers than on employees, and they gained strength in the elections later that year. From the limited money available, the sick funds must pay out doctors' fees, hospitalization costs, drug bills, and unusually generous disability allowances. Doctors' complaints about inadequate payments increased as the Depression cut the funds' incomes. The ceaseless recriminations led some funds to search for ways to relieve themselves of blame. A few, notably those in the influential city of Leipzig, offered to transfer all the available money to the associations of their panel doctors, which had originally been formed to strengthen their members' positions when bargaining for fees. A few sick funds organized themselves from the start in this manner: they established panels of doctors who would receive a lump sum and who would be free to divide the money as they pleased, and the funds then advertised for doctors willing to work on these terms.[36]

During the many decades of controversy, some persons suggested that associations of insurance doctors be organized on a *Land* or national scale as the profession's collective representative in all dealings with the funds. Such self-governing associations finally were accepted by the sick funds during the 1920's as the best way to rid themselves of the difficult task of distributing a declining amount of money. The statute of 1931 included in its reforms authority for the sick funds to pay for insured care indirectly, by turning over to groups of doctors lump sums equal to the total value of their care, and the predecessors of the present Insurance Doctors' Associations—the KLV's and

[35] I. G. Gibbon, *Medical Benefit: A Study of the Experience of Germany and Denmark* (London: P. S. King & Son, 1912); and Ludwig Preller, *Sozialpolitik in der Weimarer Republik* (Stuttgart: Franz Mittelbach Verlag, 1949), pp. 234, 284–85, 327–30, 378–80, 471–73.

[36] Gibbon, *Medical Benefit* (note 35), pp. 53–58, 247–70.

the KBV described in chapter III—were created in 1933 by decrees of both the Weimar Republic and the Nazi government.[37] These associations continued to function after the war and were established on a new legal basis by the Insurance Doctors Act, passed by the Bundestag in 1955.[38]

The emergence of the Insurance Doctors' Associations solved the problem of the status of the medical profession. The individual doctor no longer would be hired by the sick fund to help the fund discharge its statutory responsibility to provide medical care to its subscribers. Rather, the medical profession was incorporated into the scheme: the associations were made public corporations, and both the amended law and contracts between the sick funds and the associations assigned the latter full power and responsibility for administering medical care under social security.

One of the fundamental demands of the medical profession on national medical care systems, namely the free participation by all doctors, remained an outstanding issue long after the others were settled. Before the law of 1883, most sick funds had closed panels, and these arrangements continued for decades thereafter. The entire profession protested, since the power to offer a contract gave the funds strong bargaining positions with individual doctors; the physicians excluded from all panel practice were particularly indignant. The most militant association within the medical profession, colloquially called the *Hartmannbund*, was created in 1900 primarily to press for free entry. Demonstrations and sympathy strikes were common.

In 1913, the national leadership of the sick funds and the *Hartmannbund* agreed on a compromise: individual sick funds would not make their own policies and would not maintain their own small closed panels; the doctors admitted to insurance practice in a community would be freely available to all insured persons up to a certain numerical limit; applicants would be admitted to sick fund practice by a joint committee of the local medical society and the sick funds, supposedly using criteria of merit but actually giving priority to the assistants of established insurance doctors. At first, doctors could be appointed up to a ratio of one doctor for every 1,350 insured taxpayers or 1,000 covered people, and in 1931, the ratio was reduced to 1:600. Much like the use of a ratio to guide new appointments to Spain's SOE, the limit satisfied the sick funds' desire to avoid expensive and unethical competition among doctors.

After World War II, the profession continued to attack any restriction, since the growing annual output of German medical schools meant many doctors would be left with no source of income. By 1954, Germany had about 40,000 office practitioners, but about 10,000 were outside insurance practice

[37] Julius Hadrich, *Die Arztfrage in der deutschen Sozialversicherung* (Berlin: Duncker & Humblot, 1955), pp. 15–23.

[38] The postwar legislation is summarized in, Horst Peters, *Die Geschichte der Sozialversicherung* (Bad Godesberg: Asgard-Verlag, 1959), pp. 111–29, esp. 123–25.

and several thousand had entered other occupations for want of opportunities in medicine. In addition to the *Hartmannbund*, the doctors outside insurance formed another special association to press for free entry. When the Bundestag passed a new health insurance law in 1955, it rejected the doctors' demands for free entry and merely lowered the ratio to 1:500.[39] The angry doctors outside insurance work then turned to the courts; the Constitutional Court of the Federal Republic declared the limitation on entry into insurance practice in violation of the constitutional guarantee of freedom to enter any occupation and place of work.[40] Thereafter, for the first time in German history, any licensed doctor could treat insured patients in any community.

France

The ability of the medical profession to obstruct any unacceptable legislation in a democratic system is illustrated by the history of national health insurance in France. Basic reforms could be enacted only when the Parliament was suspended and when the executive ruled by decree. The conflicts between doctors and the State—and the possibility of resolving them only by authoritarian governments—have had parallels throughout the French economy.

Until recently, the French economy was organized almost wholly along proprietary lines. Shopkeepers, merchants, farmers, professionals, even many manufacturers have been owner-operators of small firms or have been completely independent practitioners without employees. Workplace and home often have been joined together, and therefore the proprietor has conducted his work in the highly personalized and extremely private spirit that characterizes French family life: customers, employees, and other work contacts either were expected to be acceptable as personal family guests, or their entry into the work context was closely observed and regulated to prevent excessive invasion of privacy. Producers, sellers, and customers have long been accustomed to highly personalized and private buyer-seller relationships. Everyone has been accustomed to widely diversified products and services, and attempts to introduce standardization by voluntary collaboration or by regulation long encountered apathy or active resistance. Private and public organizations have been expected to be defenders and not managers of private individual interests.[41]

[39] R. Jodin and Jean Mignon, "La médecine en Allemagne de l'Ouest," *Concours médical*, vol. 78, nos. 1 and 5 (7 January and 4 February 1956), pp. 82–83, 554.

[40] 1 BvR 216/51, 23 March 1960, published in *Entscheidungen des Bundesgerichtshofes in Zivilsachen.*

[41] The proprietary spirit in the French economy is described in David S. Landes, "French Business and the Businessman: A Social and Cultural Analysis," in, Edward Mead Earle (editor), *Modern France* (Princeton: Princeton University Press, 1951), pp. 334–53; and Jesse R. Pitts, "The Bourgeois Family and French Economic Retardation"

France has had doctors and medical services for many centuries, but the successful and archetypal doctors have always been typical French proprietors, and medical organization has been affected by the proprietary spirit of French society. Traditionally the physician's work sites were his private office (often located in his home) and the patient's home. Even hospitalization has been fitted into the pattern of private office practice: after many centuries, public hospital practice for most doctors is still but an interlude of a few hours in a work day centering around the private office and the patient's home; until recently, many patients who might have been hospitalized in other countries were treated in their homes, and it was the homeless or badly housed poor who went to hospitals; many hospitals today are private clinics owned by private practitioners. The social recruitment of the French medical profession reinforced its proprietary orientations; until recently, nearly all medical students had fathers in the *haute bourgeoisie*, *petite bourgeoisie*, and liberal professions.[42] No occupation had a better living standard, more social prestige, or a more stable position in the entrepreneurially organized French social system than did medicine. Among the social classes of the past, the medical profession was one of the most self-satisfied of the interest groups (colloquially called *les intérêts*); in the towns the doctor was a leading figure, *un notable*.

As a result of its own history and the social context afforded by French life generally, the French medical profession developed a highly entrepreneurial ideology and a corresponding set of professional rules. The basic principles emphasize the patient's right to choose any doctor and the doctor's right to accept any patient; the complete confidentiality of relations between doctor and patient; determination of fees and treatments by direct agreement between doctor and patient with no influence from outsiders; payment of fees directly by the patient to the doctor with no influence or knowledge by any outsider.[43] These are simply the medical analogues of the economic principles traditionally accepted by many other occupations in French society; as in other proprietary French occupations, many individual doctors and the pro-

---

(Cambridge: dissertation for Ph.D., Harvard University, 1957). The traditional attitude of French interest groups toward the state and their tactics of resistance to public authority are summarized in, Stanley Hoffmann, "Protest in Modern France," in, Morton A. Kaplan (editor), *The Revolution in World Politics* (New York: John Wiley & Sons, 1962), pp. 69–91. The passionate French mode of defending one's economic interests and ideological convictions is described by François Bourricaud, "France," in, Arnold M. Rose (editor), *The Institutions of Advanced Societies* (Minneapolis: University of Minnesota Press, 1958), pp. 473, 487, 515–16, passim.

[42] This continued to be true in the mid-1950's. Jean-Daniel Reynaud and Alain Touraine, "Une enquête sociologique sur les étudiants en médecine," *Concours médical*, vol. 79, no. 6 (9 February 1957), pp. 698–99.

[43] The profession's ideology is summarized in, Henri Hatzfeld, *Le grand tournant de la médecine libérale* (Paris: Les Éditions Ouvrières, 1963), pp. 46–68; and in the publications of the *Ordre National des Médecins*.

fession's spokesmen defended these principles as articles of faith and reacted toward encroachments with immediate vigilance and much heat. Because of their consistency with traditional French social structure and because they appear to have been successfully followed by the French medical profession for so many centuries, the ideology and action of private office practice have been more deeply planted in France than in any other country.

When criticizing proposed expansion of public medical care, the leaders of the American Medical Association use the rhetoric of private medical practice, but American medicine is no longer organized according to classical individualism. Many American doctors practice in groups, but few French doctors did until recently. Many American hospitals have extensive committee structures that exercise control over the individual doctor, but these are rare in France. America has an independent profession that governs its members, but traditionally French medicine (like many other sectors of the French economy) allowed autonomy to the individual practitioner.

Many French medical leaders believe that the country has never had anything but private office practice and fee-for-service reimbursement. Actually, some nineteenth-century doctors in rural and working class districts had capitation agreements with associations, much like the prepayment arrangements of neighboring countries. But the successful urban doctors (*les grands médecins*) were paid fees by their wealthy clients, as were many other doctors. When the first medical syndicates were founded, in the late nineteenth century, they were dominated by *les grands médecins* and were affected by the prevailing national atmosphere of economic liberalism. The syndicates made fee-for-service standard throughout medical practice and spread the belief that it had always been universal.[44]

Social security came late to France. The Church and private organizations had provided charitable services for the poor for many centuries. But when other European governments adopted social insurance legislation during the decades before World War I, France enacted no more than a statute concerning liability for industrial accidents and a permissive statute facilitating the creation of pension funds. Wars always create in France a sense of national solidarity and are followed by a brief postwar honeymoon, during which *les intérêts* are quiescent and the leaders of the Left call for a new era with national resources dedicated to the welfare of all. And so, after World War I, a comprehensive social insurance program was proposed. Suggested by the Left, such aims could be achieved only by legislation enacted by a Chamber of Deputies with a bourgeois Center-Right majority and by a Senate where conservatives were even stronger. For nearly a decade, social security bills were held up in committees or shuttled between Chamber and Senate, blocked by objections from various interest groups, including the

[44] Jean Mignon, "La rémuneration à l'acte en question?" *Concours médical*, vol. 85, no. 7 (16 February 1963), p. 1086.

doctors. In view of the medical profession's insistence on complete professional and economic autonomy, its apprehension was aroused by early drafts stating that the sick funds would pay the doctors directly, as in other European health insurance systems.

Nationwide pressure groups have arisen later in France than in many other countries, but they have grown rapidly since World War I and particularly since World War II, in order to demand or oppose national economic legislation. France's national medical association grew out of the struggle over national health insurance. When it appeared that the Chamber and Senate would finally agree on a law containing some dangerous potentialities (as they did in 1928), the local medical societies formed the *Confédération des Syndicats Médicaux Français*. Two provisions of the 1928 statute became foci of concerted opposition by the *Confédération:* the statutory option that the funds could pay either the doctor or the patient (depending on local collective contracts between the medical profession and the funds) made possible a relationship between doctor and fund instead of the traditional doctor-patient economic relationship; another clause allowed the sick fund to pay 80 per cent or 85 per cent of a fee schedule agreed upon by the local medical profession and the local sick funds, and thus allowed the sick fund to have a voice in establishing doctors' fees.[45]

The medical profession possesses much leverage in any parliamentary democracy, and the Third Republic was particularly vulnerable. Many deputies and senators belonged to bourgeois political parties (such as the Radical Socialists) dedicated to the philosophy that government should not interfere in private personal affairs, in proprietor-customer transactions, or in the expert activities of the free professions. *Les notables* in each town carried great weight with their deputies, and the local doctors had the sympathy of their fellow elites. Several dozen doctors usually were deputies and senators at any one time, and thus the profession was directly represented in the legislative lobbies. Since each government was a delicately balanced coalition of several parties and since slight changes in the vote could cause large political swings and damage many political careers, the party leaders and individual deputies were solicitious toward a respected nationwide profession like medicine. The executive was the creature of the legislature, and, consequently, no cabinet could act decisively or independently; an individual cabinet member's career could be helped by pleasing his constellation of pressure groups but would be destroyed if he risked defiance. A powerful pressure group usually could block adoption of adverse legislation; even if the

[45] The *Confédération*'s campaign to amend the statute is described in, Paul Cibrie, *Syndicalisme médical* (Paris: Confédération des Syndicats Médicaux Français, 1954), pp. 63–73. The legislative history of the first social security laws appears in, Henry Galant, *Histoire politique de la sécurité sociale française 1945–1952* (Paris: Librairie Armand Colin, 1955), chap. 1.

Left were strong enough to get a law adopted (and even if the Center thought its passage politically prudent), the pressure group could still block implementation of the law by influencing the cabinet and the budget officers, and it might obtain modifying amendments when the political winds changed. The *Confédération* won two such victories in 1930 and 1946.[46]

In 1930, before going into effect, health insurance was amended to please the doctors: the sick funds would pay the patients and not the doctors; the sick funds might pay their patients according to a reimbursement schedule, but the schedule would not bind the physicians, who could continue to charge whatever they wished. Until the French amendments of 1930, national health insurance in the world had been a way for the sick fund to pay the doctor, but the political compromise with the powerful French medical profession had created a novel system of subsidizing the patient. Normally, social security is a system of subsidies: from taxes levied on wages and employers' payrolls, the government pays pensions, unemployment compensation, maternity benefits, sick leave, etc. Usually national health insurance is fundamentally different, since payment of the doctor by a third party results in some organized regulation—direct or indirect—of the doctor's economic relationships. Adopted as one of a set of general social security laws, French health insurance at first resembled them by establishing nothing more than a subsidy to the citizen.

An exception was Alsace-Lorraine, which had been German provinces until 1919. They were allowed to retain their Germanic system of health insurance, since both patients and doctors were accustomed to direct payment of doctors by sick funds, according to the latter's fee schedules. However much the doctors might have preferred the system later adopted in the rest of France, the public had a vested interest in the German system, and the French government could not risk antagonizing its returned countrymen. The annexation of provinces with health insurance was one reason for proposing a program in the rest of France. Poland, like France, annexed former German provinces and also let them retain German-type health insurance.

The *Confédération* may have won in 1930 not only a victory for the doctor generally but also a particular victory for the specialists. The latter were just beginning to gain prominence among French doctors: although a numerical minority of the profession, they included many of *les grands médecins;* and since the syndicates were dominated by *les grands médecins*, the specialists were heavily represented on the governing board of the *Confédération*. The government finally got the co-operation of the governing board of the *Confédération* by making a concession of crucial importance to the specialists, namely allowing the *Confédération* to dominate the writing of the *Nomenclature*, which

[46] For analyses of the institutional customs of the Third and Fourth Republics that facilitated the successful defensive maneuvers of bourgeois interest groups, see Robert de Jouvenel, *La république des camarades* (Paris: Bernard Grasset, 2d ed., 1924); and Nathan Leites, *On the Game of Politics in France* (Stanford: Stanford University Press, 1959).

is the set of weights among medical procedures that are ultimately converted into cash reimbursements to the patient. As I said in chapter III, the *Nomenclature* has always benefited specialty practice. Just as in Great Britain in 1948 and 1957, the medical profession could be divided by a skillful government willing to make concessions to the specialists.

Almost from the start, French national health insurance was beset by the controversy inherent in a reimbursement system. The law said merely that the sick fund would reimburse the patient at the rate of 80 per cent of an official fee schedule, at first called the *tarifs de responsabilité*. The doctors had never agreed to charge patients other than by their individual decisions, and fees rose higher than the *tarifs*. The local medical societies wished to prevent fees from falling too low, and many issued recommended minimum fee schedules that exceeded the *tarifs*. As a result many patients found that the reimbursement from the sick fund was only a fraction of the total fee. On the rare occasions when sick funds raised *tarifs de responsabilité*, many doctors raised their fees by corresponding amounts. Health insurance was supposed to replace charitable care for the working class, but some insured persons had to continue using public assistance. Labor unions and the political parties of the Left accused the medical profession of misusing the health insurance system for private gain and of deserting their humanitarian responsibilities. But the *Confédération* and the political parties of the Center and Right blocked all proposals to force doctors to charge no more than the *tarifs de responsabilité*.[47]

World War II temporarily changed the balance of power in France. The *bourgeois* political parties of the Center (such as the Radical Socialists) were discredited because of their close ties to the Third Republic; the *bourgeois* Right was discredited along with the Vichy régime. The Resistance movement was youthful and Leftist. The medical profession as an interest group had been weakened during the war by the abolition of the *Confédération* and its replacement by a disciplinary body controlled by the Vichy government, the *Ordre des Médecins*. During 1945 and early 1946, France was ruled by Charles de Gaulle and a Left Cabinet of the three Resistance parties, namely the Communists, Socialists, and MRP (Mouvement Républicain Populaire). The Resistance was a social revolutionary movement as well as a subversive activity against the German army. Its members had foreseen a new era for France, after disasters resulting from the self-centered pursuit of economic interests. Frenchmen would become brothers, and a new social security system would assure the welfare of all.

The social security program was a greatly expanded type of public social

[47] The structure and operation of national health insurance during the 1930's are described in, Barbara N. Armstrong, *The Health Insurance Doctor: His Role in Great Britain, Denmark, and France* (Princeton: Princeton University Press, 1939), part 3; and I. S. Falk, *Security against Sickness* (Garden City: Doubleday, Doran & Co., 1936), chap. 11. The disputes are described by Armstrong, chap. 21.

insurance. Heavy taxes would be levied on wages and on employers' payrolls, the money would be administered by a new series of funds, and subscribers would be eligible for benefits. The funds administered several benefits, such as health insurance, pensions, family allowances, etc. The funds were to be run by governing boards elected by the insured persons. The initial decrees reaffirmed the outlines of the traditional relationship between doctor and insured person: the patient could select any doctor, the patient would pay the doctor, and the fund would reimburse the patient for part of his fee. The newly reconstituted *Confédération* protested against certain ambiguous language that implied restricted choice of doctors by patients, and the wording was changed. Any specific departures from traditional medical practice would have aroused the *Confédération* and, since the government hoped that all groups would eventually agree, the decrees contained nothing controversial. But some of the supporters of social security hoped that the *tarifs de responsabilité* would eventually become binding on the medical profession.

The new social security system was established by an *ordonnance* issued by General de Gaulle before the first meeting of the democratically elected National Assembly. It was to be implemented by laws passed by the Assembly, by regulations passed by the democratically elected boards of the funds, and by agreements made between the funds and the interest groups (such as the *Confédération*).[48] Some programs, such as family benefits had wide popularity and could easily be implemented. But health insurance affected the interests of the still important medical profession; as in the 1930's, health insurance created a conflict of interests between the doctors and the middle and lower classes. Created by decrees issued by the men of the Resistance, health insurance would now be enfeebled by the parliamentary processes controlled by the leaders and social classes of the prewar republic.

As soon as the Assembly began meeting in late 1945, the strong leadership responsible for the social security program ended. The parties of the Resistance—Communist, Socialist, and MRP—no longer had a monopoly of power but had only a small parliamentary majority. Premier de Gaulle could not work with the Communists, could not work with the Right (which contained many of his enemies), and soon resigned. As before, cabinets now became the creatures of a politically fragmented and intrigue-ridden legislature. The Cold War and the schools question split the Resistance parties, resulted in new Center and Center-Right cabinets, and made the leadership and constituency of the MRP increasingly *bourgeois* and conservative. The strength

[48] The writing and issuance of the social security decrees are described by Galant, *Histoire politique* (note 45), chap. 2. The philosophy of the resistance that lay behind the social security program is summarized in, Henri Michel and Boris Mirkine-Guetzévich, *Les idées politiques et sociales de la résistance* (Paris: Presses Universitaires de France, 1954), pp. 375–78; and Gabriele Bremme, *Freiheit und Soziale Sicherheit* (Stuttgart: Ferdinand Enke Verlag, 1961), pp. 136–37.

of the system was steadily drained by military defeats in Viet Nam and Algeria and by the humiliating dependence on the United States. Pressure groups like the *Confédération* reappeared and became better organized, more numerous, and more effective than before. An important and well led pressure group like the *Confédération*, thus could induce Ministers and deputies to refrain from initiating or to block any undesirable administrative or legislative action. Some cabinets (such as those led by Dr. Henri Queuille) realized that the secret of long life was inactivity.

According to decrees supplementing the October 1945 ordinance, *tarifs de responsabilité* were supposed to be set by a collective agreement between each local branch of the *Confédération* and by the insurance fund in each *département*. The patient would be repaid 80 per cent of the *tarif* by the fund. If no collective agreement were signed, the *tarifs* would be set by a National Tariffs Commission that consisted of representatives from the *Confédération*, the social security funds, and the Ministry of Labor. The doctors in each *département* were expected to charge no more than the *tarif*, unless they were professionally eminent, unless the patient were rich, or unless other special justifications were present. The Minister of Labor could abrogate fee schedules that threatened the financial solvency of the funds. The *Confédération* must deal with two separate bodies, the National Federation of Social Security Organizations (FNOSS) and the Ministry of Labor, and the locus of responsibility and power on the public side has always been ambiguous.

Between 1946 and 1958, the question of fees produced continuous and sometimes very bitter friction. At no time were more than half the insured persons covered by collective agreements. The medical societies in the most populous areas, such as Paris and Lyons, could not agree with the funds, partly because the societies wanted high fees and partly because they did not like the standardization of fees in medical communities that included many outstanding and expensive men. At times of greatest friction, the number of collective agreements diminished. Twice the government attempted to control fees but was forced to surrender. By adopting a comprehensive and highly publicized social security program in 1945, the government had assumed responsibility for the social welfare of all its citizens. But patients had to pay a steadily greater proportion of their costs. The democratic processes of the Third and Fourth Republics had failed to make national health insurance viable. The disputes were a principal reason for the public's desertion of the Fourth Republic.[49]

In May 1958 the Fourth Republic fell. The National Assembly recalled de Gaulle, gave him emergency powers to solve the Algerian crisis, and ad-

[49] Details of the disputes and of the government's futile attempts to control fees appear in Hatzfeld, *Médecine libérale* (note 43), chaps. 3–5; and in, Henry Galant, "The French Doctor and the State," *Skidmore College Bulletin*, vol. 52, no. 1 (September 1966), pp. 9–11.

journed. The Ministries were no longer controlled by traditional politicians dependent on the legislature but by a coalition of politicians and technicians responsible only to de Gaulle. The cadres in the Ministries now had the opportunity to push forward the reforms blocked by the legislative institutions of the Third and Fourth Republics; public reformers also gained the government's ear. De Gaulle and his associates welcomed the opportunity to rationalize and modernize France; they had long been political enemies of the mercenary and self-centered economic interests, and they foresaw national unity and national renewal on the basis of a new social and political structure. Consequently, during 1958 and 1959, the President's Algerian emergency powers were used to issue decrees reforming many sectors of the French economy.

Several long-debated reforms were decreed in December 1958: one ordinance created the groundwork for new teaching hospitals with full-time medical staffs and modern facilities; another reorganized the administration of the public hospitals.[50] The perennial problem of medical fees also finally was solved. Parliamentary procedures had failed to implement the de Gaulle decree of 1945, and the General was back to complete the job. During 1959 and 1960, numerous conversations were held within the Ministry of Labor and in an interministerial committee. Previously, because of the power of the legislature over the cabinet and the influence of the *Confédération* among the deputies, the question of fees was negotiated between the Ministry and FNOSS on the one hand and the *Confédération* on the other hand, and the *Confédération* had a veto. Now the decision was made by officials who, as in other Ministries, were no longer in any mood to negotiate with the pressure group leaders who had harassed them for decades. The *Confédération* was informed of some of the alternative proposals and was invited to only one meeting at the Ministry, and then only to present its views and not to negotiate.

The decree of May 1960 (setting up the payment system described in chapter III) contained old provisions that the *Confédération* had fought before and new sanctions to force signing of collective agreements. Fee schedules would bind nearly all doctors and would cover nearly all patients. A government commission could set ceilings on the negotiated fee schedules and could prescribe fees in *départements* where no collective agreements existed. If the local medical society did not sign a collective agreement with the social security fund, any individual doctor could do so. If a doctor were not covered by a collective or individual agreement, his patients would be reimbursed by the fund at much less than the usual rate. If the local medical society did not sign

[50] Haroun Jamous, Jacques Commaille, and Bernard Pons-Vignon, *Contribution à une décision politique* (Paris: Centre d'Études Sociologiques, Centre National de la Recherche Scientifique, 1967); and Paul Comet, *L'hôpital public* (Paris: Berger-Levrault, 1960).

a collective agreement, the social security fund retained the right to establish a polyclinic in the area.[51]

The *Confédération* responded with its first and only strike against national health insurance. Patients continued to be treated and continued to pay as before, but many (not all) doctors refused to fill out the receipts that patients customarily sent to the funds for reimbursement. The strike could hardly have come at a worse time. The country was worried over Algeria—during mid-1960 de Gaulle seemed to be failing—and few could sympathize with a well-paid profession's self-centered maneuvers to charge the public without limit. De Gaulle was at the peak of his popularity in large part because his régime had ended the incessant pressure group turmoil of the Third and Fourth Republics, and a strike by doctors—like the unsuccessful strike by farmers a few months before—seemed a relic of the disastrous past. The National Assembly no longer could be manipulated against the cabinet; in fact, a few weeks after the beginning of the doctors' strike, the Assembly gave the government special authority to act against another of the Fourth Republic's scourges, the private distillers. The press condemned the strike with unexpected vigor.

The strike was bound to fail and did. The working conditions and method of paying doctors gave them no weapons against the government: since the office practitioners did not have direct relationships with any public agencies, there were no services or information the doctors could withhold; since the doctors did not wish to cut off their own incomes, they had to continue treating and charging patients as before. Refusing to fill out official forms was no weapon: doctors had to give some kinds of receipts to their patients, and the funds accepted them for reimbursement. The *Confédération* could have won only if every doctor followed it: but only some of the Paris and Lyons doctors were so militant and prosperous as to practice outside social security; most others were content to accept the official fee schedules and would have signed individual agreements had not the *Confédération* surrendered and allowed the local societies to sign collective agreements. Thus most French physicians now practice according to the ground rules of social security, a situation unthinkable to the secretive independent practitioner of the past. But this decisive—even if belated—victory by the social security system was possible only because an authoritarian régime had replaced a democracy.

To some observers, the doctors did not seem defeated at all, since they retained many things they had always wanted: payment continued on a cash

[51] The preparation of the May 1960 decree is described in Hatzfeld, *Médecine libérale* (note 43), chap. 6. The *Confédération*'s experiences during this period are summarized by Pierre A. Debuirre, "Rapport du Secrétaire Général pour l'Assemblée Générale de la Confédération," *Le médecin de France*, vol. 66, no. 177 (New Series) (November 1960), pp. 1053–56.

benefits principle, it remained fee-for-service, the official fee schedule continued to be one of the world's highest, and the funds agreed not to create polyclinics that would compete with the office practitioners. But in the light of the profession's intransigent demand for full autonomy it had indeed been defeated for the moment. Medical associations prefer that they alone write fee schedules; their second preference is a negotiated settlement with the sick funds. The new French decrees gave the government full power to impose a fee schedule and its rates: the Committee on the *Nomenclature* enabled the sick funds and doctors to negotiate recommendations, but the National Commission on Tariffs consisted entirely of government officials and could adopt any fee schedule and any rates. Doctors were not completely free to ignore the rates, as the profession would have preferred: the lower reimbursements to their patients enabled the sick funds to influence the patients' choices of doctors.

If the medical profession had remained unreconciled and had continued to fight the new arrangement, the government and sick funds might have held their ground and a long period of conflict might have ensued, as in Germany. Or the medical association might have outlasted de Gaulle, and his successors might have surrendered. Instead, the medical association of France followed another course not uncommon in medical politics elsewhere: it co-operated with the new arrangements, its leadership changed from the combative advocates of the traditional autonomous model to a new and more conciliatory group of men, mutual confidence grew, and the government and funds made some fundamental concessions in the payment system. A committee was created to recommend changes in the decree of May 1960, and the medical profession's new leadership was represented. As a result, the all-governmental National Commission on Tariffs was replaced by the Tripartite Commission representing the interested parties, including the doctors. Therefore, the fee schedule and the rates would be a governmental enactment of a previously negotiated settlement. In retrospect, the medical profession had been defeated only in its unrealistic demand that it be independent of any organized national system; ultimately it had won, since the system was fashioned to please it.

Belgium

The strength of a well-organized medical association in a parliamentary democracy is demonstrated by recent events in Belgium. The problem resembled France's. The outcome resembled Saskatchewan's.

In 1964, Belgium still lacked the degree of standardization and statutory procedures for dealing with the medical profession that had been enacted in other European countries. National health insurance laws required certain classes of employees to join sick funds and regulated the procedures and benefits of the funds. But doctors were left completely free to conduct their practices and set fees; and the funds reimbursed the patients instead of paying the doctors directly. The medical profession had long resisted enactment of any more extensive organization. Demands for reform had long come from workers and others who wished ceilings on medical costs and who accused doctors of profiteering. Enactment of the social security procedures of neighboring nations was essential to permit the free exchange of labor within the Common Market.

Parliament in late 1963 finally revised national health insurance. Among other changes, the new law required doctors to adhere to fee schedules; the cash benefits system for insured patients was retained, but the doctors were no longer free to charge anything they wished. The medical profession and the government then waged one of the most bitter conflicts in medical politics in any country. The doctors struck, and many left the country temporarily. The government tried to seal the borders, called two-thirds of the doctors into the army, posted many of these physicians on hospital service, and prosecuted a few doctors for negligence leading to the deaths of patients who had failed to get treatment.

But it was not a Belgian de Gaulle who held power; it was a coalition cabinet still responsible to a divided Parliament and to a divided electorate. The Belgian government could not settle the issue by decree supported by public opinion, as did France in 1960. Rather, the Belgian régime could induce the doctors to return to work only by committing itself in advance to negotiate a mutually satisfactory arrangement and to amend the law—concessions reminiscent of Saskatchewan. And, just as in the Canadian province, the political parties that had been unable to avoid a clash and to effect an orderly solution fell from power soon thereafter. Like Saskatchewan and unlike France, trouble continued.

In the Belgian negotiations in 1964, the doctors agreed to participate in national health insurance according to certain standardized procedures in billing and remuneration, but they won numerous concessions in the actual administration of remuneration and of other aspects of the system. For example, fee schedules would take effect only if 60 per cent of the doctors in a locality agreed. The fee schedules were never binding: any doctor could charge what he wanted, but the vote of approval simply created a list of doctors following a predictable and lower schedule. The doctor and patient could agree on higher fees if the doctor practiced outside the list. The fee schedules in effect under the agreements—like many other decisions in the remuneration system—were not to be dictated by the government, and sick funds but were to be negotiated by them with the medical association.

The doctors won further concessions two years later, by restrictions on polyclinics that were providing completely free care in competition with private office practice. This dispute split the country's Center-Left cabinet and resulted in a new Center-Right cabinet more favorable to the doctors.[52]

Conclusion: How Payment Systems are Brought About

The purpose of medical pay is to motivate maximum effort from the proper physician wherever necessary. Leaders of the profession in every country try to spread and perfect whatever payment methods will serve clinical goals and will please their members. They resist procedures that might cause doctors to stint, strike, or flee. If doctors in sufficient number and with enough heat claim the methods and levels of pay are depriving them of motivation and resources, enough laymen will worry about the maintenance of care to bring about major concessions.

Most payment systems in public care schemes are simply those inherited from prior practice, since the doctors would be disturbed by changes. Most payment procedures under "socialized medicine" are simply more bureaucratized versions of the methods that were used and often even invented by the doctors under earlier private practice. The "foreign" methods denounced by one country's doctors usually are customarily accepted by the medical profession somewhere else. Some methods of medical payment that are denounced in some countries, such as salaried employment in organizations, may be welcomed elsewhere as preferable to risky conditions in the free market.

After prolonged periods of financial imbalance or inequalities in the provision of medical care, governments may impose new systems of payment. These changes are rarely as sudden as they appear, nor are they invented by laymen. Usually the plans were discussed long before and were shelved because the government lacked a firm majority willing to override the medical association. Usually the original plans were devised by committees including some doctors, and they were supported by a faction within the medical profession. Even the most authoritarian decrees customarily contain some modifications that would please the medical profession, since the government is anxious about any interruptions of medical service for which it will be blamed. Usually the significance of an authoritarian solution is to demonstrate to the medical profession that some system of rules, price ceilings, and orderly budgeting is unavoidable. The precise administrative procedures usually are

[52] John V. Craven, "A Strike of Self-Employed Professionals: Belgian Doctors in 1964," *Industrial and Labor Relations Review*, vol. 21, no. 1 (October 1967), pp. 18–30; Jean Mignon, "Les médecins et l'assurance maladie en Belgique depuis l'accord du 25 juin," *Concours médical*, vol. 86, no. 38 (19 September 1964), pp. 5175–82; "Les problèmes médicaux en Belgique: historique, difficultés actuelles," ibid., vol. 88, no. 10 (5 March 1966), pp. 1671–74; and "Le point de la situation en Belgique," ibid., vol., 89, no. 15 (15 April 1967), pp. 2986–92.

left to negotiation between the medical association and the public authorities. Once agreements are made and doctors accept the system in practice, members of the profession are assigned to administer it, with the laymen relegated to budgetary review.

Therefore authoritarian and evolutionary solutions ultimately end at the same point. Lest medical services be upset and lest they be blamed, the government and sick funds create an administrative structure and system of medical pay that is acceptable to the medical profession. Elaborate concessions are made to the profession's demands for autonomy, resources, and incentives sufficient for future recruitment. Standing consultative mechanisms are created. Shortages of money and malfunctions touch off occasional disputes, sometimes punctuated by extravagant rhetoric and strike threats, but almost invariably the doctors obtain concessions in money and procedure. Since money is limited, doctors rarely get paid as well as they would like, but usually they gain more from the public authorities than does any other private group.

VII

EFFECTS OF FEE-FOR-SERVICE AND CASE PAYMENTS: SERVICE BENEFITS

The payment system of a profession should provide the means and incentive for the members to apply their knowledge and skills for the solution of society's problems in their areas of expertise, in accordance with the precepts taught by their professional schools and other institutions. A payment system for doctors should help supply the means and incentive to give each patient what he needs in diagnosis, clinical therapy, psychosomatic support, preventive medicine, and continuity of care. The payment structure should motivate referral to the physician best qualified to do the work. Outstanding performance should be encouraged and recognized; adequate work should be suitably compensated. The doctor should be induced to learn and apply the newest effective techniques. The necessary numbers of qualified people should be induced to enter medicine, to specialize in its various fields, and to practice in parts of the country and among social classes where they are needed. A payment system should be economical administratively for both doctors and officials.

A common problem in social action is that certain features of formal organization produce effects not anticipated by the planners and at variance with the organization's official purpose. Therefore the ways that doctors are paid should not induce doctors and patients to behave contrary to the norms of professional conduct. Excessive and unnecessary care to earn money should be avoided. Patients who need attention should not be neglected because they are unprofitable. In order to earn money, doctors should not avoid making referrals and should not undertake procedures beyond their qualifications. The reward structure should produce no maldistribution of doctors and services by specialty or region. Conflicts, low morale, and interruptions of service should be avoided.

I will try to assess the effects of the different payment systems in various countries on the basis of reports from my informants in each country and a review of the literature. Certain recurrent themes will appear during the next chapters. An economic interpretation of doctors' pay would be misleading: their behavior is due at least as much to professional organization and professional values as it is to the monetary reward system.[1] How a payment system relates to the behavior of doctors and patients depends on many other considerations, such as the total organization of medical care, the doctor-population ratio, the wealth of the country, and the opportunity for supplementary income through private practice. Therefore formally similar payment mechanisms may operate quite differently in different countries. Finally, every payment system can incorporate certain safeguards that discourage its disadvantageous effects, but national medical care systems vary considerably in the skill of their architecture.

Unnecessary Work

The principal danger in fee-for-service and case payments is the performance of medically unnecessary procedures in order to collect money. Since the doctor is paid for each procedure under a fee schedule, he may order office visits, perform tests, and give treatments that the patient does not need. Profitable procedures, such as surgical operations, may be undertaken unnecessarily. In a case payment system, the doctor might place as many people as possible on his sick list and might urge them to reapply when their time periods expired. A service benefits arrangement is even more vulnerable than a cash benefits scheme. Since the patient pays nothing and may not know how the doctor bills the sick fund, the patient might not protest repetitious and unnecessary care, and the physician might bill the fund for procedures not performed. The economics of individual office practice motivates a high volume of procedures: as a practice expands, expenses level off, the unit cost of each service declines, and therefore each procedure is increasingly profitable.[2]

Conditions Producing Unnecessary Work

One cause is low fees: in order to earn an adequate income, a doctor may multiply certain procedures, particularly those that do not harm the patient,

[1] A Canadian observer's comment on his own country is more generally true: "I personally do not feel that the method of payment is as important a determinant of quality as some professional people would like to think. Experience has shown that professional people will provide a satisfactory standard of service under any method of payment, provided that the total payment is sufficient and the working conditions are conducive to independence of professional judgment and a sense of personal satisfaction in the job being done." John E. F. Hastings, "Issues and Priorities in Medical Care," in *Social Policy in the Sixties* (Ottawa: Canadian Welfare Council, 1961), p. 24.

[2] Estimates of practice expenses and of declining unit costs under German national health insurance appear in, Julius Hadrich, *Der Arztfrage in der deutschen Sozialversicherung* (Berlin: Duncker & Humblot, 1955), pp. 163–66.

such as office and home visits. This has long been suspected in the first national health insurance scheme—the system in Germany—and has contributed to the widespread belief in other countries that national medical care schemes were inherently wasteful. Since there have been no official maxima on office and home visits, an enormous number of patient contacts are possible, although care to each person would be cursory. Such doctors avoid the time-consuming patient but welcome a patient requiring frequent but simple treatments or checkups. Before the fee schedule called *Preugo* became widely used after 1924, thereby magnifying technical procedures, many insurance doctors tended to be paid on the basis of number of cases of illness and visits per quarter, and it was believed that some doctors tried to collect the entire family's patient tickets (i.e. the *Krankenscheine*) when making a home visit to one. By attracting so many insured patients, these *Kassenlöwen* (sick fund lions) could prevent younger doctors from building up a practice. Sick fund statistics several decades ago often showed that a few of the doctors in a community had nearly all the insured patients.[3]

Recently this problem has beset insurance in most of the cantons of Switzerland. Swiss health insurance is financed primarily from the subscriptions paid by employees. Employers and the State contribute little to the sick funds. Competition for members induces the funds to keep these rates low.

> The medical societies would prefer much higher fees, particularly for wealthier patients, but the sick funds try to restrict all their costs in order to keep down their membership fees. Insured persons' contributions are not fixed by social security tax laws, as they are in other countries with national health insurance, and each sick fund freely sets its own subscription rates. Since several competing sick funds exist in each canton, each fund tries to attract patients by offering satisfactory benefits at minimum subscription rates. Consequently all try to keep down doctors' fees, which otherwise would increase costs without expanding benefits. Competition among sick funds occurs in Switzerland to a greater degree than in any other country with a statutory system. Not only do most people have a choice among funds, but three-quarters of the subscribers are free not to join any fund.[4]

Therefore, one of the world's wealthiest countries has had one of the world's lowest fee schedules, particularly just before the reforms of the mid-1960's. When the ceilings on fees are set by laws rather than by bargaining

[3] The methods and superficial care of the *Kassenlöwen* are described in, Erwin Liek, *Die Schaden der sozialen Versicherung und Wege zur Besserung* (Munich: J. F. Lehmanns Verlag, 2d ed., 1928), chap. 2, sec. A passim; Rudolf Leonhärdt, *This Germany* (Greenwich, Conn.: New York Graphic Society, 1964), pp. 95–96; and "Der Wolf und die Geizer," *Der Spiegel*, vol. 15, no. 12 (15 March 1961), pp. 37–38. Statistical estimates of the work load and minutes for each service in busy practices are made by Hadrich, *Der Arztfrage* (note 2), pp. 166–68.

[4] Rolf Schlögell, "Vergleichende Darstellung der Krankenversicherung Osterreichs, der Schweiz, und der Bundesrepublik Deutschland," *Ärztliche Mitteilungen*, vol. 40, no. 32 (November 1955), p. 946.

or by standing review mechanisms, the level of fees lags behind the price level and the structure of the fees lags behind medical advances. Following were the statutory minima and maxima for home and office visits in a few cantonal statutes during the early 1960's, before the general increase in fees and before the revision of the payment system in 1964 and 1965. (All numbers are in francs, whose free market exchange rate at the time of writing is 1 fr.S. = $0.23.)

	Day Office Visit		Day Home Visit	
Cantons and Half Cantons	Minimum	Maximum	Minimum	Maximum
Zurich	3.80	5.15	5.60	7.55
Berne	5.00	10.00	6.00	12.00
Lucerne	3.00	6.00	4.00	8.00
Solothurn	2.40	4.00	3.20	5.30
Basle:				
Basle Town	—	3.20	—	4.40
Basle Country	2.80	4.20	4.00	6.00
Vaud	4.00	6.00	5.00	7.50
Valais	4.00	4.50	5.00	5.50
Neuchatel	4.00	6.00	4.40	6.60
Geneva	4.50	9.00	6.00	12.00

In 1961, Swiss office visits under the statutory rates varied between the minima of $0.46 to $1.04 to the maxima of $0.69 to $2.30. Office visits at the same time in some other European countries, ranked by GNP per capita, were: Sweden, $1.52 and $1.14; Norway, $1.68; France, between $2.00 and $2.40 for a G.P. and between $3.80 and $4.60 for a specialist; Italy, between $0.61 and $0.67. Some cantons paid surgical and other specialty procedures lower than did other European health insurance systems. Because the Swiss laws were old, some once difficult but now routine specialty procedures, such as appendectomies, enjoyed a relatively better paid position in the Swiss than in the foreign lists. For example, Zurich in 1961 paid 83.00 fr. for an appendectomy, the same as for the most difficult thoracic and cerebral operations; compared to other European fee schedules, the latter were underpaid, the appendectomy overpaid.[5]

The venal multiplication of expensive specialty procedures is not easy under Swiss health insurance. Official ethics and professional opinion strongly condemn unnecessary surgery and other medically superfluous tasks. Another conservative force is the requirement in many cantonal statutes that the sick fund approve an expensive medical procedure before it can be done under insurance. For example, thirteen of the forty-seven surgical operations on the fee schedule for Vaud during the early 1960's had to be authorized in advance. A third reason for the restraint upon unnecessary specialty procedures is that an increasing amount of specialized care is being shifted to

[5] Parts of the Zurich and Berne fee schedules during the early 1960's appear in, James Hogarth, *The Payment of the General Practitioner* (Oxford: Pergamon Press, 1963), pp. 308–11.

public hospitals from the once fashionable private clinics. The Swiss are proud and careful of the reputations of their public hospitals; the hospitals are run by powerful service chiefs who earn high incomes from legitimate private practice without exploiting the sick funds, and they are intolerant of any subordinate who does unnecessary work for money. However, optional or unnecessary specialty procedures may not have been wholly abolished: it is suspected that some well paid diagnostic tests, such as electrocardiograms, may be overdone.

Interviewed before the reforms of the mid-1960's, my informants were of the opinion that the principal way to build up income was to make many office and home visits to each patient. All who had studied and worked in America believed that compared to American doctors with similar posts, they and their colleagues saw more patients each day, worked at a faster tempo, and had less time for professional reading. This certainly appeared plausible to the visitor: in no other country did my medical informants watch the clock so anxiously, rush through our interviews, or terminate so many interviews before their conclusion on grounds of work pressure. Some of my informants in internal medicine in French-speaking Switzerland estimated that they personally saw up to sixty patients a day during much of the year, up to one hundred on some days in winter, and made more house calls than specialists in other countries. Some informants felt that an extra visit with each recovered patient "to see how he is getting along" was a common result of the Swiss insurance payment system but might not occur in private practice.

Whether Swiss doctors do in fact make many more visits than those abroad cannot be finally determined without much careful investigation. Twice during the 1950's the sick funds reported 5.3 doctor-subscriber contacts per year,[6] a figure only slightly higher than that of most other Western countries with national health insurance. In the late 1950's, Hogarth was told, the various cantons averaged between three and five doctor-subscriber contacts annually, with the higher figure prevailing in the cities.[7] But cross-national comparison would require full knowledge of the actual number of illnesses: the Swiss population is one of the world's healthiest, and possibly Swiss doctors make more visits to each *patient*.

The price paid for a high insurance income, some doctors have complained in both Switzerland and Germany, is excessive catering to patients. Since the office physician must see many patients each day to build up income, and since patients can change doctors easily, the doctor may be motivated to see any patient and encourage all to return when they wish. Some

[6] *The Cost of Medical Care* (Geneva: International Labour Office, 1959), p. 90; and "Volume and Cost of Sickness Benefits in Kind and Cash," *Bulletin of the International Social Security Association*, vol. 16, nos. 3–4 (March–April 1963), p. 57.

[7] Hogarth, *Payment of General Practitioner* (note 5), p. 319.

doctors say they would prefer fewer patients with minor or imaginary complaints, but selection would be possible only if fees were higher.[8]

Some critics of the German payment system believe it has perpetuated its own defects. The individual doctor is paid by fee-for-service. Particularly before 1964, the fees actually paid were low for each procedure, but the physician could aim for a high income. The fees were not fixed but resulted from the distribution of the lump sums held by the KLV's, according to the relative values listed in *Preugo*. The greater the number of procedures performed, the lower the fees for each, and the more difficult it was to keep fees at a level which did not tempt the physician to achieve high total income through superfluous work. When fees were low, each doctor was motivated to multiply his own procedures, thus perpetuating the low fees. Individual doctors could not afford to devote more time to each patient and have fewer patient contacts, because the system would reduce their incomes.[9]

One of the constant criticisms of German national health insurance is that patients seek and doctors grant too many sick leaves and sick benefits. Such complaints are heard far more in Germany than in any other country and have recurred for decades.[10] The benefits are said to be so generous that many persons seem to make a career of being on sick leave and collecting sick benefits. The compensation system is said to motivate doctors to issue many sick leaves without medical justification: since the patient is free to shop around among doctors, and since the large number of physicians creates a buyer's market, the doctor allegedly must please patients by doing what they ask or risk losing future customers. Malingerers are said to be profitable to the doctor, since they often return to his office for superficial checkups and the renewal of certificates.[11] Perhaps sick leaves occur excessively today: West

[8] Paul Biedermann, *Die Entwicklung der Krankenversicherung in der Schweiz* (Zurich: Buchdruckerei Davos, 1955), p. 60. The "bagatelle problem" and its supposed demoralizing effect on German medical care and health insurance have been debated for many years. E.g., Werner Bosch, *Patient, Arzt, Kasse* (Heidelberg: Quelle & Meyer, 1954), pp. 36–39; and Hans Schulten, *Der Arzt* (Stuttgart: Georg Thieme Verlag, 2d ed., 1961), p. 73.

[9] Sozialenquête-Kommission, *Soziale Sicherung in der Bundesrepublik Deutschland* (Stuttgart: W. Kohlhammer GMBH, 1966), 1: 220–23; and "Der Wolf und die Geizer," *Der Spiegel*, vol. 15, no. 12 (15 March 1961), pp. 37–40. Therefore the Sozialenquête Commission suggested abandonment of the pool system and the introduction of a planned and predictable fee schedule (first citation, this footnote), pp. 223–30.

[10] I. G. Gibbon, *Medical Benefit: A Study of the Experience of Germany and Denmark* (London: P. S. King & Son, 1912), chap. 10; Erwin Liek, *Die Schaden der sozialen Versicherung und Wege zur Besserung* (Munich: J. F. Lehmanns Verlag, 2d ed., 1928), chap. 2; and Schulten, *Der Arzt* (note 8), pp. 73–74. These arguments often are presented in favor of reforms, such as cost-sharing by patients, stronger administrative controls, and longer waiting periods before the start of disability benefits. For example, the nationwide debate during the late 1950's, reported in, William Safran, *Veto-Group Politics: The Case of Health-Insurance Reform in West Germany* (San Francisco: Chandler Publishing Co., 1967), pp. 20, 25, 48, 53, 123, 133.

[11] The allegations were true before the Weimar Republic enacted unemployment in-

Germany at present has more cases and days of disability pay per protected person than any of the eighteen other countries compared by the International Social Security Association.[12] But such statistics result not only from doctors' decisions but from cross-national differences in statutory coverage, and therefore a special study would be needed to discover whether the system of paying doctors accounts in part for the excess. German sick funds have been long aware of the danger of excessive disability benefits granted by the doctors for their own profit and that of the workers at the expense of the funds; therefore the office practitioner's renewals beyond the seventh day may be disapproved by the control doctors employed by the funds. But the control system does not reach the short sick leave.

Controlling the excessive issuance of sick leaves by doctors with mercenary motivations to please patients is not an exclusively German problem. It is one of the principal difficulties in American workmen's compensation, particularly in states where applicants have free choice of doctors in issuing diagnoses and certificates. Some physicians are alleged to attract patients by their notoriety for providing a strong medical case for the highest claims. The American funds have had to adopt some of the controls that are common abroad.[13]

Even if a country's medical profession is opposed to unnecessary charges and its payment system is carefully designed to discourage them, the sick funds may be billed for more than they think justified if the medical profession's therapeutic philosophy and economic interests coincide. For example the cautious attitudes that discourage excessive treatment in Holland also lead the country's doctors to favor prolonged observation of the patient.

---

surance in the late 1920's. Until then, sick benefits were the only possible income for an unemployed worker, and industrial unemployment was usually accompanied by rising applications. Franz Goldmann and Alfred Grotjahn, *Benefits of the German Sickness Insurance from the Point of View of Social Hygiene* (Geneva: International Labour Office, 1928), p. 54; Walter Sulzbach, *German Experience with Social Insurance* (New York: National Industrial Conference Board, 1947), chap. 3. The temptations are great for the worker today: while other countries impose waiting periods of between three and fourteen days, German disability benefits begin at once; some employers have been pressed by unions to sign contracts supplementing sick pay, so that absent workers often receive amounts almost equal to their regular wages.

[12] "Volume and Cost of Sickness Benefits in Kind and Cash" (note 6), pp. 83, 108–10; and Table 11 in each national report in *Volume and Cost of Sickness Benefits in Kind and Cash: National Analyses* (Geneva: International Social Security Association, 1963). Half the country's workers took sick leave in 1963, 16 per cent more than once. The average leave for all persons reporting sick was 19.4 days. "Krankenstand," *Pressedienst* (Institut für Demoskopie Allensbach), mid-December 1964. Some policymakers suspect that a few repeaters cause most of the abuses and the adverse publicity. Occasional investigations of applications for sick leaves have uncovered malingering. E.g., Hadrich, *Der Arztfrage* (note 2), p. 192.

[13] Herman M. Somers and Anne R. Somers, *Workmen's Compensation* (New York: John Wiley and Sons, 1954), pp. 168–77.

This bias is reinforced by the payment system, despite the variable case payment formulae that we will describe in later paragraphs. Within a few days as an inpatient, an insured person brings more money to the specialist than in several months under transfer and renewal cards. Therefore it is believed that the payment system induces specialists—particularly in the medical fields—to treat persons as inpatients rather than as outpatients. This is less true in the surgical specialties, where the doctor may have to accept a global fee for a single expensive procedure and forego daily case payments for inpatient care. Therefore, several Dutch informants suspected that the surgical specialists are more eager to discharge an inpatient promptly, in order to make room for a new patient. The sick funds have been distressed at the rising cost of hospitalization and have urged specialists to treat patients in the outpatient departments whenever possible.

The reduction of the daily inpatient case payment after the fifth day might be expected to reduce the average length-of-stay in Dutch hospitals. But this daily rate is still higher than the monthly outpatient case payments for transfer and renewal cards. And, since Dutch specialists are very busy, they may not get around to a newly admitted patient until diagnostic tests are completed; since many are painstaking, they may avoid discharging an inpatient too quickly. So for all these reasons, the average length-of-stay seems not too different in Holland than that in other countries.[14]

Payment Formulae

National medical care systems combat these tendencies by various devices. One method is to price medical procedures in ways that discourage the doctor from doing more than is necessary. Another is the creation of administrative controls that detect and penalize for medically unjustified charges.

A few variable payment formulae can be incorporated into a fee schedule. To discourage performance of too many procedures on the same patient the national health insurance system of Holland contains many sophisticated safeguards.[15] It allows the specialist to collect a full fee for the most expensive procedure performed on a patient, while all other procedures undertaken on

[14] Compare Geneeskundige Hoofdinspectie van de Volksgezondheid, "Overzicht van de Gegevens der Ziekenhuizen in Nederland over de Jaren 1958 en 1959," *Verslagen en Mededelingen Betreffende de Volksgezondheid*, no. 9 (1961), p. 734; and Simon Btesh, "Pilot Study on Hospital Utilization" (Geneva: World Health Organization, 1962, mimeographed), Tables 1 and 2. Compared to other countries, the United States has much shorter stays, in large part because much higher daily charges must be paid by patients and by private sick funds. Compare Btesh's data with *Medical Care Financing and Utilization* (Washington: Public Health Service, United States Department of Health, Education, and Welfare, 1962), pp. 158–203 passim.

[15] See the explanatory notes throughout *Tarieven voor de Honorering van Tandheelkundig-Specialistische Hulp door Algemene Ziekenfondsen* (Amsterdam: Ziekenfondsraad, 1966).

the same patient are compensated at less than the full rate. In 1966, the Dutch fee schedule (Tariff III) allowed the surgeon to collect the fee for only the most expensive procedure performed through the same wound; there would be no compensation for other procedures performed through that wound. If the surgeon performs several procedures simultaneously through different wounds, he can collect the full fee for the most expensive one and half the fee for each of the others to a limit of f. 171.50 for the additional interventions. Likewise, French national health insurance pays the full rate for the most important procedure and half the fees for other procedures performed simultaneously.

It is common for national health insurance schemes to bar separate payments for both consultations and the technical acts performed during consultations, but this is not a universal rule: for example, in some Swiss cantons multiple billing is barred, but in others it has been allowed on the grounds that fees are too low. French national health insurance will not pay for both consultations and technical procedures performed during those visits;[16] and when several procedures are performed during the same visit, only the first is reimbursed for the full rate, while the others are paid at half or less. The fee schedule for examinations and minor surgery performed on ambulatory patients in Sweden grades procedures in three groups that earn gradually higher fees; if the doctor performs two procedures in the same visit, he does not collect payment for both but merely collects the slightly higher fee for the next group.

The Swedish groups and rates were described in chapter III, *supra*. If an office visit involves two or more Group *A* procedures, they are not paid for separately, but the reimbursement is equal to one Group *B* visit. Similarly, the visit falls in Group *C* if two Group *B* procedures are performed.

Asking the patient to make frequent and unnecessary visits can be discouraged by progressively reducing the rates. In 1966 Dutch national health insurance (Tariff II) paid the specialist f. 24.70 for a first consultation and f. 9.85 for the second and following ones. The only exceptions were cardiologists, who received f. 41.10 and f. 16.40. Several other national health insurance schemes also discourage unnecessary office and home visits by the same method, although they reduce the rates at later points. For example, several of the Swiss cantons reduce the fee after the first few visits or after the first few procedures on the same patient.

Another hazard in fee-for-service systems—particularly those offering

[16] Georges Cazac, "Cumul des honoraires d'une consultation et d'une intervention chirurgicale," *Concours médical*, vol. 87, nos. 33–35 (August 14, 21, and 28, 1965), pp. 4925–26; and Georges Cazac, "Cumul C + K," ibid., vol. 89, no. 5 (February 4, 1967), p. 929.

service benefits—is unnecessary referral to another physician. The Dutch Tariff II discourages this by paying referral from one specialist to another in the same field at a lower rate than referral from the general practitioner to the first specialist. On the other hand, referral and consultation should not be discouraged; getting a justified second opinion can be good medical practice. Therefore, the Dutch referral fee is intermediate between the first and subsequent consultation fees. In 1966, the referral fee within the medical specialties was f. 16.75, while the first and subsequent consultation fees for the same doctor were f. 24.70 and f. 9.85. Some national health insurance schemes try to encourage consultations by paying for them at higher rather than lower rates: for example if a general practitioner consults another physician in France, the former is paid one and one-half times a house call and the latter one and one-half times an office visit; if two general practitioners make a home visit to a patient, each is paid *V* 1.5.

If a specialty cannot earn much of its income through the technical procedures easily itemized in fee schedules, its profits may depend on length of hospitalization. In many of the medical specialties, income depends on the number of office visits and the number of days the patient is hospitalized on the physician's service. Prolonged hospitalization might be encouraged by daily payments. Under the Dutch system, hospitalization may not be ordered by the specialist at his own discretion but must be approved in advance by the control doctor employed by the sick fund. In 1966, the Dutch Tariff IV was designed to discourage unnecessarily prolonged hospitalization in the medical specialties by paying f. 9.90 daily for the first five days and f. 1.65 daily thereafter. If the patient is hospitalized a second time in connection with the same case, the daily rate remains f. 1.65 from the start, in order to discourage frequent discharges followed by rehospitalization orders. If the rehospitalization requires much new work, the sick fund may raise the daily rate to f. 7.25 during the first five days.

In the list of technical procedures embodied in a fee schedule, most would be too harmful to the patient if they were unnecessarily repeated. But there are a few exceptions, notably X-rays. In order to discourage the unnecessary repetition of X-rays, the Dutch Tariff VIII pays only 75 per cent of the full rate for any examination repeated within two months.

Holland's case payment system for ambulatory care contains the same sort of variable rates, in order to discourage unnecessary visits after expiration of the initial period of treatment. The rate for each subsequent month is slightly less than half the rate for the first month in specialties with short-term care, such as surgery, according to Tariff I. For the medical specialties with longer treatment and recovery cycles, the payment for each renewal period is slightly more than half the rate for the initial month. The full schedule for 1966 appeared in chapter III, *supra*.

Another problem with service benefits systems based on fees or case payments is the multiplication of procedures during home visits. Called to see one genuinely ill person, the doctor might report diagnostic or therapeutic care for several members of the household, when his contacts were actually perfunctory. As I said, this was one of the weaknesses of German national health insurance. The Ministry of Labor's decree of 1924 that reorganized insurance authorized half payment for each of the additional patient-contacts performed during the same visit to a hospital, nursing home, or private residence. The doctor could collect full payment only for the first patient. Therefore, full case payments no longer could be obtained by collecting everyone's *Krankenschein* for the quarter and mailing the lot to the sick fund. Similarly, some of the Swiss cantonal fee schedules forbid paying more than one fee for a home visit, even if the doctor claims to have seen more than one patient.

All the foregoing financial disincentives are parts of the fee schedules. The doctor knows in advance that a particular procedure will be priced unprofitably. Another monetary method of discouraging the excessive performance of procedures is to keep a record of the doctor's total work and to lower the fees after he has performed certain procedures several hundred times on his total clientele. In order to counteract the fact that net profits on each procedure increase, some of the German *Kassenärztliche Landesvereinigungen* have adopted sliding scales for payment to doctors, whereby increased numbers of office visits are paid for at decreasing rates. The first few hundred visits can be paid for at the highest rate, the next few hundred by the same doctor at a lower rate, the next few hundred at a still lower rate, and so on. This method was used by the KLV in Coblenz during the early 1950's:

For Each Visit by a Doctor	Payment for Each Visit in DM
From 1 to 200	6.00
From 201 to 400	4.50
From 401 to 600	3.50
From 601 to 800	3.00
From 801 to 1,000	2.00

Another method of discouragement is to pay *all* the doctor's visits by a standard rate calculated from a sliding scale. If a doctor makes few visits the unit fee is higher than if he makes many. This method was used in Munich during the early 1950's. For each additional one hundred visits in his total, the doctor's fee for all visits would decrease by 20 *pfennig*, with a larger drop after 800 visits. Particularly for caseloads after the 40 *pfennig* decrements take effect, great increases in work produce only slight increases in income.[17]

[17] The Coblenz scale, the Munich scale, and other financial calculations to make higher work loads decreasingly profitable are listed in Hadrich, *Der Artzfrage* (note 2), pp. 168–75.

Total Number of Visits by a Doctor	Payment for Each Visit in DM
100	7.40
200	7.20
300	7.00
.	.
.	.
.	.
700	6.20
800	6.00
900	5.60
1000	5.20
.	.
.	.
.	.
1500	3.20
1600	2.80
1700	2.40
etc.	etc.

In addition to fees, some KLV's have paid basic practice allowances to the doctors practicing under national health insurance. Munich and some other associations paid the allowances under a sliding scale to discourage large volumes of visits: in Munich, at the time of the fee schedule quoted above, the maximum allowance was 525 DM for doctors with fewer than 100 visits, the allowance decreased by 75 DM as the workload expanded by each successive 100 procedures, and no lump sum was paid if the doctor made more than 700 visits.

Revaluation of Procedures

One device for discouraging the excessive performance of procedures is to reduce their value, provided the rates do not become so low that doctors are no longer motivated to provide the services when necessary. Such decisions can be made by conferees during their regular reviews of the fee schedule. For example, once office visits involving electrocardiograms were in Group 3C under Swedish national health insurance and earned the second highest possible fee. Some observers suspected electrocardiograms were being done to excess, particularly by doctors not fully conversant with interpreting them, and they pointed to an increased number of EKG's in the statistical data of the National Insurance Office. So, the 1959 fee schedule switched EKG's and some other possible overperformed diagnostic procedures into the separate schedule for laboratory tests. Instead of being paid among the office visits in Group 3B (now worth 28 kronor in Stockholm and 23 kronor elsewhere) an EKG is included in laboratory Groups E and F (now worth 15 or 20 kronor). As a result, it is now less profitable for a general practitioner or internist in office practice to buy and operate an electrocardiograph, and such tests are probably done more often by internists and cardiologists in hospital outpatient departments or in large medical groups.

In the 1950's, some leaders of the French medical profession and sick funds suspected that many procedures were done unnecessarily in radiology and electrotherapy, and that high productivity enabled radiologists to become unduly rich. Therefore, when health insurance was reformed during the late 1950's and early 1960's—as I said in chapter III—the radiological procedure (*R*) was reduced. The maximum fee for any radiological procedure was set at less than half the maximum fee for surgical and other specialized procedures.[18]

Statistical Norms and Administrative Controls

Variable payment rates are never used alone to prevent the venal overperformance of procedures. Every fee-for-service and case payment system of which I know keeps statistical records on the average number of procedures of each type performed by all doctors in the program. These are calculated from the bills filed by doctors to collect fees; in most systems, the specific act is identified on each bill by name or code number. The accounting procedure also yields a summary of the number of procedures performed by each individual doctor during the periods for which the profession's averages are calculated. An individual doctor is suspected of overperformance if his figures exceed those of the profession's averages in a manner that cannot be explained by the clinical needs of his patients and community.

In the past, these calculations required a considerable staff and were the reason why fee-for-service had much higher overhead costs than salary and capitation. Unless the numerous bills could be collected and averaged for both the profession and the individual doctor, abuse could not be prevented. In recent years, the bills have been standardized in form and computers have been introduced, making calculations faster, more thorough, and more accurate. In several countries, computers will soon enable the accounting office to send each doctor regular reports comparing his performance and the averages for comparable doctors, and this might induce many doctors to avoid deviations.

Many countries maintain efficient statistical accounting offices for detecting abuse, but not all take effective action.[19] In some countries, such as

[18] G. Suzur, "Les rapports de la securité sociale avec le corps médical et la réforme issue du décret du 12 mai 1960" (Paris: unpublished paper by the Direction Générale de la Sécurité Sociale, Ministère du Travail, 1963), p. 14.

[19] One that does not is the United States. Several private American insurance schemes —such as Blue Shield—at present keep such statistical records and can refuse to pay unjustified bills to persistently deviating doctors and hospitals. But so far the potential controls have been applied sparingly. The statistical calculations are described in *Methods of Utilization Control* (Chicago: National Association of Blue Shield Plans, 1963). As in most countries, it is believed that only a minority of doctors abuse the system. The preventive methods and penalties used by American private sick funds are summarized by J. F. Follman, Jr., *Medical Care and Health Insurance* (Homewood, Ill.: Richard D. Irwin, 1963), pp. 393–410.

Switzerland, the control doctors employed by the sick funds complain to the medical association and ask that the association press the doctor to mend his ways. If the association decides the sick fund's evidence is correct and its complaint valid, it will urge the doctor to reduce the work that appears clinically unnecessary. If he refuses, the medical association and sick fund can bring charges before a joint conciliation commission, which can then order a reduction in the insurance payments due him. In some cantons the sick funds complain directly to the commission, without the initial consultation with the medical association, although usually the funds involve the association first. These arrangements work differently in different cantons, depending on the degrees of co-operation and hostility between funds and medical associations.[20]

In several countries the control doctors employed by the sick funds have the authority to interview deviating doctors and urge them to come into line with the national statistical norms and with some reasonable standard for their practices. Sick funds send their control doctors to practitioners regularly only in the few countries where the medical association is enthusiastic about national health insurance, such as Holland. Without being bound by any requirement to file a complaint and hold hearings, the Dutch sick funds may send doctors less than the full sums requested in their bills, if the numbers of procedures and case renewal cards exceed the statistical norms without apparent justification. This happens rarely in the small towns, where work loads are less; but partial payments are commonly made to specialists in Amsterdam and other big cities.

Before the reorganization in the early 1930's, German national health insurance had the most publicized problems in controlling the unjustified overperformance of procedures. Some funds tried the Swiss method of asking the medical associations to bring the doctors into line, but they were rebuffed. Other funds tried the Dutch method of paying only those bills that seemed justified, but they were attacked by medical associations and rocked by strikes. A principal reason for the funds' acceptance of the Insurance Doctors' Associations was to be rid of the task of controlling the *Kassenlöwen*. Now the funds turn over lump sums to the KLV's, and each KLV distributes the money. Therefore, the rest of the medical profession is now pitted against the *Kassenlöwen*, whose excessive bills reduce the income of their colleagues, while the funds stand aside. Each KLV collects the patients' *Krankenscheine*, on which the doctors have listed treatments; the KLV keeps all statistical records by which every individual doctor is compared with the profession's norms; the KLV's staff detects and investigates apparent overperformance; and an Examining Committee of the KLV can order that less than all the

[20] Hogarth, *Payment of General Practitioner* (note 5), pp. 308–11.

offending doctor's bills shall be paid. This sanction was common when the KLV's could secure only limited sums from the sick funds.[21]

Besides failing to pay suspicious bills, the KLV's also had to refuse to pay a small proportion of the entire profession's bills because money was lacking. The failures to pay were approximately proportionate to the size of each doctor's practice.[22] In 1965, as part of the general agreement to modernize national health insurance and improve relations between the sick funds and the profession, the funds gave the KLV's more money. Thereafter, nearly all doctors' bills were to be paid at the full rates fixed by the KLV's after dividing the lump sums. The KLV's retained the power to reject bills when necessary. But the assumption that the sick funds could always supply enough money to pay all fees at par was unrealistic. Within a year, the sick funds claimed they lacked the money, and the KLV's again had to pay some fees at less than the full rate.[23]

Structural Conditions That Inhibit Unnecessary Work

Fee-for-service always includes formal procedures to discourage unjustified work for profit. But whether they are effective depends on other conditions. One crucial set of factors is professional values and professional organization. Most important of all, of course, are the simple beliefs that it is wrong to do any more or any less than the patient needs, that it is wrong for a doctor's professional decisions to be governed primarily by money, and that it is wrong to cheat the sick funds. In Holland and Sweden—and doubtless in other countries—the widespread assimilation of these values and the tacit disapproval of deviants are at least as effective in restricting abuse as payment formulae and administrative controls. A tradition of therapeutic conservatism is also an important preventative. For example, Dutch doctors avoid unnecessary surgery and treatments in large part out of the caution that governs their choice of necessary treatments.

The effectiveness of the sick funds' administrative controls over doctors' bills depends on the medical association's attitude. In Holland, the Royal Dutch Medical Association supports the sick funds' financial controls and actually suggested some of them. Many funds were created by the medical profession, and the medical societies are represented on the board of the *Ziekenfondsraad*. In no other country does the control doctor have so much clinical authority that it is he rather than the specialist who issues the formal hospitalization orders. Elsewhere a weaker control system often arouses the opposition of the association.

Doctors would rather earn their livelihood honestly than dishonestly, and therefore unnecessary work for money is rare when fees are high and all

[21] Ibid., pp. 241–48.

[22] The magnitude of unpaid bills from insurance and private practice is reported in "Die Kostenstruktur in der Wirtschaft: Freie Berufe 1963," *Unternehmen und Arbeitsstätten* (Wiesbaden: Statistisches Bundesamt, 1966), Fachserie C, 1/IV, p. 25.

[23] The controversy is summarized in "Panorama professionnel allemand," *Concours médical*, vol. 89, no. 12 (25 March 1967), pp. 2364–67.

doctors are busy. An example is Sweden. National health insurance is generously financed and fees are high: payroll taxes on employers and employees are high, and the national Treasury subsidizes the sick funds from general revenue. But Sweden also has the most severe shortage of doctors of any developed country: the doctor-population ratio in 1964 was 1:933.[24] The waiting list of patients makes unnecessary fees from repetitious or superfluous work on any one person, and it seems to create a pressure to move on to the next patient.

> In some cities, patients often search for an early appointment by phoning all the doctors in the telephone book in the specialty they need. As soon as his name appears in the new edition of the telephone book, any spaces in a new doctor's appointment calendar quickly fill up. Because patients with other than emergency conditions cannot obtain early appointments with office practitioners, many queue up at the outpatient departments of hospitals, where they are certain to be examined by the end of the day.

Because doctors are so busy and because the cash benefits systems may reduce demand by patients, the rate of doctor-patient contacts in office and home—sometimes inflated in service-benefits fee-for-service systems—is less than three per person per year in Sweden. It is perhaps the lowest of any developed country, is much lower than the rate in other major European countries with national health insurance, and seems paradoxical in one of the world's most health-conscious countries.[25]

Encouraging Good Medicine and Discouraging Neglect

Fee-for-service encourages the necessary performance of all procedures that are listed in fee schedules at attractive rates.[26] Its most common affliction is not underperformance but overperformance. However, every payment system—including fee-for-service—might unintentionally discourage certain procedures and care of certain patients, because they are less profitable or take a disproportionate amount of the doctor's time.

[24] The doctor-population ratio improved during the 1950's and 1960's, but an important reason was the licensing of many foreign doctors. One-fifth of newly licensed doctors are immigrants. "The Swedish Medical Association's Annual Report to the W.M.A. for 1965" (Stockholm: Läkarförbundet, 1966, mimeographed), pp. 1–3. Comparisons with other countries can be made in *World Health Statistics Annual 1962* (Geneva: World Health Organization, 1966), 3: 18–43.

[25] "Volume and Cost of Sickness Benefits in Kind and Cash" (note 6), p. 57; and Simon Btesh, "The Place of the Family Doctor," *Medical World*, vol. 98, no. 1 (January 1963), p. 11.

[26] For example, an Australian visitor to general practices in Germany and Britain thought that fee-for-service induced the German doctors to perform more thorough diagnoses than did British doctors, who were paid by capitation and lacked monetary incentives for extra effort. Hanns Pacy, "The Common Factors Affecting the Standard of General Practice," *Medical Journal of Australia*, vol. 52, pt. 2, no. 13 (25 September 1965), p. 547.

Preventive Medicine

Nearly every fee schedule in a national medical care system is a list of therapeutic procedures performed with equipment. Therefore the payment systems tend to reinforce rather than counteract the clinical and technical orientation that doctors acquire in nearly all countries from their medical education and professional journals. If the doctor feels under pressure to see many patients and perform many separate procedures that are itemized in the fee schedule, he will not spare the time to interview the patient at length about his life history, home life, anxieties, and needs. Nor will the doctor advise the patient at length about his daily schedule, work adjustments, home life, diet, etc.

Many reformers in medical care throughout the world believe that increased attention to preventive medicine is essential both for the welfare of the public and the financial solvency of the national medical care schemes. These reformers have had the chronic difficulty of devising some way to motivate practicing doctors to engage in health teaching and other preventive procedures with the citizens who come to their offices, instead of merely treating illnesses.

Physicians and medical associations often have been unenthusiastic about introducing preventive medicine into fee schedules, because of preoccupations with clinical therapy. At times they have combated programs of preventive medicine by governments and sick funds. For example, once many German sick funds sponsored for their members programs of health education, diagnostic checkups, and other types of preventive medicine.[27] But, as a condition for co-operation with the KLV's, the funds now must agree to set up no more new polyclinics or other medical establishments. Existing polyclinics, many formerly centers of preventive as well as therapeutic medicine, have declined in staff and importance. Once individual funds could pursue medical policies through small groups of doctors who believed in the preventive viewpoint or who reluctantly did preventive work in order to earn a living, but now the funds are expected to be no more than financial agencies, dealing with the medical professional on a *Landwide* basis. Once strongly influenced by the funds and by their preventive-minded allies in the trade unions, Social Democratic party, and the "social hygiene" movement, medical care since creation of the KVD and the KBV is increasingly controlled by a profession whose training, traditional viewpoint, and compensation procedures emphasize scientific medicine.[28]

[27] Goldmann and Grotjahn, *Benefits of German Sickness Insurance* (note 11), chaps. 3–4 passim.

[28] In addition, some German doctors welcomed the restriction and probable future elimination of the fund-sponsored medical installation as a destruction of a collectivist threat under the guise of preventive medicine. E.g., Carl Korth, "The Misuse of Preventive Medicine, A Basis for Socialized Medicine," in, Helmut Schoeck (editor), *Financing Medical Care* (Caldwell, Ida.: Caxton Printers, 1962), pp. 203–13.

The government and some leaders of the medical profession were concerned that the victory of the profession might lead to an exclusive preoccupation with therapy. Therefore the abortive bill to reorganize national health insurance in the early 1960's authorized the payment of doctors for periodic checkups and for courses of preventive treatment carried out in their offices. This was one of the few reforms enacted after the complete package failed in the *Bundestag*. Doctors were authorized to collect fees for examinations and tests on normal pregnant women throughout pregnancy and after delivery. Every pregnant woman could obtain this care by right. Formerly, she could have been examined and treated under national health insurance only if the pregnancy was abnormal. In order to prevent the unjustified multiplication of visits and tests for profit, the procedures were specified and the development of the experiment was supervised by a committee representing the sick funds, the KBV, and the public. At first, the maximum number of visits was limited to ten, and the doctor could earn no more than 28.50 DM every three months for each pregnant woman in his practice. Costs did not rise as much as had been expected, since more doctors than originally thought had already been conducting preventive examinations under the guise of clinical therapy. Now, instead of listing false complaints on the *Krankenschein* to describe the visit, the doctor could mention that he had conducted a preventive examination. Since the experiment suggested that preventive medicine could be encouraged under fee-for-service without venality, discussions began about adding other preventive work to West German health insurance, such as tests for cancer of the uterus.

Reformers elsewhere have pressed for inclusion of checkups of healthy persons and inclusion of preventive inoculations in fee schedules. The right to obtain nine checkups during one's lifetime was included in the decrees reforming French national health insurance in 1945 and 1966. The examintions can be performed by general practitioners and radiologists using their customary office equipment and are reported on bills as some combination of the ordinary key letters *C* and *R*.[29] Because of the key letter method of identification, no-one knows how many preventive examinations are performed in France and whether they greatly increase the costs of national health insurance.[30]

Apprehension about money and staff has delayed this expansion of insurance coverage in other countries. Inclusion of examinations and inocu-

[29] Georges Cazac, "Les examens de santé des assurés sociaux," *Concours médical*, vol. 88, no. 52 (24 December 1966), pp. 8137–38.

[30] Probably not many examinations are secured through the customary cash benefits payment system for office practitioners, since patients can substitute examinations that are completely free. Three-quarters of insured persons have been examined at some time by the doctors at their place of work. Jean-Daniel Reynaud and Antoinette Catrice-Lorey, *Les assurés et la sécurité sociale* (Paris: Institut des Sciences Sociales du Travail, 1959), appendix, Q. 53. One-sixth were examined at the offices of the sick funds. Ibid., p. 134. But probably far fewer checkups are performed than the number authorized by the law.

lations has long been favored by the Royal Medical Board of Sweden. But usually the sick funds and the government postpone a decision on grounds of costs. Not only would doctors' bills increase, but the numbers of laboratories and technicians would have to grow suddenly. For example, if every insured woman in a country could demand as a right, regular examinations for cancer of the uterus, the sick funds or government would be bound to maintain and staff new laboratories.

Home Visits

Because they enable doctors to observe the patients' physical and social environments, home visits are an indispensable part of both preventive medicine and comprehensive therapy. But home visits have become much less common than office visits in almost every national medical care system in the world, and particularly those using fee-for-service.[31] Only rarely do fee schedules rate the time-consuming home visits as much as twice the value of office visits; but during that time a doctor can perform many profitable technical procedures in his office.

The principal national health insurance fund of Italy—INAM, or the *Istituto Nazionale per l'Assicurazione contro le Malattie*—was one of the last national medical care schemes in which the number of home visits nearly equaled the number of office visits. The reason was tradition reinforced by the payment system. Italy's general practitioners were long expected to do no more than the simplest tasks and to refer everything else to the specialist.[32] The G.P.'s had neither the education to use advanced equipment nor the incomes to buy it. Therefore the fee schedule for general practice under INAM for decades referred almost entirely to office and home visits. The modest facilities in the doctor's private office made the patient's home almost as satisfactory a site for treatment, and the higher fee for home visits (once double that for office visits) created a financial inducement. But even in INAM, office visits increasingly outnumbered home visits, as the G.P.'s discovered they could complete more work in their offices.[33] The fee schedule

[31] *Volume and Cost of Sickness Benefits in Kind and Cash: National Analyses* (Geneva: International Social Security Association, 1963), Table II in each national report. It is generally believed that home visits have decreased greatly, but accurate statistics are not available from the past. Since World War II the absolute number of home visits per insured person has remained constant in nearly all countries; rates of office consultation have remained the same in some countries and risen in others. Where office visits have increased, of course, the home visits have declined relatively. The data appear in ibid.

[32] For example, until 1960, INAM expected its general practitioners to refer all injections to its polyclinics. *Bilancio consuntivo dell'esercizio 1960* (Rome: Istituto Nazionale per l'Assicurazione contro le Malattie, 1961), pp. 139–40.

[33] As a proportion of all contacts between G.P.'s and patients, home visits were 47 per cent in 1948, 42 per cent in 1956, 35 per cent in 1960, and 28 per cent in 1965. *Annuario Statistico 1964–1965* (Rome: Istituto Nazionale per l'Assicurazione contro le Malattie, 1967), based on chart facing p. 264. The references in the text to fees for home and office visits apply to the fee-for-service system used primarily in Italian cities. In the late 1960's,

changed to make office work more attractive. In the successive increases in the rates, office visits rose faster than home visits, so that by 1965 they were nearly the same. In the big cities the office visit was *L* 940 and the home visit was *L* 980. But as yet INAM did not broaden fee-for-service by allowing the G.P. to collect payments for minor surgical and medical procedures, of the sort that would make the purchase of equipment possible and profitable. Such a change would reduce referrals and greatly increase the proportion of patient contacts in the general practitioner's office.

Home visits can be increased by paying attractive fees to doctors who otherwise would have gotten none. For example, the British hospital consultant receives fees for home visits in addition to the salary for his inpatient work. Exact trend statistics are lacking, but my British informants were certain that home visits by consultants were far more numerous than before the National Health Service.[34] Before World War II, the consultant might not have gotten a separate fee for the home visit alone, but might have received a global fee only if the patient were hospitalized. Now the consultant is paid for the visit and has no financial incentive to recommend hospitalization; because of the long waiting list for beds, most consultants probably are interested in avoiding hospitalization, particularly for the chronically ill. Most home visits are requested by general practitioners to get the consultant's opinion as to whether the patient should be hospitalized. Some consultants use these occasions to suggest methods of home care for the elderly and chronically ill, and thus fees for home visits could provide the incentive for organized home care programs that would be quite novel in Europe.

Besides the loss of time, an important reason for the decline of home visits is the irritation of driving and parking in urban traffic.[35] In order to make home visits more tolerable, French health insurance in 1966 added a "special supplement for inconvenience" of two francs per home visit in Paris and one franc per home visit in designated metropolitan areas with more than 300,000 inhabitants.

The "Supportive" Specialties

Fee schedules in most national medical care schemes give the medical specialties a technical bias, when much work in these fields consists of exami-

---

the fees were changed in a direction more typical of payment schedules in the rest of the world—i.e., home visits became twice the rate of office visits—but the proportion of all office visits continued to rise. Outside of Italian cities, most general practitioners are paid by capitation, supplemented—after the reforms of the mid-1960's—by individual fees for home visits.

[34] The great increase in home visits by consultants during the first years of the National Health Service is reported in Brian Abel-Smith and Richard M. Titmuss, *The Cost of the National Health Service* (Cambridge: University Press, 1956), p. 126.

[35] Francis Peillet, "Les médecins des grandes villes autres que Paris, Lyon, et Marseille seront-ils les sacrifiés?" *Concours médical*, vol. 87, no. 24 (12 June 1965), p. 4179.

nation and advice. For example, in many countries the fee schedules' lists of procedures for pediatrics and psychiatry are confined to the use of equipment for drastic illnesses, while in practice both fields now are quite different. In developed countries the pediatrician has become a skilled teacher for mothers and healthy children as well as physician to the sick child. The average office practitioner is treating the sick child less frequently. The fee schedule usually pays the pediatrician no more than the standard rate for office or home visits, and since the fee is low and gives no rewards for extra time, he may be under financial pressure to deal with each patient quickly. Similarly, much modern psychiatric practice consists of conversation rather than mechanical procedures. But the insurance fee for a psychiatric consultation often is not much higher than an ordinary office visit for any specialist and, unlike the internist and pediatrician, the psychiatrist cannot accumulate income by seeing many patients each hour. Consequently, in most countries using fee-for-service under national health insurance, psychiatry has been performed only in private practice or in salaried jobs.

Because of protests by psychiatrists and because of the spreading appreciation of its importance, psychiatrists during the 1960's began to receive more generous fees in official schedules. For example, the older German fee schedule *Preugo* had rated a psychiatric investigation as only 6.40 DM, while an ordinary office visit to any doctor was 4.00 DM. When *Gebührenordnung* was adopted in 1965, it rated a psychiatric interview at 30.00 DM, provided it lasted at least fifty minutes. Thus psychiatrists were able to earn an income under national health insurance, but their fees remained considerably below those of the surgical specialties for procedures requiring comparable time.[36]

The payment system of Dutch national health insurance illustrates how psychiatrists' rates have been increased over the levels of ordinary office visits in some countries recently, but still are not high enough for psychiatrists to prosper without considerable private practice. In the fee schedule (Tariff III) a psychiatrist can earn f. 23.25 in 1966 for each of ten psychotherapeutic sessions of forty-five minutes each or f. 15.50 for each of fifteen sessions of thirty minutes each. In the case payment rates (Tariff I) the all-out rates for the initial transfer card were f. 18.05 for psychiatry, f. 16.75 for pediatrics and internal medicine, and considerably less for the surgical and medical specialties that rely primarily on rapid technical procedures. But psychiatrists were still not pleased, since they see far fewer patients than the recipients of slightly lower case payments. Other countries' fee schedules under national medical care systems treat psychiatry even worse.

[36] On the complexities of redesigning German health insurance to include psychotherapeutic care when needed, but without abuse, see Rolf Liebold, "Die 'Grosse Psychotherapie' in der Kassenärztlichen Versorgung," *Der Ortskrankenkasse*, vol. 49, no. 21 (1 November 1967), pp. 577–83; and Annemarie Dührssen, "Zum Problem der 'Grossen Psychotherapie' in der Kassenärztlichen Versorgung," ibid., vol. 49, no. 23 (1 December 1967), pp. 633–37.

It is difficult to alter fee schedules and pay the supportive specialties for their time. Payment systems do not change quickly, and most fee schedules were designed to pay doctors for surgical interventions and for therapies involving equipment, chemical treatments, or other manual activities. Fee-for-service is so subject to abuses from the reporting of unnecessary or non-existent work that administrators are reluctant to include procedures which cannot be unambiguously defined and timed. In practice, the supportive specialties are under-represented on the committees of doctors that write fee schedules in national medical care systems and that influence payment policies, and these groups seem oriented toward the more technical specialties. Within the medical professions of many countries, psychiatry and psychosomatic medicine have little repute, and the doctors participating in payment decisions will not fight hard for the economic interests of the supportive specialties, particularly if higher fees for the latter reduce the money available to the more influential specialties.

I had the following conversation with a doctor occupying a central role in drafting the fee schedule of his country:

> Surgery is the best paid specialty. Psychiatry and neuropsychiatry are poorly paid ones. (Do you think that any are paid too much, any too little?) That is hard to say. Actually psychiatry is dangerous in [this country]. We don't have psychoanalysis here. (If psychiatry were paid too well, do you think there would be too many psychiatric consultations?) Yes. And I want to prevent that! I don't want too much of that sort of thing in this country!

Thorough Care

Ideally, the doctor seeing any patient should learn about all factors bearing on the condition presented, and he should learn about any needs that the patient did not mention initially. But comprehensive patient care and psychosomatic support consume time, and fee-for-service pays doctors by the procedure. When fees are low—as I said earlier—physicians are motivated to see many patients and therefore to spend a minimum of time on each.

Neglect is widely believed to be a particular danger in service benefits schemes, since the doctor is paid by the sick funds and not by the patient. The need to motivate more attention to patients is a common argument for the replacement of full service benefits schemes by reimbursement systems or by partial cost-sharing by the patient. If the patient pays the doctor directly, it is contended, he will expect better service and the doctor will be more attentive. However, complaints about hasty care under fee-for-service in national health insurance are heard even in France, which has a full cash benefits system.[37]

[37] Jean-Jacques Dupeyroux, "Sécurité sociale et médecine expéditive," *Recueil dalloz* (24 February 1960), pp. 39–44; Marc Nèdelec, "Une impasse: la rémunération à l'acte,"

While some reformers favor more comprehensive patient care and psychosomatic medicine, the public is satisfied with the care it gets from office practitioners under national health insurance. A recurrent surprise in countries using fee schedules has been the results of public opinion polls: medical reformers and the press frequently say that patients are examined and treated too superficially, but overwhelming proportions of the public say their doctors give them as much time as necessary. For example, 78 per cent of the French people in 1959 thought the medical visits were the right length, 14 per cent thought them too short, and 3 per cent said they were too long.[38] But even if patients get what they want, some reformers in medicine may think they are not getting enough of what they need.

As we shall see throughout this book, surveys in every medical system usually elicit high levels of satisfaction. Unfortunately, these surveys rarely confront respondents with choices, particularly whether they think they are getting true value for their taxes and whether they would prefer other arrangements.

One method of encouraging thorough medical care under national health insurance is to pay for it. An affliction in Swiss insurance for many years was rapid work because of the low fees. During the reforms of the mid-1960's, the contract between the cantonal medical association of Bern and the sick funds experimented with extra payment for time-consuming work. In 1965, the basic payment for the first office visit with a low income patient was 8.00 fr. If he conducted a time-consuming investigation, a specialist could collect an additional 6.50 fr. If the office visit lasted more than half an hour, the doctor could collect 20.00 fr. from the fund for each additional half hour during the day and 40.00 fr. for each extra half hour at night.

Continuity of Care

A payment system should encourage rather than discourage sustained contact between patient and doctor, so that the physician gains a thorough understanding of the patient's needs and can alter treatments in the light of new findings. In practice, the medical profession tries to keep fee-for-service in a national medical care scheme as close as possible to conditions in private practice. Usually in the free market the patient can change doctors whenever

---

Esprit, vol. 25, no. 2 (February 1957), pp. 360–67; and "Note d'actualité: le projet Gazier," *Présences*, no. 59 (Second Trimester 1957), p. 30.

[38] "Les français et leur médecin," *Sondages*, vol. 22, nos. 1 and 2 (1960), pp. 49–50, 79. The French prefer efficacious medication to comprehensive health guidance, according to the data in ibid., p. 52. The high public satisfaction with the work of office practitioners is not due to France's cash benefits scheme. It is confirmed by unpublished public opinion polls in Germany and other countries where national health insurance uses fee-for-service and service benefits.

he likes, even when his treatments with one doctor have not been completed. Continuity is left to agreement between doctor and patient. Since national medical care schemes using fee-for-service are simply ways of paying the doctor, they add little to the existing incentives for continuity of care.

One of the few provisions in fee-for-service that encourages continuity is payment for a global procedure. It is common in many fee schedules: an expensive procedure obligates the doctor to give preparatory and follow-up care. For example, in France payment for an expensive procedure (*K* 10 or more) includes post-operative care for twenty-one days.

Some administrative requirements of national medical care systems make it difficult to change doctors and retain coverage, and thus they result in the continuity not specifically encouraged by the payment system. For example, in Holland a specialist is paid under national health insurance only if he is referred by a general practitioner, and the patient cannot select a new specialist under insurance without referral by the first for a good reason. In the German and Swiss service benefits scheme, the patient gives his *Krankenschein* to the doctor whom he visits at the beginning of his illness; since the issuance of a new *Krankenschein* by the fund requires effort by the patient and an explanation, probably he remains with the same doctor, at least until eligible for a new *Krankenschein*—three months later in Germany, between one and three months later in the Swiss cantons.

Some fee-for-service systems unintentionally encourage continuity of care by allowing a doctor to be paid for both simple and complex procedures. For example, in Germany any doctor may collect any fee. But, as I shall explain, the drawback is that doctors may be motivated to perform procedures beyond their training and ability. The only control over the assumption of excessive responsibility is the structure of the public and religious hospitals: usually these have closed staffs recruited from the specialties, and an office practitioner may have difficulty performing a specialized procedure requiring hospitalization unless he has a staff appointment.

If fees for both simple and complex procedures may not be collected by the same doctor, technical expertness may be satisfied at the expense of continuity of care. For example, the Dutch fee schedule lists only specialty procedures, the general practitioner cannot bill the sick funds for these and must refer the patient to the specialist. The fee schedule of INAM in Italy produces the same result by the opposite logic: only the simplest procedures are paid by fee-for-service, neither the G.P. nor anyone else can bill INAM for more complex procedures, and the G.P. must refer patients to the salaried specialists in the polyclinics and hospitals. Continuity of care is difficult to achieve by such referrals in most of the world because of the gulf between general practitioner and specialist: in most countries they constitute two distinct classes within the medical profession, rarely do they communicate about a patient by more than charts and brief letters, and rarely does the specialist invite the general practitioner to see their common patient in the hospital. When a G.P. has referred a patient to a specialist, usually he cannot collect any fees for visits to the patient or for consultations with the specialist, until the specialist has referred the patient back.

Holland's case payment system for ambulatory care by a specialist probably achieves greater continuity of care than does fee-for-service. The specialist is responsible for all necessary care in that field for a month at a time, and transfer to a new specialist is difficult administratively. But the continuity holds only for specialty treatment: the division between general practitioner and specialist is at least as wide in Holland as elsewhere.

Preferential Treatment for Private Patients

The introduction of national medical care schemes in the world was supposed to eliminate differential treatment of patients because some could pay the doctor more money than others. Thereafter the physician's efforts were supposed to vary with the patient's needs and not with his purse. But private practice survives in every country with national health insurance: some patients are not covered by social security; others are covered but think that direct payments will obtain earlier appointments, longer attention, and better care. Private fees are an important part of the incomes of many doctors: for example, in West Germany in 1963, private practice provided at least one-fifth of the incomes of general practitioners and at least one-third of the incomes of specialists in office practice, while the remaining money came from direct insurance payments.[39]

The medical profession usually insists on retaining rights of private practice lest it become completely dependent on the official medical care scheme and lest its income be reduced. Under fee-for-service schemes, usually any patient covered by national health insurance may see any doctor either under insurance or privately. The doctor may bill either the sick fund or the patient, but not both. In some countries, such as Holland and Sweden, the government tries to motivate the doctors to see as many patients as possible under insurance rather than privately by offering the hospital outpatient department, nursing service, and laboratories at a very low rental for this part of their practice. In Germany, the powerful chiefs of service—even in many nonteaching hospitals—have secured use of hospital facilities completely without charge or at low rental for inpatient and outpatient care of both their insured and private patients.

When a national medical care system uses fee-for-service—and particularly when it uses cash benefits rather than service benefits—it differs from

[39] "Die Kostenstruktur in der Wirtschaft: Freie Berufe 1963" (note 22), p. 21. Official reports underestimate the value of private practice to an unknown extent, since many doctors conceal private fees from the tax collector.

private practice within that country, not so much in procedure but in the size of the fees. Except for a few poor people not covered by insurance and not receiving public charitable care, most private patients pay more than the official fee schedule. The absence of research comparing insured and private practice by the same doctors makes it difficult to estimate whether the private patients get more and better care as a result of money rather than their clinical needs. Probably the discrepancy is less in countries using fee-for-service than in the national medical care systems using salary and capitation. In the countries based on fee-for-service, all my informants believed that private patients received preferential treatment by obtaining earlier appointments, longer visits, and more thorough examinations.[40] But, they thought, insured patients received just as good clinical therapy as private patients, because of the standards of the medical profession. Treatment probably is most comparable in the countries where the official fee schedule is closest to private fees, such as Holland and Sweden.

Before the spread of official medical care schemes throughout entire countries, the medical profession's fees usually followed sliding scales according to each doctor's judgment of the patient's ability to pay. Usually national medical care schemes standardize payments for all patients, regardless of affluence. But, largely because of the medical profession's pressure to continue to earn more money from the wealthier patients, a few countries have retained the sliding scale in their official schemes. In Germany, doctors receive different fees for the same work done on patients from different funds, because the funds represent different occupations and classes with unequal incomes.[41]

In particular, the *Ersatzkassen* pay higher fees because they have more money. Since their members are white-collar workers, administrators, and employed professionals, the *Ersatzkassen* collect higher premiums. Since the employers often continue to pay the salaries of these employees during sick leaves, the *Ersatzkassen* have to pay fewer disability benefits and can use all their money for medical treatment.

It is widely believed that some doctors give better care and more time to patients from the better-paying funds, but actual evidence is lacking. Usually the office physician does not have patients from several statutory funds—i.e., he usually has patients from an *Ortskrankenkasse* or from a *Betriebskrankenkasse*, but usually not from both—but he may have patients from both a statutory fund and from at least one *Ersatzkasse*. A belief that doctors will give them better care for higher fees induces persons to join *Ersatzkassen* instead of the statutory funds. A belief that this actually occurs explains why

[40] Confirmed by Roul Tunley's interviews in Germany. See his *The American Health Scandal* (New York: Dell Publishing Co., 1966), p. 187.

[41] Differences in payments are documented in *Statistisches Jahrbuch der Kassenärztlichen Bundesvereinigung* (Cologne: Kassenärztliche Bundesvereinigung, 1965), p. 45.

leaders of the statutory funds have long campaigned for abolition of the *Ersatzkassen*, or at least a reduction of their fees, so that the subscribers to the statutory funds will be treated equally.

Because Switzerland lacks strong legislation requiring mass coverage and standardizing the procedures of the sick funds, the doctors have been able to retain many customs from private practice. Since the basic fees for the population are low, doctors have pressed for the right to earn more money from the wealthier insured patients. Therefore, Switzerland is the only country incorporating the sliding scale into its official payment system. By 1961, half the population was covered by cantonal contracts between sick funds and medical societies allowing fees differentiated according to patients' incomes, and the amendments to the national health insurance law made this universal after 1964. In each canton, the wealthiest insured persons—constituting up to 10 per cent of all the insured—can be charged any fees that they and their doctors agree upon. In addition, many cantonal contracts between the sick funds and the medical associations distinguish between fees of the middle-income and lower-income persons. For example, in Bern, the official fees for middle-income patients have been 45 per cent higher than the fees for the less affluent. Most sick funds pay—either by cash benefits or service benefits—more money for the care of the middle-income patients than for the lower-income patients, on the theory that the subscription rates have brought the funds more money from the middle-income patients. The funds do not reimburse the wealthy patient more than the official maximum for that canton: therefore he must pay directly most of the high fees that the doctor may charge him. Similarly, if a cantonal contract allows the doctor to charge any fee of a middle-income patient, the fund may not be obligated to reimburse the insured person more than the official maximum. My informants believed that Swiss doctors are more *attentive* to the more profitable patients but try to give the same *quality* of treatment to all. However, no studies have been done comparing the care associated with different fees.

Regulating Particular Procedures

Leaders in clinical medicine believe that certain procedures are safe and efficacious while others are not. In most countries the payment system does not affect these clinical decisions. The profession insists that the administrative structure of the Ministry of Health and sick funds avoid influencing the doctors' clinical judgments. Rather, the profession wishes to restrict such controls either to professional institutions alone—such as the staffs of hospitals or the disciplinary machinery of the medical association—or to individual doctor-patient agreements.

But a fee schedule can be designed to influence clinical decisions, since it rewards certain procedures more than others. Therefore the medical representatives from the sick funds and the professional associations occasionally decide to price procedures so that dangerous or useless procedures have no monetary value, or much less than the approved techniques. For example, a few procedures are omitted from the French *Nomenclature* or are given low coefficients because the Committee on *Nomenclature* believes them medically undesirable. Most of chiropractic is omitted. Reduction of hernia by hand pressure was dropped from the list in 1960, because the Committee believed it dangerous and preferred surgical intervention. Acupuncture steadily declined and now has the lowest coefficient (*K* 2 per consultation), to the distress of the physicians who specialize in it. Homeopathy is reimbursed by social security—dropping it completely would stir up too much public contention, including some devotees in high places—but a homeopathic treatment is rated no higher than an ordinary office visit. French medicine has had an old tradition of clinical freedom, and disapproved or esoteric treatments may continue to be given freely in private practice for higher fees than those earned from social security practice.

Assignment of Tasks

Ideally a payment system should not encourage a doctor to assume more work than his time and qualifications warrant. If he has substantially more work than other equally qualified doctors, he should refer the patients, so that each patient will receive maximum professional attention. If the doctor lacks the training and experience to understand certain conditions or perform certain procedures, the payment system should not motivate him to diagnose and treat the patient, but he should be willing to refer the patient to the best qualified physician.

The Blurring of Specialties

In practice, most fee-for-service systems lack any mechanisms for encouraging referrals. Usually medical professions press national health insurance schemes to avoid any regulations or payment procedures that alter the conventional flow of work in medical practice. Therefore the sick funds usually agree that any licensed physician may treat their patients and perform any procedure under the fee schedule, regardless of whether the procedure is in a specialty for which he has postgraduate credentials. As in private practice, the decision to perform the procedure is left to the physician, the patient, and the norms of the medical profession. If a doctor earns a satisfactory income from patients with problems exclusively in his special field, he may not bother with conditions in other specialties. But if fees are low, if doctors are numerous and must seek all possible sources of livelihood, the physician is motivated to perform any procedure for which he has the equipment and which is not risky. The results are considerable technical skill among general practitioners, a reduction in the usual technical and economic gulf between general practitioners and specialists, and a greater versatility among the specialists in office practice.

For example, the payment system of German national health insurance has been affected by the scientific and technical tradition of German medicine and tends to perpetuate it. Nineteenth-century and early twentieth-century Germany initiated modern scientific medicine, using elaborate equipment and chemicals in diagnosis and therapy, a tradition subsequently continued by the United States and Sweden. The scientific viewpoint has long been the foundation of undergraduate medical education and postgraduate hospital training; expert surgeons and other technically innovative doctors have been heroes within the profession and with the public. The average German office practitioner seems better qualified and more eager for these tasks than his foreign counterpart: until the elimination of the quota on entry into insurance practice in 1960, many young doctors awaited openings by serving in hospitals, where all learned advanced techniques and where some remained the four years necessary for certification as specialists.

The German payment system does little to discourage any office doctor from performing advanced and profitable procedures. The fee schedule gives its highest payments to procedures which call for the use of equipment, or surgical intervention. Any doctor may perform any procedure and collect the full fee, regardless of possession of specialty credentials. Hospitals have small outpatient departments and offer much less competition to the office practitioner than do hospitals in many other countries. Hospital doctors may see social security patients during their private hours in the hospital, but usually only on referral from an office practitioner, a custom that reduces competition with the latter. Contracts between sick funds and KLV's bind the funds to reduce their once extensive polyclinic installations and to leave all ambulatory care to the office practitioners. In order to attract patients in a competitive market, to impress other doctors, and to bolster his confidence that he is practicing modern German medicine, the office doctor is motivated to buy modern equipment and to use it.

Parenthetically, in countries with technically oriented fee schedules, the doctor may be motivated to select from among alternative procedures the one that uses equipment or physical intervention. For example, injections are itemized in the German fee schedules while oral medication is not, and some of my informants suspect that German doctors tend to prefer injections. Physicians in neighboring Holland are believed to prefer oral administrations because of the absence of any financial incentives and the presence of a heritage of clinical caution.

As in Germany, fee-for-service in Switzerland encouraged a technical orientation and a mixture of specialized and unspecialized work. The effects were accentuated in the past by the low fees for visits. The need to see many patients each day has led many doctors to mix specialty and general practice. Usually only the leading specialists can earn high enough private fees to prosper from thorough treatment of a limited number of patients in their fields. Except in a few cantons, any doctor can perform any procedure; thus general practitioners often do specialty procedures without referring patients to specialists, and many office specialists have general practices in addition to their specialty work. Since all doctors get postgraduate hospital training now, and since Swiss medical schools and hospitals follow the technical and scientific traditions of Germany and of the United States, many office practitioners have learned advanced techniques. Since Swiss doctors try to give all necessary care for ambulatory patients in their office, hospitals are basically for inpatient care, and Swiss outpatient departments appear quieter than those in many other countries. Possessors of specialty credentials (the F. M. H. certificate [Federatio Medicorum Helveticorum]) have a competitive advantage over G.P.'s in attracting patients of all sorts, and in recent years specialty training has become very popular: at present over half the office practitioners are licensed specialists, and the proportion will greatly increase.

In Sweden, too, any licensed physician may perform any procedure under the fee schedule. This is essential in a large geographical area with few doctors. Therefore, in a survey performed by the Swedish Medical Association, only a minority of the respondents pictured themselves as full-time general practitioners. Many of the office physicians were specialists, and many others thought of themselves as part-time G.P.'s and part-time specialists.[42]

Underdevelopment of Specialties

If the payment system does not require that certain acts be referred, entire specialties can fail to grow within the medical profession. For example, one of the quirks of the German payment system is that it causes anesthesiology as a specialty to be underdeveloped while the science of anesthesia is highly developed. The insurance system allows the operating surgeon to collect fees for anesthetics administered under his direction. As a result, most surgeons hire salaried assistants or salaried nurses to give all anesthetics, they themselves bill the sick fund for each anesthetic, and they keep the profits. Consequently very few physicians can make a living as anesthesiologists and few enter the field, an anomaly in a country whose surgeons have been among the world leaders in many difficult thoracic and cerebral operations requiring advanced anesthetics and whose equipment companies have developed some of the world's most advanced methods. In early 1965, Germany's 94,503 practicing physicians included only 260 anesthesiologists—one of the

[42] "Sveriges läkare och deras verksamhet i statistisk belysning," *Svenska Läkartidningen*, vol. 53, no. 49 (1956), pp. 3256, 3262.

lowest proportions in any developed country—and 236 were primarily or exclusively salaried staff members of public or religious hospitals.[43] Since so many give complicated anesthetics during their hospital training, surgeons probably know more about this field in Germany than in any other country. Perhaps the practice of German anesthesiology has been affected in some way by its domination by surgeons instead of by partially autonomous anesthesiologists.

Throughout this book, I identify the possible effects of payment systems, but I do not claim the latter to be exclusive causes. For example, the underdevelopment of anesthesiology is due also to hospital structure and not to the insurance payment system alone. Most German hospitals have full-time staffs with few of the part-time salaried appointments that would allow an anesthesiologist to make a living at several smaller hospitals. Few hospitals have enough work for full-time anesthesiologists, and thus job opportunities are limited.

Similarly, any licensed doctor may collect fees for X-rays under German national health insurance, and therefore most take and interpret their own X-rays. As a result, fewer doctors make their careers in radiology in Germany than in other developed countries.[44]

Although Americans assume that obstetrics is a large and busy specialty, this is not true in most countries. Elsewhere, normal deliveries often are performed by nurse-midwives, while obstetricians manage the complicated cases. An increasing number of normal deliveries are now referred to obstetricians in private practice—often in private clinics—but the national medical care scheme still recognizes the role of the nurse-midwives. Based on custom, these assignments are perpetuated by the organization of the hospital and the payment system: the obstetrical services of public and religious hospitals have several salaried nurse-midwives but only small staffs of obstetricians; the fee schedule under national health insurance pays the obstetrician only for his gynecological work and for complicated deliveries. In Holland, the fee schedule reinforces this division by including the work of the midwife: only she can collect fees from the sick funds for normal deliveries. As a result, most other countries have fewer doctors in obstetrics than does the United States.[45]

While low pay may suffice to damage recruitment into a specialty, high pay is not enough to increase it. The field must also be interesting and respected. An example of the failure of pecuniary incentives is radiology in

[43] Gerhard Wolff, "Zahl der Ärzte steigt weiter stark an," *Deutsches Ärzteblatt-Ärztliche Mitteilungen*, vol. 62, no. 49 (4 December 1965), p. 2734.

[44] 1.6 per cent of German doctors specialized in radiology and radiotherapy in 1963. In other developed countries, the figure was higher—often double or more. *World Health Statistics Annual 1962* (Geneva: World Health Organization, 1966), 3: 122–29.

[45] Ibid.

France. The French fee-for-service system gives radiology by far the highest gross income. Radiologists can perform many procedures in a short time, and demand for their work mounts steadily. But young doctors prefer other fields, apparently because they prefer more contact with patients and dislike the efficient but *qua si* industrial atmosphere of laboratories. Some French radiologists foresee an imminent crisis in the field.[46]

Referral Inducements

A few national health insurance schemes with fee-for-service encourage or require referral of specialized procedures to fully qualified doctors by refusing to pay fees to anyone else. The patient still may be treated by a physician who does not meet the standards, but he must pay the doctor privately. The alternative is to allow national health service to support the performance of highly technical procedures by doctors not fully trained in the work. This is a widely criticized custom under private health insurance and private practice in the United States.[47]

One device in official schemes is an abbreviated fee schedule that includes only the basic procedures that every doctor is qualified to perform. The sick fund will pay only for those specialized procedures performed in polyclinics and hospitals. When the patient reports to one of these organizations he is referred to an appropriate department and is seen by a salaried specialist. This method is used by INAM in Italy. For the more advanced procedures in each specialty, the same method is used in Sweden—i.e., while any doctor may perform any procedure in the fee schedule, the list covers only the less complex work, and the more advanced procedures can be treated under insurance only by the salaried specialists in the public hospitals.

It is also possible to forbid anyone to collect a fee for a specialized procedure under a national medical care scheme unless he is fully qualified in the specialty. In Holland, a surgeon cannot collect a fee for an anesthetic given under his direction; such payments go only to an anesthesiologist—i.e., only to a physician specialized in the field. Thus surgeons cannot collect an extra fee, give the work to salaried nurses and salaried assistants, and pocket the profits, as they can in some other countries. The surgeon is not compelled to use an anesthesiologist for an insured person, but the anesthesia fee is paid only to an anesthesiologist. No anesthesia fees appear in the fee schedule for procedures where it is presumed that the specialist himself will give a local anesthetic. Such unusual regulations are possible only because of

[46] The income figures are in, Inspection Générale de la Sécurité Sociale, *Rapport annuel 1964* (Paris: Inspection Générale de la Sécurité Sociale, 1965), pp. 212–13. The problems of radiology are summarized in, M.-C. Montin, "L'avenir de la radiologie," *Concours médical*, vol. 88, no. 52 (24 December 1966), pp. 8141, 8143–44.

[47] Milton I. Roemer, "On Paying the Doctor and the Implications of Different Methods," *Journal of Health and Human Behavior*, vol. 3, no. 1 (Spring 1962), pp. 6–7.

the close understanding between the Royal Dutch Medical Association and the sick funds: they are united in a common concern about financial abuse. They are also apprehensive about the effects in neighboring Germany of a more permissive way of paying for the administration of anesthetics.

A second rule in Dutch national health insurance is that an anesthesiologist can collect fees only for anesthetics that he personally administers. Thus he cannot collect fees for several operations simultaneously, where the anesthetics are actually given by salaried nurses or salaried medical assistants—a profitable tactic in some other countries.

A method of discouraging—rather than forbidding—procedures by a doctor outside his specialty is to pay him less than a fully qualified specialist. For example, in Dutch national health insurance a specialist without credentials in radiology can perform any of the numerous diagnostic and therapeutic procedures in the fee schedule for that field (Tariff VIII). But unless he is fully qualified in radiology, he collects only 90 per cent of the full fee.

Availability of Services

Ideally a payment system should induce doctors to work in geographical areas in which they are needed. In practice in nearly every country physicians concentrate in the cities, where they find the largest numbers of hospitals, private patients, colleagues, and personal amenities.

Because of the medical profession's insistence that official medical care systems reproduce as much as possible the conditions in private practice in the absence of public intervention, fee-for-service usually encourages rather than discourages the gravitation of doctors to the cities. Instead of paying higher fees to draw personnel into under-doctored areas, the fee schedules with regional differentials give the higher rates to urban practitioners. In some countries, such as Germany and Switzerland, this differential results from the absence of an equalization mechanism among the sick funds. The funds in the cities usually get more money from their subscribers and can afford higher fees.[48] Therefore the urban doctors—and particularly those in

[48] An exception is the canton of Basel. Its cantonal government and sick funds were long dominated by Socialists who kept subscribers' premiums low, who wished to spend the funds' income for purposes other than medical fees (such as hospitalization), and therefore kept the fee schedule lower than that in most rural districts. The sick funds and medical societies were bitterly opposed and several strikes were called. The turmoil and the economic disincentives probably reduced the once heavy concentration of doctors in Basel. In 1944, the city had the sixth highest doctor-population ratio of any Swiss city; by 1962 it was twenty-third. Compare Roger Stupnicki, *Die soziale Stellung des Arztes in der Schweiz* (Bern: Verlag Paul Haupt, 1953), pp. 127–128, and "Ärztestatistik," *Schweizerische Ärztezeitung*, vol. 42, nos. 40–41 (1962), pp. 14–15.

the largest cities—collect the highest fees and earn the highest incomes. Such national health insurance operates much like a completely private market of individuals: farmers and residents of small towns earn lower incomes, their lower purchasing power results in lower fees to doctors, and they could attract more doctors only by deciding to allocate a much higher proportion of their incomes to medical care.

Even when national health insurance has an equalization account and national standards, the medical profession often presses successfully for differentials in favor of the largest cities. They argue that the metropolitan doctors must pay the highest practice expenses and the highest living costs. For example, the French and Swedish fee schedules quoted in chapter III give higher rates for doctors in Paris and Stockholm than in the rest of the country, despite the fact that the rural-urban imbalances in both countries are serious policy problems.[49] Instead of reversing the urban concentration in France, national health insurance may have contributed to it: the imbalance has steadily increased during the twentieth century.[50] Spokesmen for the medical profession have cited the concentration of doctors in Paris to justify even larger monetary differentials in favor of Paris: many doctors in the capital are said to earn too little because of the competition, and therefore each patient should bring more money than in the provinces. But the commission revising the payment decrees in 1965 rejected this argument and endorsed smaller differentials.[51]

Position of the Medical Profession

Critics of national medical care systems warn of the degradation of the medical profession. Medical care supposedly will fall under the control of laymen who are hostile to the medical profession and who aim to provide medical services at the lowest cost. Therefore, it is predicted, doctors' pay will drop under national medical care schemes, their social prestige will

[49] The doctor-population ratios are 1:485 in Paris and 1:1,100 in the rest of France, according to Alain Laugier and C. Besson, "L'espace médical français," *Concours médical*, vol. 83, no. 23 (10 June 1961), pp. 3355–62. The doctor-population ratios are 1:450 in Stockholm and 1:1,400 in the rest of Sweden, according to *Public Health Service in Stockholm* (Stockholm: Stockholms Stads Sjukvårdsstyrelse, 1960). A critique of the geographical distribution of French doctors appears in, Pierre Grandjeat, *La santé gratuite* (Paris: Éditions du Seuil, 1965), pp. 84–87. Grandjeat's maps show the maldistribution of doctors among the neighborhoods of Paris as well as throughout the entire country.

[50] The city-dwellers were insured before the residents of towns and rural areas. As coverage widened, more and higher fees could still be collected in the cities. The historical trend in the concentration of doctors is summarized in, Alain Laugier and Jean Bui-Dang-Ha-Doan, "La concentration médicale en France," *Cahiers de sociologie et de démographie médicales*, vol. 1, no. 2 (October 1961), pp. 7–41.

[51] "Rapport de la Commission de l'Article 24 du Décret du 12 Mai 1960," *Notes et documents*, no. 17 (First Trimester 1965), pp. 43–45.

diminish, fewer people will enter medical careers, and the quality of recruits will decline.[52]

However, theories of wage determination—whether in a market economy or under socialism—list certain variables that might predict a favorable position for doctors in income and in social prestige as medical care becomes more extensively organized. These determining variables are: the occupation's functional importance to the survival and work of the rest of the economy; the amount of skill, responsibility, and preparatory education; the scarcity of the required skills in the economy relative to the public's effective demand; the occupation's in-group controls over the supply of manpower and over price competition; deference by the rest of the population; and influence with decisionmakers.[53] The income and status of the medical profession should decline only if the introduction or expansion of a national medical care system is associated with the profession's decline on these determining variables.

In practice, the income and prestige of the medical profession remain high in countries with national health insurance and national health services. This results from the profession's continued high rating on the factors that determine income and prestige. Doctors' work is indispensable to the survival and efficiency of people in every social system. Skills and judgment of such a high order are scarce, require much training, and attract general respect from the public and from leaders of the government. Organizations of the profession influence recruitment and prices. In practice, the medical profession acquires a powerful voice in the policies and management of national medical care systems in addition to the clinical services that are its recognized preserve. Consequently, the medical profession eventually manages to ensure that these systems do not operate to its disadvantage in any way.

Income

Medicine is one of the highest paid occupations in every country, regardless of whether the medical services are public or private and regardless of the method of payment. Fee-for-service seems particularly advantageous to doctors. To a much greater degree than salary and capitation, physicians

[52] E.g., Matthew J. Lynch and Stanley S. Raphael, *Medicine and the State* (Springfield: Charles C Thomas, 1963); Melchior Palyi, *Compulsory Medical Care and the Welfare State* (Chicago: National Institute of Professional Services, 1949), esp. chaps. 8, 9, 14 and 15; Cecil Palmer, *The British Socialist Ill-Fare State* (Caldwell, Ida.: Caxton Printers, 1952), chap. 2.

[53] David W. Belcher, *Wage and Salary Administration* (Englewood Cliffs, N.J.: Prentice-Hall, 1962), chap. 3 passim; and Lloyd G. Reynolds, *Labor Economics and Labor Relations* (Englewood Cliffs, N.J.: Prentice-Hall, 3d ed., 1959), chap. 18.

TABLE 5. MEAN INCOMES IN 1963, GERMAN OFFICE PRACTITIONERS

	Average Income in DM		Proportion of Income from Insurance	Income from Each Patient in DM		Number of Doctors
	Gross	Net		Insured	Private	
All office doctors	65,373	42,975	77	13.94	35.74	(1,377)
General practitioners	64,701	43,905	80	14.67	36.52	(839)
Internists	92,210	49,940	64	25.09	71.90	(137)
Pediatricians	62,040	40,933	77	13.04	31.34	(49)
Urologists	85,144	47,138	59	34.02	95.52	(13)
Ophthalmologists	77,036	53,793	79	12.14	23.77	(56)
Orthopedists	111,253	61,573	77	24.43	59.51	(36)
Radiologists	148,099	65,505	77	33.03	57.80	(20)

can increase incomes by their own efforts.[54] (If an individual doctor increases his practice unduly, the control system under fee-for-service concludes that he is out of line; but if all doctors perform more procedures, the statistical norms and incomes rise for everyone.) As the technical level of medicine rises and new therapies are introduced, more numerous and more expensive items are added to fee schedules, and doctors can treat many conditions more profitably. The complexity of fee schedules usually leads to the creation of standing review bodies, and therefore most schedules are modernized regularly and the fees are increased in the light of changes in the country's living costs and wage structure.

For example, despite the persistent furor over pay, German doctors depending on insurance practice do not earn substantially less than other professions. A national survey of German doctors yielded the data reported in Table 5.[55] The figures for orthopedists and radiologists show that considerable sums can be earned even when a large part of the practice is

[54] Accurate comparisons of the effects of payment systems on the incomes of the same doctors performing identical work are rare. But it is widely believed that fee-for-service results in higher incomes than salary or capitation. Support from American research is cited by Roemer, "On Paying the Doctor" (note 47), pp. 7–8, 12.

[55] "Die Kostenstruktur in der Wirtschaft: Freie Berufe 1963" (note 22), pp. 20–23. 1 DM = \$0.25. Because the original data were published in categories, the average is the mean within a category containing the median for all doctors, G.P.'s and internists; and the averages are the means for all other specialties. Means are higher than medians, since they are affected by the small numbers of very high incomes. Because salaries constitute such a large component of their incomes, the survey excluded the chiefs-of-service of hospitals and medical administrators. Because their incomes result from profits of an organization, the survey excluded owners of private clinics. As in many studies of incomes by European governments, the figures in Table 5 may be low because of evasive responses. The sick funds reported to the International Social Security Association that the average doctor contracted to them had a gross income of 87,000 DM in 1964 and had a net income of 58,000 DM after deduction of office expenses. But these estimates depend on one's partisan position: the KBV's sample survey of doctors' earnings in 1964 suggest that the average gross income under insurance was 40,000 DM. Mario Alberto Coppini and Franco Illuminati, *The Relationship between Social Security Institutions and the Medical Professions* (Geneva: International Social Security Association, 1967), p. 42. Even the lowest estimates show medicine at the top of the country's income distribution.

insured and follows the official fee schedule. The total incomes for ophthalmologists are high even when the earnings from each individual patient under insurance are low.

Compared to the rest of the German economy, these figures are high. During 1963, the average annual wage for male industrial workers was 8,953 DM; the average annual salary for industrial engineers and technicians was 12,228 DM; the average annual salary for industrial administrators was 10,068 DM; the average income from all sources of a household of four members was 11,706 DM; and the highest annual salary in the federal civil service was 29,724 DM.[56] Less than one per cent of all German wage-earners are in the same net income bracket as the doctors.[57] In 1953, even before the recent increases in fees and before creation of a more regular mechanism to review fees, the ratio of medical income to the average economically active person's income was much higher in Germany than in all seven Western countries used for comparison, including the United States.[58]

The ability of doctors to attain the top of a country's income structure under national health insurance paying fee-for-service is confirmed by data from Holland. Table 6 shows the median incomes for men, according to a sample survey.[59] The specialists, who are paid predominantly by fee-for-service and case payments, earn higher incomes than do other groups, except for the small number of self-employed engineers.

Income differentials are narrower in Holland than in most developed countries. In the annual review of fees, doctors try to preserve their existing relationship to other occupations, with corrections for the rise in living costs, and they do not press for special advantages. The control process and therapeutic caution discourage sudden increases in income through the rapid growth of medical procedures. Therefore, ironically, health insurance may be less profitable to the specialist relative to nonmedical incomes in Holland than in other European countries beset by louder complaints about the underpayment of doctors.[60]

[56] *Statistisches Jahrbuch für die Bundesrepublik Deutschland* (Stuttgart: W. Kohlhammer GMBH, 1964), pp. 501, 512, 517, 523, 529.

[57] Compare the earnings estimated for 1958 by Hogarth, *Payment of General Practitioner* (note 5), p. 259; and the income distribution in *Handbook of Statistics for the Federal Republic of Germany* (Wiesbaden: Statistisches Bundesamt, 1961), p. 168.

[58] *Cost of Medical Care* (note 6), p. 149. Additional information about the incomes of German doctors from national health insurance and other sources are summarized by Bosch, *Patient* (note 8), pp. 27–31; and Michael Brunner, *Wer soll das bezahlen?* (Essen: Industriedruck A.G., 1959), p. 58. Estimates of incomes from all sources and from insurance alone at intervals during the twentieth century appear in Hadrich, *Der Arztfrage* (note 2), pp. 147–56.

[59] A. I. V. Massizzo, *Rapport Statistisch Onderzoek Intellectuelen 1966* ('s-Gravenhage: Federatie Organisaties Intellectuele Beroepen, 1968), p. 34. The exchange rate is f. 1 = $0.28.

[60] *Cost of Medical Care* (note 6), p. 150.

Table 6. Median Net Incomes after Deduction of Expenses (The Netherlands, 1966—in Guilders)

Professions and Skilled Occupations	Self-Employed	Salaried Employees of Industry	Salaried Employees of Government	Number of Respondents Self	Number of Respondents Industry	Number of Respondents Government
Physicians:						
Specialists	74,400	34,760	33,460	(124)	(57)	(153)
General practitioners	52,640			(152)		
Accountants	62,500	29,610	29,000	(49)	(52)	(43)
Lawyers	35,710			(43)		
Engineers	85,000	32,460	32,140	(26)	(263)	(43)
Teachers:						
University graduates			29,060			(359)
Lacking university degrees			26,240			(317)
University graduates not in professions	65,000	31,220	29,450	(27)	(161)	(235)
Other persons lacking university degrees	42,200	33,620	23,310	(69)	(258)	(330)

Not only do Dutch specialists earning fees and case payments obtain more than other occupations, but they earn more than doctors paid by other methods. Dutch general practitioners are paid by the capitation system. The spread between specialists and G.P.'s is wider in Holland than in Germany, where the general practitioners are paid under the same fee schedule as the specialists. According to the foregoing Dutch data, the self-employed specialists earn considerably more than the physicians who receive full-time or nearly full-time salaries from hospitals, public health agencies, industry, and other organizations, even after the deduction of practice expenses.

Despite the low fees in Switzerland in the past, and despite the absence in most cantons of standing review procedures for continually modernizing the rates, Swiss doctors have always been able to earn satisfactory incomes under fee-for-service. Hogarth was told that the average income from insurance practice alone fell between 30,000 fr. and 35,000 fr.[61] In some of the cities, I was told in 1961, the average practitioner grossed between 60,000 and 70,000 fr. annually from all sources (insurance and private) and netted between 40,000 and 60,000 fr. The relationship between the average gross medical income from all sources and the national income per economically employed person in Switzerland is one of the most favorable in the world.[62]

As in other European countries, the clinical professors of medicine earn the highest incomes, but they rarely treat insured patients. In some of the cities, I was told, they received salaries of about 50,000 fr. for teaching and for being chief of service in the university hospital in 1961, and private practice brought between 50,000 fr. and 100,000 fr. more.

[61] Hogarth, *Payment of General Practitioner* (note 5), p. 316. 1 Fr.S. = $0.23.

[62] *Cost of Medical Care* (note 6), pp. 148–49, 203. This was true in the 1940's as well. See Stupnicki, *Die soziale Stellung* (note 48), pp. 114–20.

National health insurance has brought many economic benefits to doctors: more patients visit them and uncollected bills are much less common. While doctors—and particularly general practitioners—are better off financially, so are other occupations, and therefore medicine may not have improved its relative position. The spread of national health insurance and national health services has coincided with economic stabilization and higher incomes for all. Therefore, some occupations have improved even more than medicine. For example, once the German doctor netted more than the lawyer, but more recently he has netted slightly less.[63] But the trend is not the same everywhere. In Switzerland, despite the controversy over rigidities in the rates, doctors were able to earn steadily rising incomes under fee-for-service, so that they gained relative to the rest of the economy.[64]

Prestige

Public opinion surveys ranking the prestige of doctors place them at or near the top in every country, regardless of how they are paid and regardless of their employment conditions. Payment by fee-for-service has no effect on their popularity and respect. Nor does conflict with the government and sick funds lower the prestige of doctors, a fact that may help the medical profession win so often. Their high pay probably is a more important determinant of their high prestige than their method of payment.[65]

If any occupations rank ahead of medicine, this seems due more to cultural tradition than to any effects of the payment system. For example, some German studies of prestige and of public valuation have ranked medicine first, while a few have ranked it second to the university professor, who is a government employee paid by salary.[66] If a poll includes very prestigious

[63] Compare Fr. Thieding, *Das soziale Mozaik* (Hamburg: Hamburger Ärzte Verlag, 1956), pp. 142, 144; and *Royal Commission on Doctors' and Dentists' Remuneration 1957–1960: Report* (London: H. M. Stationery Office, Cmnd. 939, 1960), p. 320.

[64] *Cost of Medical Care* (note 6), pp. 148–49.

[65] Income is one of the strongest correlates of social prestige in public opinion polls—at least in the American studies that have examined the basis of ranking. Medicine is high on all the values of respondents that correlate with prestige, such as social contribution, special training, moral and intellectual requirements, and profit. A. F. Davis, "Prestige of Occupations," *British Journal of Sociology*, vol. 3, no. 2 (June 1952), p. 146.

[66] Friedrich Weltz, *Wie steht es um die Bundeswehr?* (Hamburg: Henri Nannen Verlag, 1964), pp. 13 and 104; "Am meisten geachtet: der Arzt," *Informationsdienst* (Institut für Demoskopie Allensbach, May 1965); and Alex Inkeles and Peter H. Rossi, "National Comparisons of Occupational Prestige," *American Journal of Sociology*, vol. 61, no. 4 (January 1956), pp. 329–39. The UNESCO Institute's survey of West German villagers placed medicine above sixteen other occupations for reasons independent of income and payment method. The respondents respected doctors because of their skill, social importance, and occupation. Gerhard Wurzbacher and Renate Mayntz Pflaum, *Das Dorf im Spannungsfeld industrieller Entwicklung* (Stuttgart: Ferdinand Enke Verlag, 1961), pp. 33–34. Similar results are reported in, G. Mackenroth and K. M. Bolte, "Bericht über das Forschungsvorhaben 'Wandlungen der deutschen Sozialstruktur (am Beispiel des Landes Schleswig-Holstein)'," *Transactions of the Second World Congress of Sociology*, vol. 2 (1954), pp. 95–96.

titles held by a few public leaders—such as ambassador or prime minister—they may outrank doctors, but medicine is usually rated first, or nearly first, in the list of occupations.[67]

Recruitment

Controversies over the payment system and the levels of pay often are accompanied by predictions that recruitment will suffer in quality and quantity and that shortages will develop. These forebodings have often been heard in Germany during the frequent disputes in the past, but they have never been borne out. In many countries, enrollment in the nonmedical faculties has been rising faster than in the medical faculty, but the opposite has been true in postwar Germany.[68] Instead of discouraging their children from following in their footsteps, German doctors encourage them: one-quarter of West Germany's medical students come from physicians' families.[69] So many students graduate from medical schools each year that Germany has more doctors for its population than nearly any country in the world,[70] competition has long enabled the sick funds to keep fees low, and some doctors emigrate. Administrative restrictions on entry into medical school have been discussed for some years, but such a drastic break with German tradition has not yet been made.[71]

Nor have the service benefits system and the level of fees hurt recruitment in Switzerland. Applications to medical school and the numbers of doctors have risen without interruption.[72]

Conclusion: The Effects of Fee-For-Service

As in every payment system, how fee-for-service works in practice depends on the prosperity and ethics of the medical profession. If a country has a

[67] Kaare Svalastoga, *Prestige, Class and Mobility* (Copenhagen: Glydendal, 1959), pp. 62–67, 123–27.

[68] Alfred Heim, "Ärztebedarf und ärztlicher Nachwuchs," *Deutsche Medizinische Wochenschrift*, vol. 86, no. 30 (28 July 1961), p. 1443. During the twentieth century, the absolute number of students in medicine has risen in Germany and in most other countries. Because other curricula are now available, the *proportion* of university students in medicine is smaller than it was earlier in the century. Figures for Germany and other countries are in Joseph Ben-David, "Professions in the Class System of Present-Day Societies," *Current Sociology*, vol. 22, no. 3 (1963–64), pp. 266–67.

[69] Fritz Beske, "Der ärztliche Nachwuchs im Bundesgebiet und in Berlin," *Ärztliche Mitteilungen*, vol. 46, no. 19 (1961), pp. 1069–72.

[70] *World Health Statistics Annual 1962* (Geneva: World Health Organization, 1966), 3: 18–42. Annual recruitment figures and the steady growth of the German medical profession since the beginning of health insurance appear in Hadrich, *Der Arztfrage* (note 2), pp. 137–38.

[71] The problems of overcrowding, the futility of recent measures to discourage entrants, and the possibility of a *numerus clausus* in medical school are discussed in "Der weisse Traum," *Der Spiegel*, vol. 16, no. 34 (22 August 1962), pp. 28–37 passim; and "Medizin-Studium: Auf der Wildbahn," ibid., vol. 20, no. 35 (22 August 1966), pp. 37–39.

[72] "Ärztestatistik 1966," *Schweizerische Ärztezeitung*, vol. 47, no. 46 (18 November 1966), pp. 1217, 1231.

high national income and effective taxation capable of supporting generous health insurance, fees and doctors' incomes may be high; but in a poor country, medical incomes and morale may be low, and the payment system may be denounced as the scapegoat. Regular consultation between the medical association and the public agency are essential to morale and peace. Regular machinery to review rates is necessary to modernize them as the incomes of the doctors' social peers rise.

Fee-for-service systems (whether using service or cash benefits) have common characteristics. Whether or not the authors of the fee schedule so intended, better paid procedures tend to be more frequently practiced than poorly paid, and the former may be substituted for the latter—for example, injective instead of oral administration of drugs—if they are interchangeable. Fee schedules must be changed in accordance with modern trends in medicine, lest simple procedures be overpriced in accordance with their past rather than their present technical difficulty. Failure to pay for certain procedures satisfactorily can result in the underdevelopment of an entire specialty in the medical profession. Fee-for-service benefits the surgical specialties more than the medical and preventive specialties, since the surgical specialties' procedures can easily be itemized and priced. If any doctor can be paid for any procedure, general practitioners become more alike in skills and income, and specialists become more versatile. Low fees do not inevitably produce low incomes, if each doctor can have many patients and do many tasks.

Fee-for-service systems using service benefits present special problems. If the patient pays nothing, neither he nor the doctor will thereby be deterred from medically unnecessary work that gives the doctor extra income and that gives the patient the feeling that the money he paid in taxes isn't wasted. Most service benefits schemes enable the doctor to bill the funds without the patient's knowledge, so the only witness to the work provides no control over the doctor's claims. Doctors' morale may be lowered by economic pressures to do medically unnecessary work, and therefore abuses may be fewer in systems with shortages of physicians and with high fees. Fee schedules can be written with variable payment formulae that discourage the unnecessary multiplication of work, but the problem is to prevent these formulae from discouraging justified long-term care. Effective and acceptable administrative controls over the venal multiplication of procedures requires the co-operation of the medical association.

Under fee-for-service, the doctors' income depends on whatever problems patients present to him. Usually patients are not bound to one particular doctor. Therefore, compared to other payment systems, doctors more often must cater to patients.

VIII

EFFECTS OF FEE-FOR-SERVICE: CASH BENEFITS

When national health insurance is introduced into a country with many well-established private office practitioners, the medical profession often presses for a cash benefits system. The doctors believe the arrangement will preserve their autonomy in full: since the patient and not the physician communicates with the sick funds, the profession believes the funds can never limit its fees, regulate its clinical decisions, or influence the choice of doctors by patients. The physicians believe they will have no obligations beyond their customary professional duties, except to give the patient a receipt for transmission to the fund. As this chapter will demonstrate, these utopian hopes are realized only if the medical profession has considerable self-discipline and co-operates closely with the funds.

At times, critics of service benefits schemes recommend cost-sharing by patients in order to increase the resources of the funds and deter unnecessary use.[1] The patient pays the doctor a sum additional to the one he collects from the fund; or the patient reimburses the fund for part of its payment. But cost-sharing would not change the basic system of direct billing of funds by doctors. In some countries beset by controversies, doctors occasionally propose the complete abandonment of service benefits and the substitution of cash benefits schemes.[2]

[1] This is the principal issue described in, William Safran, *Veto Group Politics: The Case of Health Insurance Reform in West Germany* (San Francisco: Chandler Publishing Co., 1967). A convenient summary of the arguments for and against cost-sharing appears in, Bernhard Külp, *Hauptprobleme der Krankenversicherungsreform* (Paderborn: Verlag Bonifacius-Druckerei, 1959), chap 5. Cost-sharing was recommended by the representatives of British general practitioners in order to discourage clinically unnecessary burdens on the family doctor. *Abuse and Misuse: A Critical Problem in the Family Doctor Service* (London: General Practitioners' Association, 1965), pp. 49–56.

[2] E.g., the resolution adopted in "British Medical Association: Annual Representative Meeting, Swansea 1965," *British Medical Journal Supplement* (17 July 1965), pp. 67–68.

Swiss doctors long sought adoption of cash benefits, in order to charge the higher income patients much higher fees and avoid dictation of their charges by cantonal legislatures. The amendments to the federal health insurance act in 1964 established the cash benefits principle for the wealthiest insured patients throughout the country, unless the cantonal medical association and the sick funds decided otherwise. Some cantonal contracts distinguish between middle and lower income persons and create a reimbursement system for middle income people. Cash benefits prevail if the doctors and funds cannot agree on a contract, but the cantonal statute specifies the rates for funds' reimbursements to the patients.

Encouraging Good Medicine

Close Relations between Doctor and Patient

One common argument in favor of reimbursement schemes is that the cash nexus leads to improvements in the doctor-patient relationship. Since the patient must invest his own money, he is said to expect conscientious performance by the doctor and is more careful to pick a good one. Since he receives money from the patient, the doctor is supposed to be more attentive than if he were paid by an impersonal sick fund. Poor work by the doctor results in the sanction of an unpaid bill, just as in private practice.

It is difficult to conclude that the cash relationship ensures more conscientious performance by doctors. The levels of satisfaction reported by patients using the French cash benefits scheme are no higher than among populations covered by service benefits.[3]

In most public opinion polls, satisfaction with the respondents' doctors is high, regardless of payment system. But a serious limitation of all these polls is that they rarely ask about alternatives, such as whether the patients would prefer another arrangement, even if they had to pay more. Valid cross-national comparisons of levels of public satisfaction are difficult to make, because the questionnaires and samples differ. Comparisons—when possible—often cannot be published, since many national polls were commissioned privately by medical associations and by sick funds, and they can be examined but not cited by scholars.

Whether a fee-for-service system is based on service benefits or cash benefits seems to make no clear difference in the provision of high-quality care. More decisive influences are the values and traditions of the medical profession, taught in medical school and enforced by the institutions that affect the practitioner in his daily work. And, of course, the technical level of clinical science in a country is also crucial, regardless of payment system.

[3] The principal French survey is "Les français et leur médecin," *Sondages*, vol. 22, nos. 1 and 2 (1960), pp. 43–44, 75–79.

Delays in Seeking Care

The principal criticism of reimbursement systems is that needy patients might be deterred if they had to provide enough cash initially to see the doctor. This might occur most often under schemes that reimburse only part of the fees actually paid. The danger of postponement and neglect also is cited against cost-sharing proposals under service benefits.[4]

National medical care schemes using cash benefits usually have safeguards against financial discouragement of the poor. In both France and Sweden, persons below a certain income bracket can be exempted from the usual procedure. The subscriber in France can collect the reimbursement from the sick fund in advance of his visit to the doctor, and he can ask the doctor to bill public charitable offices for the remainder of his fee. Poor patients in Sweden can ask a social assistance office to pay the office practitioner's fees on their behalf, or they can go to the salaried district medical officer for completely free treatment. These options might not be used in every possible case, since the patient is thereby classified differently from other insured people. Perhaps some patients may be deterred by the means test, if not by the need to pay.

Very expensive procedures might be postponed unduly, since the patient must have a large sum available at a time when illness may have decreased his income and increased his living costs. To prevent this, French national health insurance repays in full the medical costs of patients suffering from long-term illnesses, such as tuberculosis, mental illness, cancer, poliomyelitis, and others designated by agreements between the local fund and the local medical society. (The usual patient recovers only 70 per cent of the cost of medical procedures.) But the patient still must have enough cash to make the initial payment to the doctor. Sweden avoids the problem by excluding the more expensive procedures from the fee schedule and from cash benefits: they are performed by the salaried staffs of the public hospitals, and the insured patient pays nothing.

The available studies show that the need to pay the doctor causes postponement of care, particularly the more expensive work. For example, in mid-1956, nearly all French insured patients had to pay their doctors considerably above the planned fee schedule, so that they were recovering much less than 80 per cent of their payments to doctors. Over one-third of all respondents—half the low income groups, and half the people with three or more children—said that the need to pay doctors parts of the total fees

[4] Substantial minorities of British patients said they would contact doctors less often if charges were introduced for home and office visits. *Abuse and Misuse* (note 1), pp. 69–70.

caused them to postpone visits.[5] Specialists' fees were higher and more likely to deter visits than were general practitioners' fees.[6] In 1956 insured and uninsured persons were equally likely to go to G.P.'s; but, because of reimbursement, the insured persons were more likely to consult specialists than were uninsured members of the same income groups.[7] That the initial payment by the patient inhibits utilization was confirmed by administrative experiments during the early 1960's: when certain funds paid doctors directly, use of the doctor and expenses increased and exceeded the levels in funds still using cash benefits. By this time, the unreimbursed part of the fee had been reduced to 20 per cent; this expense plus the need to make an initial payment may have reduced each patient's costs of utilizing doctors by over one-fourth.[8]

One cannot be sure of the extent of postponement or complete omission of care due to Sweden's reimbursement system. The country has a lower frequency of ambulatory and domiciliary medical care than any other with national health insurance or with a national health service.[9] One important reason is the shortage of doctors and the difficulty in getting an early appointment. Another reason might be the good health of the population. The magnitude of the financial deterrent is unknown.

Making the payment system easier for the patient will not guarantee early consultation in all necessary situations. Health surveys of the population in countries with comprehensive service benefits schemes show substantial minorities of the population not using the freely available services. Their conditions were less critical than those who consulted the doctor, but some had serious conditions with symptoms that at first were misleadingly minor. Their delays were due to apathy and to reluctance to alter work and family routines.[10]

[5] Jean-Daniel Reynaud and Antoinette Catrice-Lorey, *Les assurés et la sécurité sociale* (Paris: Institut des sciences sociales du travail, 1959), pp. 17, 22–23. Reimbursement was at the rate of 80 per cent before October 1967, and 70 per cent thereafter.

[6] Jacques Vallette, "Compte rendu global de l'enquête," *Présences*, no. 59 (Second Trimester 1957), p. 63.

[7] Philippe Michaux, "Le revenu du groupe médical," *Révue économique*, no. 1 (January 1959), p. 97.

[8] Pierre Grandjeat, *La santé gratuite* (Paris: Éditions du Seuil, 1965), p. 40.

[9] "Volume and Cost of Sickness Benefits in Kind and Cash," *Bulletin of the International Social Security Association*, vol. 16, nos. 3 and 4 (March–April 1963), pp. 57, 62, 77; and vol. 18, no. 1 (January 1965), p. 26.

[10] Political and Economic Planning, *Family Needs and the Social Services* (London: George Allen & Unwin, 1961), pp. 78, 102–05; Nuffield Provincial Hospitals Trust, *Problems and Progress in Medical Care* (London: Oxford University Press, 1964), pp. 7–9; *New Frontiers in Health* (London: Office of Health Economics, 1964); J. M. Last, " 'Completing the Clinical Picture' in General Practice," *Lancet* (6 July 1963), pp. 28–31; Arie Querido, *The Efficiency of Medical Care* (Leiden: H. E. Stenfert Kroese, N.V., 1963), pp. 49, 111–21. So important are motivational variables, other than the mere availability of services, that the utilization rate in a country with predominantly private payments may be higher than in any country with service benefits under a universal public care scheme. Osler L. Peterson et al., "What

Preventive Medicine

Reimbursement schemes are thought particularly detrimental to preventive care: patients might make an initial investment in treatments to relieve pain, but they might consider preventive examinations and inoculations to be luxuries that could be postponed. Preventive medicine requires periodic re-examinations, and many patients may feel the regular payments burdensome.

Therefore reimbursement systems usually do not include preventive care, which is offered instead on a service benefits basis. Some proposals to abolish service benefits systems, or to introduce cost-sharing, exempt preventive medicine lest utilization be discouraged by any billing of the patient.[11]

But a great deal more than free availability seems necessary to induce insured persons to use preventive services. For example, the social security of France offers its subscribers completely free examinations as well as treatments under its separate cash benefits régime. The utilization rate in a survey conducted in 1956 was much lower than that for the medical treatments requiring initial payments.[12] Apathy is at least as important as financial barriers in determining the use of preventive services.

Encouraging Superior Work

Ideally a payment system should reward outstanding performance. But a dilemma in fee-for-service and in the capitation system is that the rates are the same for all doctors, regardless of quality. A defense of fee-for-service might be that the better doctors attract more patients and thereby earn more. But the fallacy is that high incomes necessitate rapid work, and good care often is painstaking. Therefore the best doctors might earn the least, instead of the most, under standardized schedules. For this reason, many eminent physicians in the world avoid practicing under national health insurance and take only private patients paying high fees.

If it does not attempt to control the fees actually charged patients, a cash benefits system might solve the problem of enabling the ablest doctors

---

Is Value for Money in Medical Care? Experiences in England and Wales, Sweden, and the U.S.A.," *Lancet* (8 April 1967), pp. 771–76; and Roul Tunley, *The American Health Scandal* (New York: Dell Publishing Co., 1966), p. 189. A slightly larger proportion of illnesses may be brought to the doctor after the introduction of national medical care schemes, but this may be due to the secular trend for increased utilization in all societies. See the ratios between consultations and illness that can be calculated from William P. D. Logan and Eileen Brooke, *The Survey of Sickness 1943–1952* (London: H. M. Stationery Office, 1957), pp. 44, 50–62.

[11] E.g., R. K. Allday, *On Medicine in Britain and the National Health Service* (Bristol: John Wright & Sons, 1962), pp. 49–52.

[12] Reynaud and Catrice-Lorey, *Assurés et sécurité sociale* (note 5), compare pp. 133–36, 219–22.

to treat insured patients. They could charge any fees commensurate with their time and talent: the patients would be reimbursed in part according to the sick funds' standard rates. The only drawback is that poor patients might not be able to afford the best care, even though they are insured. This apparently simple solution often fails in practice: enough doctors believe they deserve high fees so that price levels rise, and subscribers complain about inadequate reimbursement. Therefore sick funds try to limit doctors' charges so their subscribers will not lose too much money. Then the eminent doctors—and their less eminent but equally expensive brethren—try to practice privately as much as possible.

How to incorporate the leading physicians into national health insurance has been one of the principal problems of national health insurance in France. Before 1958, when the government began to curb charges, the eminent doctors charged whatever they wished, and their patients recovered the standard reimbursement from the funds. Many of the most skilled and most fashionable physicians led the opposition to the decrees requiring adherence to a fee schedule as a condition for adequate reimbursement to patients. Because so many practiced there, Paris, Lyons, and Nice were among the few *départements* where the medical syndicates refused to sign collective agreements with the sick funds. So that patients of their less fashionable colleagues would not suffer, a compromise evolved: in the *départements* without collective agreements covering all doctors, doctors could guarantee the standard reimbursements for their patients by signing individual agreements pledging to charge no more than the official fee schedule. The remaining doctors could charge what they wished, but their insured patients would be reimbursed by the funds at considerably less than the standard rates. Therefore by the mid-1960's the doctors outside the official system were only the *grands médecins* and specialists in fields that believed they were so underpaid by the fee schedule that they must work privately, such as psychiatrists and practitioners of acupuncture.[13]

But the decrees of 1960 provided a mechanism for including the *grands médecins* in social security practice without depressing their fees. The funds were allowed to designate a few eminent doctors who could charge more than the standard fee schedule. Social security would not subsidize them—the patient would be reimbursed only according to the official fee schedule and would pay the balance—but social security would not penalize them by reimbursing their patients at the lower rates aimed at doctors who practiced outside the conventions.

To adapt an official fee-for-service scheme in this way was unprecedented

[13] Within and near Paris, the number of individual contracts roughly corresponded inversely to the income level of the *arrondissement* and of the suburb. See Grandjeat, *Santé gratuite* (note 8), p. 106.

and would offer lessons to other countries. To implement the idea was very difficult, since the medical profession opposed any classification of doctors, whether by a nonprofessional organization like social security or by the executives of the medical association. State intervention into realms of individual independence was exactly what the profession had always feared from national health insurance. The office practitioners and chiefs of hospital services had always resisted controls from organized medicine too in all areas except professional ethics.

A further complication—and one that led the medical associations to delay implementation of the scheme for several years—is that the ratings of doctors are inevitably public. As we shall see in the next chapter, the award of higher salaries to outstanding British specialists is confidential. But secrecy is possible only when the State or sick funds pay the doctor. France has a cash benefits scheme, and all patients must know which of the available doctors are included and excluded from the list. In order to reduce the publicity gains from inclusion and in order to allay the invidious distinctions between the members and others, the wording of the decrees was amended. The July 1960 decree called it *la liste de notoriété*, but these words were dropped in the amendments of 1965, and the privileged doctors were said to have only *le droit permanent à dépassement*. In addition, the criteria for selection were made as unevaluative as possible.

A central problem in any quality rating system is whether judgments should be made with discretionary criteria. As we shall see in the next chapter, Britain's distinction awards are given to specialists by a committee and by advisors making judgments rather than automatically counting formal characteristics. The French decrees in 1960 authorized the exercise of such discretion, but an agreement between the medical associations and the sick funds in 1967 limited the criteria to automatically applicable ones that the doctor could acquire through his own efforts. Higher fees could be charged by three groups: first, professors in medical schools, chiefs of service in hospitals, and some *anciens internes* who had served in major hospitals; second, a few clinical scientists who had produced well-known work; and third, doctors who had taken recognized postgraduate and refresher courses.[14] For the bulk of the profession, superiority was now operationalized to mean a record of postgraduate training. The payment system therefore created a powerful incentive for continuing education.

Administering the criteria and creating the lists are the responsibilities of regional commissions drawn from the medical societies and the social

[14] "Droit permanent à dépassement," *Concours médical*, vol. 89, no. 9 (4 March 1967), pp. 1759–60. The reliance on continuing education as the fundamental criterion of excellence for the majority of the profession was anticipated by Jean Mignon, "Le droit permanent à dépassement et le perfectionnement professionnel," ibid., vol. 88, no. 6 (5 February 1966), pp. 881–88.

security funds. Over-all supervision to achieve uniformity in selection and procedure is given to a new *Commission National Paritaire*. The regional commission may issue its list only after seeking the advice of the medical society primarily concerned with professional and ethical matters, the *Ordre des Médecins*.[15]

Unnecessary Work

The bugbear of national health insurance schemes using fee-for-service payment is the medically unnecessary multiplication of procedures from financial motives. In theory in a cash benefits scheme, social security has direct relationships only with the insured patient and not with the individual doctor: the fund is supposed to be reimbursing the patient and not paying the doctor, and therefore the clinical and economic relationships between doctor and patient are supposed to be exactly the same as in purely private practice. In effect, the fund is accepting the patient's judgment about whether the doctor is giving the right quantity and quality of care, since the patient is the only observer of the doctor's performance while the fund is a purely fiscal agency and does not participate in the clinical relationship between the doctor and patient. In theory, the fact that the patient must pay the doctor should motivate him to beware of abuse. The fund's status as an outsider in French doctor-patient relations is underscored by the indirect method of communication between doctor and fund by means of a payment receipt bearing only code letters and numbers concealing the specific treatments from the fund. Thus a cash benefits system seems to leave the question of medically unnecessary and financially motivated treatment where it was under purely private practice, namely an ethical problem of the profession and a private problem of doctor-patient relationships; a service benefits system clearly makes this a salient problem of the sick funds themselves.

Administrative Controls

Actually medically unnecessary and financially motivated procedures are a problem of reimbursement schemes, even if the folklore of private practice persists in the thinking of doctors and officials. Since the patient will be reimbursed, the patient may not be so thrifty and vigilant, and the doctor is not inhibited by the patient's financial position.

Most reimbursement schemes do not repay the patient the full charge by the doctor. The margin of cost-sharing is supposed to motivate the patient to resist un-

[15] The procedure is described in "Rapport de la Commission de l'Article 24 du Décret du 12 Mai 1960," *Notes et documents*, no. 17 (First Trimester 1965), pp. 46–50, 95, 97, 101–3, 107–9. A thorough commentary is Jean Garagnon's "La notoriété médicale: une notion périmée?" *Droit social*, vol. 28, nos. 7–8 (July–August 1966), pp. 443–48.

necessary treatments. But French social security authorizes full reimbursement of medical procedures that are very expensive and that indicate that the patient will suffer a great reduction in income. By 1964, these payments constituted nearly half the national health insurance expenditures for physicians' services, and some observers suspected that certain work was performed unnecessarily. A few observers recommended cost-sharing for all items, regardless of expense, in order to inhibit abuse.[16] Others favored more effective administrative controls instead, so that persons experiencing truly catastrophic illnesses would not have to bear medical expenses too.

If a visit to the doctor results in no loss of wages but enables the patient to collect disability allowances from the sick fund, he may earn a profit from clinically unnecessary visits to the doctor, despite only partial reimbursement of the doctor's fee.[17] A cash benefits scheme is vulnerable to fraud: doctor and patient could conspire to write receipts for expensive but nonexistent care and then split the reimbursement.

Therefore, a paradox of French social security is that, at the same time it supposedly does no more than pay the patient and leave the doctor-patient relationship untouched, the funds employ salaried full-time control doctors who review the work of practitioners, detect medically unjustified procedures, and advise the funds not to pay some reimbursement claims. The powers and procedures of the control doctors frequently have been revised, vary from one *département* to another in practice, and have always been among the principal irritants between the medical profession and social security.[18]

The control doctor (*médecin conseil*) in each *département* performs other medical work determining payment decisions of the local fund. He examines applicants for sick benefits and patients requiring unusually expensive treatments that the private doctor can give only with the prior approval of the fund. But in these other tasks, there is more of a division of labor between control doctor and the private clinician; the control doctor is not over-ruling the clinician's judgment after work has been completed, and he is not condemning him.

If the French experience can be generalized, a cash benefits system creates ambiguity and trouble. On the one hand, the individual doctor and the

[16] E.g., *Assurances maladie et la presse d'information* (Paris: L'Association pour l'Étude des Problèmes Économiques et Humains de l'Europe, 1966).

[17] Housewives and some other low income or unemployed persons in Sweden are thought to have made medically unnecessary visits to the doctor's office or to the outpatient departments of the hospitals for this reason. Birger Herner, "Hittills gjorda erfarenheter av den allmänna sjukförsäkringen," *Svenska Läkartidningen*, vol. 52 (11 March 1955), pp. 597–605; and Leonard Brahme, "Quo vadis?", ibid., vol. 53 (3 February 1956), pp. 295–99.

[18] Dr. XXX, "Réflexions sur le contrôle médical de la sécurité sociale," *Droit social*, vol. 16, no. 1 (January 1953), pp. 48–51; Dr. Villey, "Le contrôle médical, essai de définition, ses buts, ses limites," ibid., vol. 16, no. 8 (September–October 1953), pp. 485–93; and Barbara N. Armstrong, *The Health Insurance Doctor: His Role in Great Britain, Denmark, and France* (Princeton: Princeton University Press, 1939), chap. 24.

local medical society may claim that the system is supposed to preserve the confidentiality of doctor-patient relations, leave the doctor completely autonomous to prescribe what the patient needs, and allow the fund to deal only with the patient. On the other hand, the fund claims it has the exclusive power to pay the patient and cannot honor unjustified claims. Special conditions in France have made the role of the control doctor particularly controversial: the medical profession by world standards has been extraordinarily committed to the traditional model of private office practice and particularly sensitive to any State controls; the French medical profession is extremely devoted to the principle of professional secrecy; popular election of social security fund boards has placed Communists and left-wing Socialists in charge of some, they have often been hostile to the conservative medical profession, and some practitioners seem to have perceived the control doctors as the turncoat agents of the political enemy.

Control doctors attempt to judge medically unnecessary procedures by methods commonly used in the service benefits schemes of other countries. Some French social security funds calculate statistical norms for procedures, on the basis of the payment receipts submitted by patients. FNOSS and the *Confédération* have agreed on norms suggesting reasonable average hourly numbers of office consultations. A doctor performing far more than the norm in his field arouses suspicion.[19]

The control system is much more cumbersome than in service benefits schemes, because the reports and payments pass between funds and doctors indirectly via the patient. The control doctor's statistical information is not as inclusive as in other countries, where the sick funds get a complete record of treatment on the payment receipt sent directly by the doctor. Probably the statistical method can detect over-performance more easily among general practitioners than among specialists, since *C* and *V* are more understandable than *K*, which refers to no specific procedure. Control doctors may examine patients before reimbursement, and some funds have used examinations to detect medically unnecessary over-performance or fraud.[20] But second-guessing is resented by the practitioners; its frequent use in Paris and Lyons during the 1930's succeeded in restraining costs but boomeranged by causing much lasting resentment by the doctors against the funds. The local doctors are particularly sensitive to any procedure that might sow doubts in patients' minds against their regular practitioners, and so the control doctor cannot question the patient too freely when investigating a physician's work.

When sick funds or national health services pay salaries, capitation fees, or other fees directly to the doctor, they can penalize him promptly and quietly by fines or by nonpayment of doubtful receipts. But a cash benefits scheme has no direct monetary relationship with the doctor and a refusal

[19] James Hogarth, *The Payment of the General Practitioner* (Oxford: Pergamon Press, 1963), pp. 168, 180–81.

[20] E.g., Armstrong, *Health Insurance Doctor* (note 18), pp. 217–19.

to pay can penalize only the patient in the short run. If the practitioner does not heed the exhortations of the control doctor, the fund has a choice between retreat and filing a complaint according to several highly formal procedures. One is the complaints machinery sponsored by the disciplinary association of doctors, the *Ordre des Médecins*. The *Ordre* sets up special tribunals for insurance cases, with nonmedical as well as medical members, but the *Ordre* reviews their decisions and administers penalties. (Aggrieved private or insured patients can appeal to the *Ordre* but, because French patients seem not yet to have lost their past reverence for medical omniscience and since the French legal profession has not yet discovered the bounties of malpractice cases, few complain.) The other method available to the funds is to file charges before local conciliation committees composed of representatives from the funds and from the *Confédération's* local branches.[21]

In practice, all this machinery has been used sparingly. Formality involving complaints and tribunals may inhibit use. The social security funds and the *Ordre* often have been on bad terms, since the *Ordre* even more than the *Confédération* has been the organizational stronghold of the proponents of traditional liberal medicine, and the *Ordre* has been unenthusiastic about most complaints against doctors. The difficulty in using the *Ordre* to enforce the financial rules of social security is one reason why the local conciliation commissions (with *Confédération* representatives) were given disciplinary powers during the 1960 reforms. But the new disciplinary machinery developed slowly during the 1960's: the local conciliation commissions are the local organs of consultation between the *Confédération* and the social security, and therefore their time is occupied by many other matters; the *Confédération* representatives cannot discipline too many doctors on behalf of social security lest they alienate their constituents; the basic presumption remains that the patient has the principal responsibility for deciding whether treatments are needed.

A study commission in 1964 recommended a more effective system of medical control for the entire national health insurance system. All the funds would follow the same procedures, thereby ending the regional variations in methods and in relations with doctors that had long upset the system. On the basis of research, statistical norms of practice would be maintained by all funds. Close relationships would be maintained between the control doctors and the treating doctors. Many questions would be resolved after they examined a patient jointly.[22]

As in other countries with national health insurance, the Swedish sick funds employ control doctors to police abuse. If any doctor performs medi-

[21] Procedures in the decade before creation of the *Ordre* are described by Armstrong, *Health Insurance Doctor* (note 18), chap. 25. Recent procedures are described in Hogarth, *Payment of General Practitioner* (note 19), pp. 150–53, 169–70, 181.

[22] "Rapport du Haut Comité Médical de la Sécurité Sociale sur le fonctionnement et l'organisation du contrôle médical," *Notes et études documentaires*, no. 3088 (9 May 1964), esp. pp. 10–28.

cally unnecessary or excessively repeated medical procedures for money over the statistical norms calculated by the National Insurance Office, the control doctor could ask him to desist. The same dilemmas arise as in France. The fund could refuse to reimburse the patient, but it usually shrinks from sanctioning the doctor by striking at an innocent third person. The control doctor can file charges with the Swedish Medical Association, but this action is unusual.[23] The control system is hardly used in Sweden, since the economics and ethics of Swedish medicine produce little unnecessary work: because of the severe shortage of doctors, the profession is kept busy doing what is clinically necessary.

Payment Formulae

As in the fee schedules in service benefits schemes, procedures under cash benefits may be priced to discourage unnecessary work. For example, as I said in chapter VII, the French doctor cannot expect his patient to be reimbursed if he charges for both procedures (*PC* or *K*) and a visit (*C* or *V*), he cannot expect full reimbursement for multiple procedures during the same visit, and he knows the patient will not recover separate charges for postoperative care if a major procedure (*K*) is very expensive. If the doctor is covered by a collective or individual contract with social security, he is bound to follow these billing rules. Similarly, if a French doctor covered by a contract has visited an insured patient at home and sees his relatives too, he can charge for only one home visit (*V*), and the other examinations are paid at the rate of office visits (*C*).

Likewise, as we said in chapter VII, Swedish health insurance limits reimbursement for procedures that might be performed unnecessarily for money.

Conditions that Produce Unnecessary Work

In theory the patient's initial payment should discourage unnecessary work, but on the other hand, patients may defer to doctors' judgments and will be reimbursed. Doing unnecessary procedures that harm the patient has long been condemned by French professional opinion as unethical, but other abuses (such as frequent office visits) that harm the fund without harming the patient may appear less reprehensible. High rates for professional consultation may be unusual but could be medically useful. It is

[23] Hogarth, *Payment of General Practitioner* (note 19), pp. 69–70, 75–77. The statistics on average utilization of each category in the fee schedule by community and by type of physician are published annually by the National Insurance Office in a mimeographed volume entitled *Statistisk undersökning rörande de allmänna försäkringskassornas utgifter för läkarvård m.m.*

difficult to estimate the frequency of abuse in France. Complaints were common during the 1930's and were heard again during the 1950's,[24] but I encountered fewer during my visits in the 1960's.

The French system may be vulnerable in one important respect. When specialty procedures are done in the principal hospitals owned by governments and religious associations, abuses are usually discouraged by the disciplined medical staff structure and the salaried system of payment. In order to earn money, the hospitals owned by medical specialists ("private clinics") may do unnecessary work. In many countries, private hospitalization is competitive, occupancy is low, and the temptation therefore is strong. For this reason, national health insurance funds usually resist paying hospitalization costs and medical fees in private clinics. But the French social security system has made several concessions to the specialists in the past, in order to obtain agreements with the medical profession. And a crucial concession was to authorize payment of hospitalization costs and medical fees to the private clinics owned by specialists, provided they met minimum standards of staffing and equipment. The specialists said that the extension of social security to care in private clinics was an essential part of the principle of free choice: the doctor and patient should be able to select whatever site and facilities they deemed best. If social security payments had not been available for private hospitalization, middle class subscribers would have protested: many French public hospitals still have only the unattractive open wards originally designed to house the poor, and the middle classes have never used them.

For several decades, the position of the specialists was so strong that social security paid even higher daily hospitalization payments to the private clinics than to the public hospitals, and specialists collected higher fees for procedures performed in private clinics than for those done in public hospitals. Consequently, specialists had incentives to hospitalize patients in their private clinics rather than in the public hospitals where they were part-time chiefs of service. The preferential situation of the private clinics was reduced during the reforms of the 1960's: the higher fee schedule for private clinics was abolished, and every physician in a private clinic authorized to treat insured patients had to follow the official fee schedule in all of his insured practice. But unnecessarily expensive and repetitious work was still believed by many to be done in the private clinics in minor surgery, in X-rays, in the use of other equipment, and in certain manual procedures.[25]

[24] Armstrong, *Health Insurance Doctor* (note 18), chaps. 24 and 27 passim; I. S. Falk, *Security Against Sickness* (Garden City, N.Y.: Doubleday, Doran & Co., 1936), p. 234; and Walter A. Friedlander, *Individualism and Social Welfare* (New York: The Free Press, 1962), p. 182.

[25] For example, suspicions about too many appendectomies were voiced by Dr. Maurer at the meeting of the *Confédération*, reported in *Le médecin de France*, vol. 66, no. 178 (December 1960), p. 1197.

Disputes Over Charges

In addition to the ambiguity over how to control the excessive performance of procedures for money, cash benefits schemes may suffer from disputes over the charges actually collected from patients by doctors. The medical profession demands cash benefits under the assumption that its freedom to charge patients should never be regulated by laymen and on the assumption of permanent preservation of the individual doctor's autonomy. Officials of governments and sick funds may make such oral promises in order to obtain the profession's co-operation at the commencement of national health insurance; some officials may fail to anticipate a widening gap between charges and reimbursements.

But there is an inherent danger of a large difference between the patient's payment and his reimbursement. A reimbursement system attempts to mesh the private and public sectors of the economy: but prices and incomes tend to rise faster and earlier in the private than in the public sector. In an expanding economy, sellers may increase prices quickly to cover higher costs and to earn incomes commensurate with their peers. But payments by public agencies can rise only slowly, since resources are limited by tax rates that change infrequently, and since increased resources must be spread over an expanding population. When fees set by doctors in the free market outrun the fixed reimbursements from the sick funds, patients complain that social security fails to prepay their costs in the intended way. The sick funds may claim the responsibility to protect the economic interests of their subscribers. The medical profession may retort that the spirit and perhaps even the letter of the original agreements with the government and sick funds gave the funds no such power but reserved complete freedom to the doctor.

The funds cannot guarantee both complete pricing freedom to all doctors and high reimbursement to all patients. This would eliminate the price elasticity of demand for medical services, make income elasticity of demand irrelevant, invite monopolistic pricing by the doctors, and result in steady and large increases in fees. The funds cannot increase payments so fast, because the social security taxes cannot rise indefinitely, and the Treasury would not guarantee additional subsidies without limits. If the patients stopped complaining about higher fees, they would start complaining about higher taxes.

Therefore cash benefits systems of national health insurance may tend toward a method of standard charges negotiated between the funds and the medical association. The individual doctor loses his pricing freedom in insurance practice and can raise fees only when the profession and the funds agree on collective price changes. When the fee schedule acquires this binding property, a cash benefits method from the standpoint of the medical profession differs very little from a service benefits system.

France

National health insurance in France was racked by conflicts over charges for decades, until the decrees of the de Gaulle government in 1958 and 1960 made the doctors' conformity to the fee schedule a condition for adequate reimbursement to the patient. During the 1930's and 1950's—as I said in chapter VI—individual doctors raised fees beyond officially agreed levels, and bitter controversies ensued. During periods when charges far exceed reimbursements, patients suffer many of the disadvantages of completely private payment. French public opinion polls showed that many people were angry about paying so much money, when they were also covered by national health insurance.

Eighty-seven per cent of a sample of the insured French urban public interviewed in mid-1956 said they had to pay the doctor more than the 20 per cent difference between the standard charges and reimbursed rates in the collective agreements between the *Confédération* and the public authorities. Insufficient reimbursement was their principal complaint against the social security system. In 1956, less than one-third of the population's total payments to doctors were reimbursed by social security. Even among occupations covered by social security, less than half of all payments were reimbursed.[26]

Many doctors had collection problems, just as if health insurance did not exist.[27] The Fourth Republic's inability to impose a solution was one of several matters that demonstrated its impotence and led to its downfall. A surprising number of people blamed the system rather than the doctors for their medical costs.[28]

Under the new arrangement, doctors were not required to follow the fee schedules negotiated by the social security, government, and medical association. But if they did not, their patients would recover so little from social security that the patients would be motivated to consult doctors whose charges followed the collective agreements. After the abortive strike threat described in chapter VI, the medical profession quickly came to terms with the new arrangement and found that it continued to prosper.

[26] The survey of the public is in Reynaud and Catrice-Lorey, *Assurés et sécurité sociale* (note 5), pp. 13–20. The estimate of the proportions of payments that were reimbursed appears in Monique Chasserant, "La consommation médicale des ménages d'après l'enquête de 1956 sur les budgets familiaux," *Notes et documents*, no. 1 (First Trimester 1960), p. 39.

[27] Jean-Jacques Gillon, "Les difficultés professionelles les plus importantes," *Concours médical*, vol. 78, no. 47 (24 November 1956), pp. 4929–30.

[28] Reynaud and Catrice-Lorey, *Assurés et sécurité sociale* (note 5), pp. 20–22; Vallette, "Compte de l'enquête" (note 6), pp. 81–82. This response by public opinion may be widespread and explains why the disputes over doctors' pay do not diminish the prestige of medicine. The British public blamed the system and not their embattled general practitioners in the surveys reported in *Abuse and Misuse* (note 1), p. 74; and in *Gallup Political Index*, no. 60 (May 1965), p. 52, published by Social Surveys (Gallup Poll), of London. However, this

Sweden

Skyrocketing charges and bitter conflicts are not inevitable in every cash benefits system, but the seeds of trouble are never wholly absent. The events in France have not yet been duplicated in Sweden for many reasons. The medical profession does not bear such hostility to the State, many doctors are State employees, and many voluntarily conform to State policy. High and steeply progressive income taxes dampen the urge to raise fees. Individual venality at the expense of patients and insurance funds is considered bad form by the profession. Doctors have come to accept insurance as the basis of a standardized payment system for most groups in the population: therefore they rarely use a sliding scale of fees based on insurance plus the patient's wealth.

On its side, the government has not drawn the lines over doctors' charges. It has not yet officially guaranteed that insured persons shall pay reasonable charges, but it has only guaranteed limited reimbursement. Throughout the social services, the government has preferred to act by subsidies (such as paying whatever the doctors want) instead of by controls. The *krona* is not a major international banking currency, the country's balance of payments has always been stable, and the Ministry of Finance has not yet had to cope with serious problems of price inflation and capital outflow. Disagreements between the government and private groups are, if possible, settled by private conferences with a minimum of public haranguing from either side.

The government does not entrust the entire insurance system to the voluntary restraint of the medical profession. It restricts the pricing of certain groups of doctors and could extend its regulations if charges suddenly rose. The physicians in public hospitals and the district medical officers outside Stockholm must conform to the fee schedule as a condition of their appointment. Junior hospital doctors in Stockholm must conform to the fee schedule during their outpatient hours, and possibly the ceilings might be extended gradually to the higher-priced chiefs as well. Some municipalities have offered space for medical groups, on the implied condition of charging no more than the official fees.

The DMO's collect salaries for the hours in which they treat poor patients without charge and conduct public health clinics. The rest of their day is devoted to office practice, like other doctors. The DMO's in Stockholm must follow the fee schedule for some of their hours and may exceed it during other hours.

But government control of all the profession's pricing decisions is as little welcome in Sweden as elsewhere. Therefore, in order to retain control

response is not invariant. Despite the normal popularity of general practitioners in Holland, their high pay demands in 1966 were opposed by a public long accustomed to a stable national wage policy. "Publiek kiest zijde van zienkenfondsen in het konflikt tussen huisartsen en ziekenfondsen," *NIPO, het Nederlands Instituut voor de Publieke Opinie en het Marktonderzoek: Bericht No. 1147*, 13 December 1966.

TABLE 7. CHARGES BY SWEDISH DOCTORS (IN KRONOR)

	Stockholm				Rest of Sweden			
Tariff Groups	Tariff	Charges by All Doctors	Charges by Hospital Chiefs	Charges by Office Practitioners	Tariff	Charges by All Doctors	Charges by Hospital Chiefs	Charges by Office Practitioners
1	8.00	9.97	9.62	10.13	6.00	6.37	5.98	6.94
2	15.00	20.57	22.88	21.40	10.00	11.41	11.08	13.47
3a	20.00	28.17	30.23	28.93	15.00	17.22	16.46	20.20
3b	25.00	33.18	35.37	33.84	20.00	21.75	20.95	24.81
3c	30.00	39.88	41.62	41.43	25.00	27.54	27.80	32.33
Average medical bill		23.71				13.74		

over their own fees, some office practitioners have formed groups and have erected their own buildings with the help of the Swedish Medical Association.[29]

Table 7 shows the fees actually charged patients in 1963 by all Swedish doctors and by full-time office practitioners, based on a one per cent sample of all receipts filed with the National Insurance Office.[30]

The Swedish patient is reimbursed three-fourths of the official tariff. Since charges exceed the fee schedule, reimbursement of actual payments is lower. Not only does Stockholm have a higher fee schedule than the rest of the country, but its doctors exceed the official rates by larger amounts. Therefore, patients are reimbursed a smaller proportion in Stockholm than in the rest of the country—less than three-fifths in Stockholm, over three-fifths in the rest of Sweden.

The government has been watching the charges by chiefs-of-service in Stockholm and by private office practitioners, since these uncontrolled groups might incite public protests if they raised their fees sharply. The selective regulations described earlier did not prevent fees from inching upward, even while the official schedule remained the same, but probably they slowed the pace. Charges have risen gradually and have not generated a crisis: they rose by about 5 per cent between 1955 and 1958 and by 15 per cent between 1958 and 1963.[31] Although fast enough to invite official consideration of wider controls, these increases were slower than those in France and in some other cash benefits systems during periods of growth and infla-

[29] Dag Knutson, "Annual Report of the Swedish Medical Association," *Svenska Läkartidningen*, vol. 59, no. 22 (1962), pp. 1653 et seq. (reprint); Dag Knutson, "Annual Report for the Year 1962" (Stockholm: Läkarförbundet, 1963, mimemographed), pp. 2–4; and *Läkarhus* (Uppsala: Läkarhus A.B., n.d.).

[30] *Statistisk undersökning rörande de allmänna försäkringskassornas utgifter för läkarvård m.m. 1963* (Stockholm: Riksförsäkringsverket, 1966), pp. 15–16.

[31] The figures for 1958 and 1963 are in ibid. The figures for 1955 and 1958 are in *Statistisk undersökning rörende de allmänna sjukkassornas utgifter för lakarvård m.m. 1958* (Stockholm: Riksförsäkringsanstalten, 1960), pp. 42–43.

tion. A rise in charges could lead a government to conclude either that its fee schedule was obsolete or that profiteering existed. In 1958 the government concluded that the problem presented a little of both: it raised some fees slightly and thereafter extended price controls over provincial hospital chiefs and some others. The adoption of formal collective bargaining in 1965—described in chapter III—was supposed to introduce a regular mechanism for resolving these disputes. But these contracts could govern the fees only of the doctors with part-time public appointments, and they left untouched the charges by the increasing number of full-time private practitioners.

Position of the Medical Profession

Income

Under any service benefits system—whether fee-for-service, salary, or capitation—pay rates lag behind prices in the free market, particularly during economic expansion. The pay rates are tied to statutes or formal contracts and are ultimately limited by the rates of social security taxes. Therefore pay rates change irregularly and by large increments, instead of by steady accretions following the market. In private practice and in unregulated cash benefits systems, doctors have greater freedom to try to set fees in accordance with general price movements and their own income goals.

The difference between statutory and private fees was demonstrated in France during the 1950's. The fees set by official procedures as the basis for reimbursement lagged behind price rises in the economy. But doctors' charges were not controlled and kept pace with price rises for other services and commodities.[32] The widening discrepancy between charges and reimbursements led to the public protests described earlier. The success of a cash benefits scheme, with controls over charges, depends on the stability of prices throughout the economy. One reason for the French medical profession's harmonious adjustment to controls over charges during the 1960's was the price stability achieved throughout the country by means of the de Gaulle government's "hard money" policies.

Even after charges are controlled, doctors can earn considerable incomes under cash benefits systems based on fee-for-service. Table 8 shows gross incomes estimated from insurance practice by French office practitioners in 1963, according to a study of the receipts filed with sick funds. Their true net incomes are slightly higher: doctors' total gross incomes may be

[32] Michaux, "Revenu du groupe médical" (note 7), p. 102; and Alain Vessereau, "L'évolution des dépenses médicales en 1957 et 1958," *Notes et documents*, no. 1 (First Trimester 1960), p. 24.

TABLE 8. GROSS INCOMES OF FRENCH OFFICE PRACTITIONERS, FROM NATIONAL HEALTH INSURANCE, 1963 (IN FRANCS)

	Lower Quartile	Median	Upper Quartile	Number of Doctors
All office practitioners	25,000	45,000	85,000	(5,181)
General practitioners	15,000	35,000	65,000	(3,420)
General surgery	35,000	85,000	125,000	(314)
Neurosurgery	50,000	70,000	100,000	(16)
Obstetrics and gynecology	25,000	65,000	125,000	(144)
Anesthesiology	35,000	65,000	125,000	(41)
Pediatrics	15,000	45,000	75,000	(117)
Cardiology	40,000	75,000	95,000	(85)
Gastroenterology	25,000	55,000	125,000	(63)
Rheumatology	7,500	25,000	65,000	(37)
Urology	15,000	65,000	125,000	(29)
Thoracic medicine	25,000	45,000	95,000	(109)
Ophthalmology	35,000	65,000	95,000	(162)
Otorhinolaryngology	25,000	45,000	125,000	(141)
Stomatology	25,000	40,000	65,000	(115)
Dermatology and venereology	35,000	55,000	75,000	(54)
Neuropsychiatry	15,000	35,000	65,000	(137)
Radiology	55,000	125,000	175,000	(197)

as much as 20 per cent higher than the figures in Table 8, because of private fees not reported through social security; but between 20 and 35 per cent of gross incomes are spent on practice expenses.[33] One-quarter of the doctors earned less than the figure for the "lower quartile"; half earned less than the "median," and half earned more; one-quarter earned more than the "upper quartile." Fee-for-service works to the advantage of the specialties that can perform inexpensive procedures very rapidly—such as radiology, ophthalmology, and otorhinolaryngology—and specialties whose procedures are few but expensive, such as surgery and obstetrics. The low earnings for neuropsychiatry, pediatrics, and rheumatology illustrate how fee-for-service works to the disadvantage of the supportive specialties.

French doctors earn considerably more than the rest of the population, more than higher administrators in business and industry, and more than salaried professionals in government. The comparative figures are in Table 9.[34]

[33] Inspection Générale de la Sécurité Sociale, *Rapport Annuel 1964* (Paris: Inspection Générale de la Sécurité Sociale, 1965), pp. 212–13. The free market exchange rate is 1 F = $0.18. The data were grouped in the published source, and therefore the medians and quartiles are estimated by taking the mid-points of the groups containing the median doctors and the quartile doctors.

[34] Mean incomes for doctors are taken from ibid., pp. 212–13. The figures for business and industrial occupations appear in, R. Padieu, "Les salaires dans l'industrie, le commerce et les services en 1963," *Études et conjonctures*, vol. 20, no. 11 (November 1965), pp. 19, 51. Except where otherwise indicated in Table 9, the business and industrial employees are men employed full time. The nonmedical mean incomes are estimated from the reports submitted by employers to the tax collection office of the government at the end of 1963.

Table 9. Annual Incomes in Medicine and Other Occupations, France, 1963 (in Francs)

	Mean Incomes
Gross incomes of doctors from National Health Insurance:	
All office practitioners	60,000
General practitioners	47,500
General surgery	94,900
Obstetrics and gynecology	78,500
Pediatrics	51,000
Radiology	131,900
Salaries and wages in industry, commerce and services:	
All employed persons, including women and part-time persons	9,952
All male employed persons	10,343
Highest ranking managers	41,194
Middle managers	31,409
Engineers	30,957
Technicians	15,264
Administrators	19,176
White-collar workers	9,627
Skilled workers	9,035
Blue-collar workers	6,384
	Salary Scale in Largest Cities
Salaries of professionals in government:	
University professor	34,940
Director of a *lycée*	13,820–34,940
Professor *agrégé* in a *lycée*	13,495–34,940
Elementary school teacher	8,245–17,340
Judges:	
Maitre des requêtes, Conseil d'État	27,390–34,940
Auditeur, Conseil d'État	13,495–25,585
Greffier en chef, Cours de cassation	29,150
Magistrate of first grade	26,140–34,940
Magistrate of second grade	16,645–34,940

The capacity of fee-for-service operating on a cash benefits principle to produce very high incomes by national standards is illustrated also by the figures from Sweden. Table 10 compares the median incomes of physicians and other economically active persons, according to the government tax records for 1959. Either fees or salaries, or both, give doctors an unusually

The salaries for professionals employed by government were calculated by Mme. Denise Walbert from *Classement hiérarchique des grades et emplois des personnels civils et militaires de l'état: régime général* (Paris: Ministère d'État Chargé de la Réforme Administrative, Direction Générale de l'Administration et de la Fonction Publique, 7th ed., Brochure no. 1042, 18 November 1963); and from Ministère d' État Chargé de la Réforme Administrative, "Décret No. 63–1146 du 19 novembre 1963 portant majoration des rémunérations des personnels civils et militaires de l'État," *Journal officiel de la République Française*, vol. 95 (21 November 1963), pp. 10372–73.

Table 10. Median Incomes in Medicine and Other Occupations, Sweden, 1959

	Median Incomes (in Kronor)	Number of Doctors in Sample
Physicians:		
Full-time private practitioners	46,000	(876)
District medical officers	52,000	(461)
Chiefs of service in hospitals	68,000	(934)
Lower ranks in hospitals	41,000	(1,046)
All economically active persons:	9,248	
Employers and self-employed		
All persons	8,454	
Mining, manufacturing, etc.	9,988	
Commerce	11,399	
Professions	11,244	
Salaried employees and wage-earners		
All persons	9,387	
Mining, manufacturing, etc.	10,381	
Commerce	7,380	

good position in Sweden. The highest pay is earned by the service chiefs and DMO's who collect both fees and salaries. Even the junior staff members of hospitals—who are paid entirely by salary—achieve very high earnings by Swedish standards: in order not to lose doctors to private practice, the government must pay salaries comparable to the net earnings from fees earned by the private practitioners.[35]

Whether fee-for-service results in wide or narrow income differences depends partly on how it is administered and also on many special conditions of medical practice. The introduction of national health insurance tends to standardize the charges of the medical profession for particular acts, but the official fee schedule is not sufficient to standardize incomes.[36] Inequalities are greater within the French than within the Swedish medical professions, as Table 11 demonstrates. A reason arising from the payment system is the freedom to perform specialty procedures: in France only licensed specialists may perform procedures in that field for reimbursement under social secur-

[35] *Sjukhus och öppen vård: betänkande av öhs-kommittén* (Stockholm: Kungl. Inrikesdepartmentet, Statens Offentliga Utredningar, 1963, Number 21), p. 398; and *Statistisk årsbok för Sverige* (Stockholm: Statistiska Centralbyran, 1961), p. 287. Only one per cent of the labor force earned more than 50,000 kr. annually, but probably every hospital service chief, every professor of medicine, and many private practitioners were included. The distribution by income brackets appears in *Statistisk årsbok för Sverige* (1962 edition), p. 300. The free market exchange rate has been 1 kr. = $0.19.

[36] The widespread uniformity of charges is reported in a French survey of general practitioners, "Une enquête sur le budget des familles médicales," *Concours médical*, vol. 83, no. 51 (30 December 1961), pp. 6803, 6805. The survey also reports the wide spread in work loads that leads to a great range in incomes among French doctors.

TABLE 11. INCOME DISTRIBUTIONS OF OFFICE PRACTITIONERS, FRANCE AND SWEDEN

Incomes of Private Office Practitioners, in Francs or Kronor	France 1963	Sweden 1959
Under 10,000	15%	
10,000–19,999	9	15%
20,000–29,999	9	
30,000–39,999	9	22
40,000–49,999	9	21
50,000–59,999	9	18
60,000–69,999	8	10
70,000–79,999	6	
80,000–89,999	6	
190,000–99,999	4	14
100,000–149,999	11	
150,000 and over	5	
	100%	100%
	(5,181)	(876)

ity, while any Swedish doctor may perform any procedure under the fee schedule. Consequently, the more remunerative acts and the work load are spread less evenly across the profession in France than in Sweden. Another reason for the different income distribution is the doctor-population ratios in the two countries. France's more numerous doctors earn considerably less than their fully employed Swedish counterparts if they work in overdoctored areas, whether they are young or old. Finally, another cause of the difference in distribution might be incentives. In contrast to France, Sweden has had a more steeply graduated income tax to pay for its generous social services and national defense; its tax collections are more effective, and hard work and high fees may be discouraged.[37]

Fee-for-service under the cash benefits systems of France and Sweden results in distinct differences by age, according to Table 12.[38] The middle-aged earn more than the young or old. We do not know whether the individual's career earnings follow the same cycle, since the data compare different age groups at the same time and do not trace career curves.[39] The

[37] Based on Inspection Générale de la Sécurité Sociale, *Rapport Annuel 1964* (note 33), p. 213; and *Sjukhus och öppen vård* (note 35), p. 398. The franc and krona exchange nearly at par. The data are sufficient for a comparison of distributions but are not identical: the Swedish figures report all income, the French figures are only the total fees processed under social security. A measure of spread in a numerical distribution—the semi-interquartile range—is much larger for the French than for the Swedish data. Measuring half the difference between the upper and lower quartiles, this statistic is 30,000 F for France and 12,500 kr. for Sweden.

[38] Inspection Générale de la Sécurité Sociale, *Rapport Annuel 1964* (note 33), p. 217; and *Sjukhus och öppen vård* (note 35), p. 398.

[39] Cross-sectional surveys usually show that the old earn less than the middle-aged, and many economists have concluded erroneously that career cycles follow this curve. But the

TABLE 12. INCOMES OF DOCTORS BY AGE, FRANCE AND SWEDEN

Ages of Doctors	France (Means in Francs), 1963		Sweden (Medians in Kronor), 1959, Private Practitioners
	G.P.'s	Surgeons	
29 and under	16,000	—	
30–39	50,000	78,000	
35–44			47,000
40–49	52,000	108,000	
45–54			49,000
50–59	50,000	102,000	
55–64			49,000
60–69	35,000	87,000	
65 and over			42,000
70 and over	18,000	37,000	

distribution of medical incomes is less unequal in Sweden than in France. Perhaps the career cycle has a narrower amplitude in Sweden.

Under fee-for-service in private practice, a distinguished physician can earn a much higher than average income by charging higher fees, by doing more work, or both. If national health insurance uses service benefits or cash benefits with controls, the leading doctors usually prefer to practice outside. Their patients can be reimbursed by the sick funds only if no controls exist on any doctor or if they are exempted from the usual fee schedule. As we said earlier, France is now attempting to induce the leading physicians to practice under social security contracts by allowing them to charge as they wish. At the time of the survey of social security receipts in 1963, two *départements* in the sample were experimenting with this method. The results foreshadowed the wider income distribution that would probably arise under any national health insurance scheme that enforced controls over some but gave complete freedom to the doctors who were already earning more in private practice. On the average, the leading doctors earned 40 per cent more than the others. The differentials were widest in obstetrics and gynecology, dermatology, gastroenterology, and pediatrics.[40] The survey does not report whether these doctors were even more prosperous than they might have been under completely private practice. Under social security, probably they had fewer collection problems.

Recruitment

Both France and Sweden have cash benefits systems that result in a high income for the average doctor. But recruitment into the medical profession

few studies of career earnings often show that individuals earn steadily more during their working lives or level off after middle age. Gary S. Becker, *Human Capital* (New York: National Bureau of Economic Research, 1964), pp. 139–42.

[40] Inspection Générale de la Sécurité Sociale, *Rapport Annuel 1964* (note 33), p. 224.

differs markedly. France has always enrolled many medical students and has a large number of doctors; Sweden's profession is small. France does not welcome foreign doctors into its practice; Sweden needs many foreign-trained doctors to staff its hospitals and to fill some of the rural district medical officer posts. France has long debated whether a surplus of doctors was real and permanent and whether medical school enrollments should be reduced; Sweden has long debated how to expand the medical schools.

The different situations show how many causes besides doctors' pay affect the actual operation of medical care. In both countries, the pay is sufficient to attract numerous applicants to medical school. But French education affords less intensive scientific training and clinical practice, and therefore both the entering and graduating classes are larger. Sweden's medical education provides more thorough laboratory and clinical supervision, and class size is limited at entrance. France has a larger labor force, and all its organizations and occupations may be staffed more liberally than Sweden's.[41]

Conclusion: The Dilemmas of Cash Benefits Systems

Medical associations sometimes press for cash benefits schemes in the hope doctors will be completely free of any scrutiny and regulation by the sick funds and government. But it is utopian to think that the patient's relations with the doctor can remain in a completely unregulated private market, while his relations with the source of money are a regulated public transaction. Disputes and public intervention will be avoided only if the medical profession voluntarily restrains all its charges, but such unanimity and harmony may not be easily preserved for long. Cash benefits schemes may merely postpone and not eliminate trouble.

Sometimes cash benefits schemes were initiated under a vague agreement that doctors' charges should be reasonably related to reimbursement rates, but this receives competing interpretations when a rise in the national price level brings about wider differentials between doctors' charges and the funds' payments to the patients. Pressures may arise for restraint of doctors' fees: patients may complain they are not getting their money's worth; managers of funds, the trade unions, and the political parties of the Left may claim the original statute conferred upon the funds a responsibility to

[41] The debate over a possible surplus of doctors in France is summarized in, Henri Hatzfeld, *Le grand tournant de la médecine libérale* (Paris: Les Éditions Ouvrières, 1963), pp. 253–56. The shortage in Sweden and the recent increases in medical school enrollments are described in "The Swedish Medical Association's Annual Report to the W.M.A. for 1965" (Stockholm: Läkarförbundet, 1966, mimeographed), pp. 1–3. Compared to nearly all other developed countries, Sweden long had fewer medical schools relative to its population; compared to many developed countries, each Swedish medical school has smaller annual admissions. The statistics can be found in *World Directory of Medical Schools* (Geneva: World Health Organization, 1953, 1957, and 1963).

insure full care at fair costs; the government may worry about the erosion of public confidence in the social services; the Ministry of Finance may be searching for all possible levers to restrain rising prices in the economy. A bitter conflict can result, if the medical association replies that the public system has relations only with the patients and not with the doctors, that guarantees of economic freedom were a condition for medical participation, and that any change is a breach of a commitment. However, peace can be established if the medical association and funds agree to negotiate a schedule of reimbursement and if the doctors co-operate. But the resultant system is hardly different from a service benefits scheme using fee-for-service.

At the time of their creation, cash benefits schemes seem to promise fewer controls and less paper work than service benefits methods. It is assumed by doctors that they will have no dealings with the sick funds and government, that their billing and collections will be a private relationship with the patient, and that their own books will be secret. But if the doctor is expected to conform to a fee schedule, the sick funds may have to communicate their policies and complaints to the individual doctor, get full information about each of his bills, and investigate his practice to determine the justice of doubtful charges. This unexpected intervention may be greatly resented by doctors. The amount of investigation and communication may be less in a service benefits scheme: where the funds pay the doctor directly, they know much more about his individual fees and total finances; under service benefits, the doctor takes for granted regular contact with the funds. Sanctions against the doctor under cash benefits are indirect, public, and clumsy: since the fund pays him nothing, it can hurt him only by refusing to pay his patients and by warning all subscribers not to visit him. Under service benefits, the funds can withhold some payments to the doctor without affecting care and without notifying the public.

A cash benefits scheme has an important advantage over service benefits in that important and expensive physicians can participate in health insurance. Under a service benefits system, their fees would be too high, and patients could see them only privately. But under cash benefits, their high fees would not bankrupt the fund, and a patient would recover some of his expenses from the fund, as he could not under service benefits. The problem is to restrict the number of eminent doctors; if too many charge too much, the public may demand higher reimbursement than the funds can afford.

Cost sharing by the patient (whether under service benefits or cash benefits schemes) and the patient's initial payment under reimbursement systems are often commended as devices to discourage unnecessary work by physicians. But the danger is that the need to pay will cause some patients to postpone seeking needed care. The poor can be specially exempted. But this remedy reintroduces the "means" test that national health insurance was supposed to eliminate.

IX

EFFECTS OF SALARIES

Salaried methods of payment are preferred by many officials because they are easy to administer. Personnel costs can be predicted during the next fiscal year; they increase only if the administrator decides to grant overtime or pay raises, and they do not fluctuate according to the efforts of doctors or the demands of patients. Paper work is minimized, since the doctor does not bill the patient or the fund for each procedure.

Salaried methods also are said to benefit both patient and doctor. The patient pays the doctor nothing, is not burdened by fees in times of trouble, and is not deterred by financial barriers. The doctor has no collection problems, and his income is easily predicted.

Encouraging Good Medicine and Discouraging Medical Neglect

Thorough Care

Salaries are paid for spans of time. If work increases during those hours, the doctor does not gain; if work is slack, he does not lose. Therefore salaried systems may be vulnerable by not providing enough incentive for extra effort and by omitting effective penalties for neglecting patients' needs. Salaried methods are not self-regulating. However, salaries usually are paid to persons who work in organizations with rules and with a hierarchical arrangement of positions. Therefore the structure and operation of the larger organization can supplement the simple mechanics of payment by providing methods for reviewing the doctor's performance, rewarding extra effort, and penalizing neglect. Whether salaried doctors give good care depends on the size of their salaries, how the hospital or polyclinic is administered, and the values of the country's medical profession.

Salaried pay and the shortage of doctors might be expected to lead to hasty examination and treatment in (for example) the hospitals of Sweden. But several factors militate against it. The salaries earned by the full-time and nearly full-time doctors are very high. The chiefs-of-service are allowed a part-time private practice in the hospitals' outpatient departments in return for an obligation to work conscientiously during their salaried hours. The lower ranks are filled by a select number of young aspiring specialists who learn good medicine by practicing it and who need to impress the chiefs in order to gain help in their careers. Professional controls of this sort govern the younger hospital doctors throughout Europe and apparently result in conscientious care at their ranks, particularly in the teaching hospitals, and even when the salaries are lower than in Sweden.

The hierarchical medical staff organization can lead to performance that is even too conscientious. One of the complaints by some office practitioners in Sweden is that hospital residents ignore their diagnoses and, in order to impress their service chiefs, perform complete workups of referred patients.

Satisfaction with the doctor depends on a population's customary expectations. Therefore even when an observer may think doctors are working too quickly, many patients may be satisfied. Some of my informants in Sweden thought that hospital doctors had to hurry because of very heavy work loads, particularly in urban outpatient departments, where many patients come because local office doctors have excessive waiting lists. But most patients may not think doctors neglect them, since they are accustomed to the fast tempo of urban life; many people hurry throughout the society because of labor shortages and the widespread understaffing of organizations, and relations in organizations customarily seem far more impersonal than in many other countries. Of the hospital inpatients interviewed by Israel, three-fifths said they had as much contact with the medical staff as they wanted, and over two-thirds said that doctors had enough time to talk to them.[1] (Nevertheless, these levels of satisfaction are not as high as those in surveys in some other countries, and critics of salaried pay and of Swedish medical organization may think the proportions of complaint too large.)

The fact that patients' satisfaction depends on their expectations is further illustrated by Poland. One might predict that Polish doctors should be very hurried and Polish patients should be very critical. The country has always been short of doctors, and the profession was decimated by the Nazi extermination of the Jews.[2] The government's austere economic policies have

[1] Joachim Israel, "Vad Tycker Patienterna?" *Tidskrift för Sveriges Sjuksköterskor*, vol. 28, no. 22 (November 1961), pp. 856–57. Surveys of patients in other countries record even higher levels of satisfaction with the work of the salaried hospital doctors. E.g., *Family Needs and the Social Services* (London: George Allen & Unwin, 1961), pp. 113–21; and Gordon Forsyth, "Is the Health Service Doing Its Job?", *New Society*, no. 264 (19 October 1967), p. 547. But a substantial minority in England would prefer more thorough communication and more personalized care by the doctors. Ann Cartwright, *Human Relations and Hospital Care* (London: Routledge & Kegan Paul, 1964), chap. 7.

[2] Marcin Kacprzak and Boguslaw Kozusznik, *Health Care in People's Poland* (Warsaw: Polonia Publishing House, 1957), pp. 10–14, 25–26.

kept doctors' salaries low. Some periodicals that express the viewpoints of the liberal professions claim that the underpayment of doctors results in hasty care for most patients and under-the-table payments by anyone seeking adequate attention.[3] But Polish patients seem satisfied. Of the inpatients in a Cracow hospital interviewed by Csorba, 93 per cent said they had complete confidence in their doctors' ability, 90 per cent said that doctors' care in that service was superior to any treatments they could have gotten elsewhere, and 76 per cent said that the doctors were interested in them. Most patients thought that the doctors' knowledge and efficiency were more important than bedside manners.[4]

As in Sweden and Poland, the doctors of the Soviet Union may devote to their patients enough attention to keep them healthy and satisfied. The time schedules of Soviet doctors seem to be a function of the doctor-population ratios and of Russian work habits rather than an automatic consequence of salaried payment. One sometimes reads complaints of hurried work and brusque behavior.[5] Some polyclinics with personnel shortages once attempted to reduce patients' waiting times by setting work norms, so the *vrach* must see a certain number of patients each hour and must avoid excessive time to one.[6] Today many urban polyclinics and hospitals have numerous doctors, the work pace actually appears more leisurely than in the West, and doctors (particularly hospital specialists) may have more opportunities for personal conversations with patients than do their Western counterparts.[7] One reads about excessive time devoted to writing records instead of working with the patient.[8] The complaints come from doctors and from the lay newspapers and magazines that often publish overstated criticisms of the medical services in order to keep the Ministry of Health on its toes. But possibly these criticisms are exaggerated, since the objective reasons may not exist. The Soviet Union has simpler patient records than all but one of the countries that I have visited, and Soviet doctors should have much less paper work than do Westerners.

[3] For example, Wilhelmina Skulska, "Sluzba Zdrowia I Co Dalej?" *Kultura* (5 December 1965), pp. 5, 9.

[4] Helena Csorba, *Szpital-Pacjent: System Spoleczny Kliniki Internistycznej* (Wroclaw: Zaklad Narodowy Imienia Ossolinskich, 1966), pp. 292–300.

[5] E. g., "Vie ne pravii, Tovarich Minister: po povrei otvieta chitatielam," *Literaturnaya Gazeta*, 11 June 1960, p. 6; and Vladimir Dyagilev, "Vrachebnye oshibki i zhiznennye sledstviia," *Oktyabr*, no. 9 (September 1968), pp. 175–87. These complaints were common during the 1930's, when the country suffered from a shortage of doctors.

[6] Mark G. Field, *Doctor and Patient in Soviet Russia* (Cambridge: Harvard University Press, 1957), pp. 134–44, 197–98.

[7] Observations by C. Fraser Brockington, "Public Health in Russia," *Lancet* (21 July 1956), p. 140; R. S. Saxton, "Soviet General Practitioners and Polyclinics," *British Medical Journal Supplement* (17 August 1957), pp. 95–97; T. F. Fox, "Russia Revisited: Impressions of Soviet Medicine," *Lancet* (9 October 1954), pp. 752–53; and by myself.

[8] Field, *Doctor and Patient* (note 6), pp. 138–42.

The doctor in most urban polyclinics today has little reason for hasty work. His patient load is not too high. A *vrach* is assigned an *uchastok* of about 4,000 people and only sees the adults regularly. The polyclinic's pediatricians see the children. The polyclinic and its connected hospital have many specialists with some or much advanced training, and *vrachi* seem to make many referrals. Receptionists at the polyclinics send some patients directly to specialists, instead of to their *vrachi* first. The specialist at a polyclinic may have had three or six months training in his specialty. Actually he is a former *vrach* with additional qualifications, and his polyclinic function is to deal with referrals beyond the competence of the typical *vrach*. Soviet hospital specialists, like those in other countries, have had many more years of hospital training than do the intermediate specialists. Sometimes the hospital assigns one of its better trained specialists to help in the polyclinic. As an example of staffing patterns in 1961, I visited a *rayon* in Kiev with 44,000 people, of whom 40,000 used the polyclinic. The combined hospital-polyclinic had 128 doctors, of whom eleven were *vrachi* responsible for eleven *uchastoks*. 11,600 of the residents were children, so the average *vrach* had a panel of about 3,500 patients. This is not an excessive number, since he has few time-consuming patients: he has no children, he has few elderly people, and accidents at work usually are treated by the factory's doctor.

Soviet doctors give fewer diagnostic tests and treatments than Westerners,[9] but this may be due less to salary than to a clinical tradition arising out of shortages of equipment, technicians, and laboratories. Therefore, even if payment by salary were replaced by fee-for-service in the U.S.S.R., there still might be fewer X-rays, blood tests, other diagnostic procedures, and optional treatments than in Western countries.

Even the severe personnel shortages and time pressures during the 1930's and during World War II may not have produced as much hasty care and public discontent in the U.S.S.R. as one might expect. The Harvard Russian Research Center interviews with Russian escapees shortly after the war revealed a remarkably high level of satisfaction with the doctor-patient relationship. Soviet medical services were one of the most popular accomplishments of the régime and one of the features fewest would recommend changing. Escapees in America preferred Soviet socialized medicine over the American system. Most thought Soviet doctors would not have treated them better under private fee-for-service arrangements. As one would expect from the paucity of rural medical services during the 1930's and 1940's, the escapees from the countryside were more critical than former city dwellers, but even a majority of them were favorable.[10]

But Soviet salaried medical practice is not perfect. Its limitations are reflected by the presence—and apparently heavy use—of several dozen polyclinics operating on a fee-for-service basis. The polyclinics are owned

[9] Milton I. Roemer, "Highlights of Soviet Health Services," *Milbank Memorial Fund Quarterly*, vol. 15, no. 4 (October 1962), pp. 381, 385; and J. B. Harman, "Hospital Medicine in Russia," *Lancet* (4 April 1959), pp. 726–27.

[10] Field, *Doctor and Patient* (note 6), chaps. 11–13; and Alex Inkeles and Raymond A. Bauer, *The Soviet Citizen* (Cambridge: Harvard University Press, 1959), pp. 59, 236–39, 349.

by the government, apparently originated as experiments, and employ doctors who spend most of the day in full-time salaried jobs in the regular health service. The reasons given by the patients in a survey reflect some of the complaints about the free polyclinics, where they saw their usual general practitioners. One-fourth preferred the paying polyclinic because its doctors were older and more experienced. (As I shall say later, the salary structure used in the Soviet Union gives both the incentive and the opportunity to move into specialty practice and administration, and the G.P.'s are young.) One-fourth liked the paying polyclinic because—if they wished to pay personally—they could get multiple opinions. National medical care schemes usually prevent patients on their own initiative from getting several opinions on the same matter, a necessary financial control that is one reason for the survival of private practice in many countries. Many patrons said they came to the paying polyclinic because of the free choice of doctor.[11] In other words, they occasionally visited the paying polyclinic because of limitations in how the salaried polyclinic was administered, not because of neglect arising out of the salaried method of payment.

Some of the predicted malfunctions of salaried pay occur in underdeveloped countries, but remuneration alone is not a sufficient explanation. The performance of doctors in public services in these societies is affected by many circumstances that could produce the same results as deficient motivation due to a salaried service and low pay. For example, the visitor may see hurried and impersonal care by a salaried doctor in a hospital outpatient department, but this may be due less to the salaried system than to the very large number of patients relative to the supply of doctors. If some doctors are pessimistic about the possibility of helping patients, a more important reason than money is the fact that many patients in underdeveloped countries come at late stages of their illness. The visitor sees little of the communication between doctor and patient that he expects in the West, but an important reason is the wide social class differences between doctor and public patient. Many public hospital chiefs-of-service avoid their rushed and uncomfortable outpatient departments; the junior doctors on duty often are forced to diagnose superficially by symptoms and must treat hastily.[12] Raising pay might elicit improved performance, but other social and medical reforms would be necessary to motivate the doctor as well.

[11] Varvara Karbovskaia, "Otniud ne lirika," *Literaturnaya Gazeta*, 12 October 1965, p. 1.

[12] On the professional frustrations of the public hospital doctors when treating lower class patients in underdeveloped countries, see Ahmed Kamel Mazen, "Hospital Administration in Egypt," *Journal of the Ministry of Health* (Cairo), vol. 1, no. 3 (January 1960), p. 62; Ahmed Kamel Mazen, *Development of the Medical Care Program of the Egyptian Region of the United Arab Republic* (Stanford: dissertation for Ph.D., Stanford University, 1961), p. 276; and William A. Glaser, *Medical Organization and the Social Setting* (New York: Atherton Press, 1970), chap. 4.

Attendance

In return for a salary, the doctor must spend designated hours in the public hospital or in the polyclinic. Where salaries are high and professional organization is strong, doctors come and go as scheduled. Even in less affluent countries such as Spain and Italy, the salaried specialists in polyclinics come for their fixed hours, since their absence would leave large waiting lines of patients and would be too obvious.

But in many countries—such as the southern European and Middle Eastern countries that I visited, and other underdeveloped countries—a common problem is behavior of the chiefs-of-service in the public hospitals. The proportion of the service chief's time devoted to public practice does not match the proportion of income from that source, and problems of priority arise. Public hospital appointments obligate the service chiefs in urban hospitals of most countries to spend half or more of each work day in the hospitals. Also, since they are service chiefs, they are supposedly on call at all other times. But profits from private practice often have risen faster than public salaries, and many of my informants said that three-fourths or four-fifths of their incomes came from private practice. The imbalance was largest for surgeons and obstetricians. Usually the imbalance is greatest in the poorest countries with the lowest salary scales.

As a result, many lay administrators, nurses, and junior hospital doctors in southern Europe and the Middle East told me that service chiefs often came late, left early, and spent part of their official time in nonmedical activities, such as lunch. Also, they said, service chiefs were rarely called back to the hospital after official hours; the chief resident would be responsible for emergencies and, at most, the service chief would give advice by phone. Since the service chief is supreme in his field, he risks no sanctions: in most countries he is more powerful than the hospital director; the governing body (whether a local board or a national Ministry) customarily gives him total professional freedom, and his subordinates (such as younger doctors on his service and nurses) avoid antagonizing him.

Certainly one should not make blanket generalizations about all service chiefs: there are conscientious doctors who, despite low official salaries and the temptations of private practice, give maximum attention to their public hospital services. But the problem in hospital administration is to adopt a system that will standardize obligations and that will provide appropriate incentives and rewards. Then conscientious attendance will not be an individual choice. Several countries with these difficulties, such as France, have raised salaries and have made the chiefs' obligations more explicit. The problem for Spain, Italy, Greece, and the less affluent countries on other continents is to raise enough money to pay salaries commensurate with the chiefs' net earnings from private practice.

If adequate salaries replace low or no pay, attendance and performance will improve. An example is Great Britain. Care to public patients probably is more regularized today than before the National Health Service. Since the consultant is paid for a certain number of sessions, he is expected at the hospital at specified times. The hospital administrator must certify to the Regional Hospital Board periodically that all doctors were present in accordance with their contracts and that absences were justified. In case of prolonged absences, the consultant is replaced by a *locum tenens* paid on a sessional or weekly basis. Therefore, organization and salary have introduced work discipline and accountability. Before the National Health Service, when most consultants were not paid for their hospital work and when hospitals were much less systematically organized, consultants usually had no fixed hours and might come and go as they wished. A consultant could send an assistant in his place but cannot now.

The introduction of salaries for younger British doctors may have changed their orientations toward the patient. Before the appointed day, registrars and house officers were badly paid trainees getting free specialty training. Now they are paid to give service. Once they may have been concerned with what the patient could teach them, but now they have official obligations to the patient. Once the ward patient was the object of the doctors' charity; now he is the taxpayer, fully aware that he is paying the doctors' salaries. Because of the salary grades and more formalized rank structure, possibly the consultants screen their subordinates more carefully now before recommending promotions and delegating higher clinical responsibilities.

Office and Home Visits

Logically one would expect contacts between doctor and patient to be minimized by salary payments. The doctor gains nothing financially by working harder during his fixed hours; instead, he should be motivated by a desire to conserve effort.

But type of payment does not correlate directly with the frequency of contacts between doctor and patient. Among countries with salaried ambulatory care, one can find both high and low rates for office and home visits. Factors other than the payment method may be at least as important, such as the number of available doctors, the demands of the population, and the clinical customs of the medical profession. Although the statistical data for reliable comparisons are lacking, I suspect that Soviet general practitioners have a higher frequency of contacts with each patient and make more home visits than their Polish counterparts, despite the formal similarities in the methods of payment and patient assignment. The essential difference is that

Soviet cities have many more doctors than Polish cities. Therefore the Polish G.P.—in his need to cope with a heavier patient load—may use more time-saving devices, such as referral of time-consuming patients to the polyclinic's specialists or to the outpatient departments of hospitals. Because the Polish polyclinic doctor is less able than the Soviet *vrach* to cope with the full work load during his salaried hours, private practice after the official work day is far more common in Poland than in the U.S.S.R.

The Soviet *vrach* makes many referrals because he is expected to do so for clinical reasons. Compared to the Polish general practitioner, he may make fewer referrals—for time-conserving reasons—of patients whom he is competent to treat. As I said earlier, Soviet polyclinics have many specialists with less than a year of postgraduate training who are there to help the *vrachi*. Polish medical leaders prefer Western forms of training and licensing, have no intermediate grades of specialists, give specialty ratings only after several years of hospital training, and assign most of their specialists to hospitals. The Soviet polyclinic is part of the hospital, and the *vrach* is expected to refer difficult patients to his superiors in the medical hierarchy. But the Polish polyclinic is a separate organization, the Polish G.P. is more autonomous in clinical matters than the *vrach* (although less so than the Western G.P.), and he is expected to exercise more clinical responsibility than the *vrach*. As in the U.S.S.R., the Polish general practitioner is one of several G.P.'s and specialists assigned to a polyclinic. The city is divided into districts, and the general practitioner automatically is assigned all patients in his district.

Israel illustrates how the demands of a population can force a salaried medical service to maintain a high level of work. Israel has the world's highest utilization rates for general practice: *Kupat Holim* of *Histadrut* has over eight visits per subscriber each year, and some smaller sick funds have even higher rates; most countries average between four and five, and Sweden has less than three.[13] Some polyclinics may have been rushed during large

[13] Utilization rates of Israeli sick funds are published in the annual *Statistical Abstract of Israel*. Comparisons between Israel and other countries appear in, Judith Shuval, *Doctor-Patient Relationships in a Bureaucratic Medical Organization in Israel*, forthcoming; and Simon Btesh, "The Place of the Family Doctor," *Medical World*, vol. 98, no. 1 (January 1963), p. 11. A few countries, such as Germany, have higher rates of patient-doctor contacts, since national health insurance allows patients to go directly to specialists. "Volume and Cost of Sickness Benefits in Kind and Cash," *Bulletin of the International Social Security Association*, vol. 16, nos. 3–4 (March–April 1963), p. 57. The high demand by the Israeli population has several causes. Jews in much of the world—including Israeli immigrants from Europe and *Sabras* descended from Europeans—may be very attentive to their physical and mental feelings, quick to seek professional help, and eager for multiple medical opinions. See David Mechanic, "Religion, Religiosity, and Illness Behavior: The Special Case of the Jews," *Human Organization*, vol. 22, no. 3 (Fall 1963), pp. 202–8. Several of my informants believed that many Israelis feel that they have paid for medical services and that the money would be wasted if they didn't go to the doctor. Since most Israelis work on salary, a visit to the doctor does not cause a financial loss; some of my informants thought some urban patients used brief visits to the polyclinic as the opportunity to take the day off from work. Shuval's survey suggests that the less assimilated and lower-class Israelis have unusually high rates of visits, because the clinics are the most accessible sources of help during their difficult adjustment to a new society. *Doctor-Patient Relationships* (this footnote).

waves of immigration, but now enough doctors work in nearly all parts of the country—and possible surpluses exist in Tel Aviv and Jerusalem—so that time pressures have diminished. Some hospital doctors may be more rushed than they like—some *Kupat Holim* hospitals have patient loads exceeding 100 per cent of bed capacity—but the visitor hears few complaints that they minimize care because they get the same pay regardless of effort.

There exist two powerful moral forces militating against neglect of the patient in Israel. One is the high standards of the medical profession. Laxity by polyclinic or hospital doctors is strongly disapproved by the profession generally and by the doctors' immediate superiors. In some sick funds, if a G.P. is suspected of poor quality work or neglect, he may be kept out of solo practice and assigned a job under supervision, such as in an urban polyclinic. The Israel Medical Association and its members have long been hostile to the *Kupat Holim* of *Histadrut* and to some of the smaller sick funds, and therefore the profession is reluctant to donate to the funds time and effort beyond the obligations in the contracts. But the minimum duties to the patient are scrupulously honored.

The second important control over the quality and thoroughness of care is the Israeli patient, particularly the European immigrants and the *Sabras* of European lineage. Several hospital officials and medical administrators told me that they felt under continuous observation and pressure from the public and that any lapses would immediately arouse those common Israeli reactions, namely complaints to highers-up and criticism from the press.

Comparing Israelis with the populations of other countries he had visited, one administrator told me:

> The Jewish patient is different from the Gentile in approaching questions of health. Proverbs like "nothing too expensive for health" are typical. Thus our hospitals couldn't be built with unequal quality, or our patients wouldn't go to the poor ones. Even if we build a small hospital in the north with a small maternity ward with six beds, we have to equip the unit with full services, like a blood bank. . . . Competition among sick funds promising to give potential members the best facilities [results in such services]. . . . If our Jewish patients had to wait for a hospital bed [as long as in England], our doctors would be stoned in the street.

Capitation or salaried systems elsewhere may induce general practitioners to refer many patients to outpatient clinics of hospitals, particularly if they have many patients, since thereby doctors economize on their time. This may occur particularly if the G.P. is a solo practitioner, since he can claim that the hospital O.P.D. is better equipped than his office. Israel illustrates how the organization of medical care can deter unnecessary referrals to relieve the treating doctor of time-consuming patients. Urban general practitioners do not work alone but work in polyclinics possessing most necessary facilities for ambulatory care. The outpatient clinics of

Kupat Holim hospitals do not appear as elaborately equipped or as busy as in some other countries, because it is assumed that ordinary ambulatory care is rendered in the polyclinic. Since several *Kupat Holim* hospitals operate at more than full capacity in inpatient care, the hospital doctors would protest to the polyclinic management or to higher officials if any G.P.'s were burdening them further with unnecessary referrals. Therefore my interviews uncovered little evidence of over-referral in Israel.

However, the high levels of effort under salaried payment do not extend to home visiting in Israel, since the disincentives of pay coincide with clinical tradition. Home visits have long been a small fraction of all contacts. Today *Kupat Holim* has one of the lowest rates of home visits of any national health insurance scheme, namely one out of ten contacts between patient and general practitioner.[14] Attempts to manipulate the payment system and the work load to increase home visiting have been fruitless. For example in the 1960's each urban general practitioner was given a list of no more than 1,400 subscribers, a work load easier than in England and Holland. During part of his day set aside for the purpose, the G.P. was supposed to make home visits. But many doctors reduced their work hours under their contracts. As before, home visits were performed for fees in the private practices conducted by these doctors after work in the polyclinic.

Preventive Medicine

Fee-for-service rivets doctors' attention on the diagnostic and therapeutic procedures that can easily be itemized. Usually preventive medicine is not sufficiently rewarded in fee schedules, and the average therapist in those countries with fee schedules does little of it. But salaries can give large rewards and an adequate position in the medical profession to specialties where work cannot easily be itemized. Therefore most specialists in public health and preventive medicine in the world are salaried functionaries of governments or of other organizations.

Salaried systems can be adapted to any set of job definitions. Therefore salaries can be paid to ordinary doctors for the performance of both therapeutic and preventive procedures. If fee-for-service were used, the doctor might neglect the preventive part of his work, since it would be less profitable. With the aid of salaried remuneration, the Soviet Union seems to have developed the most public-health-minded medical profession in the world. Hospitals and polyclinics include public health education and sanitary inspection in the daily work schedules of many of their clinicians. The hospital and polyclinic doctors are supposed to do much health teaching of

[14] Compare Table II in each national report in *Volume and Cost of Sickness Benefits in Kind and Cash: National Analyses* (Geneva: International Social Security Association, 1963). The Israeli figures are on p. 126.

patients who report ill, in addition to the usual diagnoses and treatments. One feature of the compensation system reinforces interest in preventive medicine: among the few payments by procedure available to the ordinary *vrach* are the fees for public health lectures given after his regular work hours.[15]

Sick Leaves

A professional is supposed to solve society's problems by means of his expert knowledge. The doctor is supposed to cure his patients and thereby solve the society's problems of staffing and stability. But it is not self-evident that society's needs can be met by thorough treatment of every individual complaining of discomfort. Perhaps society would gain more if some patients with minor or psychosomatic illnesses were urged to stay at work. Absenteeism might hamper urgent production. Therefore at times a doctor must choose sides in conflicts between patients and society.

In completely private practice using fee-for-service, the doctor's obligations appear to rest entirely with the cure of the patient by all available means. The payment system reinforces the doctor's belief that the cure of the individual patient has the highest priority: it is the patient and not the society at large that retains and pays the doctor; if the doctor bids the patient return to his family and job at once, he loses money. Fee-for-service under national health insurance or a national health service also makes the doctor patient-oriented, since his income rises as he performs more numerous and more complex diagnostic and therapeutic procedures.

However, payment by salary may confront the doctor with the conflicting goals that are hidden by other payment systems. The doctor is paid not by the patient but by an organization responsible for managing the society. His pay is not reduced if he decides that the patient should not be treated but should conform to other social requirements. The doctor may be rewarded through bonuses and promotions if he economizes in the use of medical services and if he induces patients to fulfill other social obligations.

These role conflicts are often experienced by salaried members of national health services when granting sick leaves, particularly during wars or rapid industrialization. Supervisors may chide doctors who grant too many sick leaves, and they may disallow some. The treating physician himself may easily absorb the idea that maximum production has priority over the patient's comfort, particularly if his office is in the plant. In the U.S.S.R. during war and during industrialization, absenteeism was condemned and

[15] Descriptions of the preventive work by the ordinary doctor appear in, John Burton, "Health Education in the U.S.S.R.," *Public Health*, vol. 69, no. 7 (April 1956), pp. 152–55; Brockington, "Public Health in Russia" (note 7), p. 140; and Roemer, "Soviet Health Services" (note 9), pp. 383–86.

doctors in the polyclinic and plant were urged to grant sick leaves sparingly.[16] Polish industrial physicians experienced similar role conflicts during the period of industrialization under the Stalinist government between 1951 and 1957.[17] Supplements to the basic salaries sometimes reinforced the reluctance to grant sick leaves. Often the Soviet and Polish industrial doctors shared in the factory-wide bonuses distributed for exceeding output norms, and therefore they had a direct personal interest in keeping workers on the job.[18] These role conflicts are not peculiar to Eastern Europe or to socialized medicine but can be found in any Western medical institution where the doctor has a double allegiance both to the patient and to an organization that pays him directly.

Rewarding Superior Performance

Excellent work is supposed to be recognized by higher pay, but remuneration systems do not bring about these results automatically. Under fee-for-service using direct payment, that doctor earns the highest income who performs the largest number of expensive procedures. He is the best doctor only if patients are wise enough to flock to him, and only if he is so unusual that he combines skill and speed. But often the highest incomes under fee-for-service are earned by fast workers in fields with high fees, particularly in regions with shortages of doctors. A cash benefits scheme can give high incomes to the better doctors, if their charges are not controlled and if patients are willing to pay a large difference between the doctors' charges and the official reimbursement. But patients may pay high fees to doctors who are fashionable, while the profession may have different judgments concerning their medical skill.

An unembellished salary system would give the highest pay to those doctors in the highest ranks and with the greatest seniority. Rank could relate to clinical skill, but seniority need not. However, salaried payment is the method that can most efficiently be designed to reward the superior doctor. And it is the method that can give the greatest power to the profession itself in identifying and rewarding superior performance. In fee-for-service

[16] Field, *Doctor and Patient* (note 6), pp. 162–80 passim; and Solomon M. Schwarz, *Labor in the Soviet Union* (New York: Frederick A. Praeger, 1952), pp. 311–15. Disability allowances are administered to discourage unjustified or prolonged sick leaves. The trade unions are responsible for social insurance, and their delegates periodically visit patients on sick leave, check whether the workers are still disabled, and review whether they are following doctors' orders. Gaston V. Rimlinger, "The Trade Union in Soviet Social Insurance," *Industrial and Labor Relations Review*, vol. 14, no. 3 (April 1961), pp. 412–15.

[17] Brunon Nowakowski, Magdalena Sokolowska, and Adam Sarapata, *Lekarze Przemyslowi* (Warsaw: Ossolineum, 1965).

[18] Magdalena Sokolowska, "Socjomedyczne Problemy Zakladu Przemyslowego," *Kultura i Spoleczenstwo*, vol. 7, no. 2 (1963), p. 145.

and capitation, the informal referral network is the only way for the profession to reward the superior doctor.

The most formalized method of designing salaries to reward ability is the "distinction awards" for consultants in the National Health Service of Great Britain. One purpose is to induce the leading specialists to practice in the service's hospitals. Another purpose is to prevent seniority alone from determining income.[19] Differentiating conditions present in other countries' structures are absent in England: after the age of forty-four in England, the annual pay increments end; medical staff structures are much more egalitarian in English than in most foreign hospitals and therefore lack rank differentials among consultants to provide the basis for salary grades.

A consultant is responsible for forty (or fewer) beds in a hospital. In many foreign countries, the hospital chief-of-service heads a department comprising between one hundred and three hundred beds, plus other facilities. Under the foreign chief usually comes a series of other fully qualified specialists holding various ranks at different salaries; into the English consultant category fall only the trainee grades and occasionally a senior hospital medical officer. An English doctor's consultantship comes at a much younger age than a European's appointment as chief-of-service. Except for distinctions between senior and junior partners in some large two-man firms and except for a few bureaucratically and hierarchically organized departments (such as pathology and radiology), all English consultants are considered equal in rank.

The Spens Committee recommended that consultants' salaries vary by quality of work, as judged by a predominantly professional body, and merit pay has existed since the beginning of the hospital service.[20] These "Distinction Awards" are paid to the consultant annually in addition to his basic salary. Once he is awarded a higher pay rate, the consultant keeps it every year until his retirement, and it becomes the base for calculating his pension; the selection committee can raise him to an even higher rate but cannot demote him if his performance declines. For many years, two-thirds of the consultants received the basic rate and one-third were distributed among three higher rates for distinction. The Royal Commission placed numerical ceilings on the number of persons receiving distinction awards and added another rate for unusually meritorious doctors.[21] The awards recommended by the Review Body in 1969 were: [22]

[19] Another unstated reason is to ensure that many consultants earn substantially more than the general practitioners, their habitual rivals in the politics of British remuneration. Gordon Forsyth, *Doctors and State Medicine* (London: Pitman Medical Publishing Co., 1966), pp. 30–34.

[20] *Report of the Inter-Departmental Committee on Remuneration of Consultants and Specialists* (London: H. M. Stationery Office, Cmnd. 7420, 1948), pp. 10–12.

[21] *Report of the Royal Commission on Doctors' and Dentists' Remuneration* (London: H. M. Stationery Office, Cmnd. 939, 1960), pp. 83–84.

[22] *Review Body on Doctors' and Dentists' Remuneration: Tenth Report* (London: H. M. Stationery Office, Cmnd. 3884, 1969), p. 15.

100	A plus awards of	£5,275
340	A awards of	£4,000
1,030	B awards of	£2,350
2,110	C awards of	£1,000

To evaluate and reward the elite of English medicine, an unusually distinguished selection committee was picked, including current and former presidents of the Royal Colleges, a representative of the university vice-chancellors, a representative of the Medical Research Council, a former Treasury civil servant, and others.[23] The chairmen and vice-chairmen usually have dominated the committee's decisions by thorough work, but at times the committee has met often and scrutinized recommendations critically. The first chairman and vice-chairman traveled often to solicit advice and meet likely prospects. The second chairman organized a series of advisory committees throughout the country.

One of the prewar structural defects to be corrected by the National Health Service was the excessive concentration of consultants—usually the ablest men—in London teaching hospitals. This reflected the concentration of income and consumer demand in London, as well as the concentration of teaching and research facilities. The distribution of distinction awards has aimed to make service attractive outside of London and in nonteaching hospitals. Consequently, no attempt is made to place all consultants in a single national ranking, but the awards are distributed according to regional quotas, and a consultant is picked if he surpasses other candidates for available openings in his region: since about half of England's consultants work in London, half of each year's new distinction awards are given in London; the remaining awards are distributed among ten regions in the provinces, in proportions matching the distribution of all consultants, with slight variations if one region has more competent candidates one year than does another. Thus for any year, the committee knows how many awards of each type will go to each region, and the numbers are manageable: for example, Region X might receive an A plus award, no A award, two B's, and four C's. Active members of the selection committee visit each region, get nominations from respected local consultants, and make inquiries. In some regions the selection committee now has standing advisory groups; elsewhere informal grapevines are used. Extra efforts locate possible nominees in the nonteaching hospitals of London; because of the capital's impersonality, geographical size, and

[23] The distinction award system is described by Rosemary Stevens, *Medical Practice in Modern England* (New Haven: Yale University Press, 1966), chap. 15. The reasoning of the selection committee was summarized by its then chairman, Lord Moran of Manton in *Minutes of Evidence Taken before the Royal Commission on Doctors' and Dentists' Remuneration* (London: H. M. Stationery Office, 1958), pp. 171–208. The procedure is summarized by the Royal Commission, *Doctors' and Dentists' Renumeration* (1960) (note 21), pp. 72–82.

preoccupation with the teaching hospitals, such doctors are less well known to the professional community and might otherwise be overlooked.

When the selection committee makes its decisions, it acts on the basis of the candidates' *curricula vitae*, the candidates' publications, the advice of several local medical leaders, and the impressions gained by its own members during visits. Different standards of judgment are used for different fields: for example, research and publication are more important when evaluating a pathologist than a gynecologist; an interest in the newest methods is considered particularly crucial for a thoracic surgeon but perhaps less decisive in some less fluid fields. Since the selection procedure relies upon the grapevine and the judgments of the local leaders among consultants, it readily identifies the ablest mature doctors and the brilliant young ones. According to Lord Moran's testimony before the Royal Commission, one of the greatest problems is to identify the good but less brilliant men destined for C Awards; the committee's greatest anxiety is that it may be overlooking some unspectacular but worthy doctors in their mid-fifties, who may then lose forever their just rewards. Since the system emphasizes merit and not seniority, a doctor's chances of getting his first distinction award decline after his peak work years.

The deliberations and decisions are secret. Only the committee and the recipient know that he obtained an award, but of course the professional grapevine can make intelligent guesses. (Some of my informants have cultivated the art of diagnosing hospital budgets, to detect the presence of distinction awards in various departments.) One reason for secrecy is to prevent conflicts within the medical staffs: senior consultants might be irritated at their juniors with higher awards; senior doctors without awards might feel humiliated if the listings were public. Primarily, secrecy is maintained to prevent the distinction awards from becoming a form of advertising that would attract private patients to the recipients.

About one-third of the consultants hold distinction awards at any one time. According to statistical probabilities, 43 per cent will receive awards during their careers. The proportions of consultants possessing awards varies greatly by specialty: in the more glamorous and publicized fields (such as surgery and internal medicine), over half the consultants receive this extra pay; in the fields which are less prestigious within the medical profession (such as psychiatry) and whose members are less generally publicized among clinicians (such as anesthesiology and radiology), one-fifth or fewer receive awards. As one would expect, the distribution of awards is related to affiliation with teaching hospitals: although the quota system intentionally divides the *total number* of distinction awards equally between teaching and non-teaching hospitals, almost 90 per cent of the A plus awards and over 80 per cent of the A awards are held by consultants at teaching hospitals.

Besides Great Britain, the Soviet Union is one of the few countries that formally recognize merit in the payment system.[24] Some physicians are awarded the title "Honored Doctor of the Republic" while some teachers (including members of Medical Institute faculties) are named "Honored Teacher of the Republic." Each designee receives ten rubles a month in addition to his basic salary and may wear a small decoration on his lapel. The awards are distributed by committees of leading doctors, within the totals set by the all-Union and Republic Ministries of Health. Both clinical expertise and conscientious performance seem to be recognized. It is so difficult to motivate physicians to practice in the countryside that many who make their careers in rural areas receive the awards.

Other supplements in the Soviet Union are intended to motivate post-graduate training. Any doctor who has taken courses and passed the examinations for the degree "Candidate of Medical Sciences" receives permanently ten rubles a month besides his basic salary. The additional study and examinations for the degree "Doctor of Medical Sciences" earn an extra twenty rubles a month for life.

A few official posts that denote clinical leadership bring higher pay. Soviet medical services have numerous administrative and clinical committees. Some committees are groups of experts who examine and prescribe for difficult cases; others set policy and provide advice for the conduct of clinical services. The chairmanship is a mark of professional distinction that brings an additional ten, seventeen, or twenty-two rubles a month, depending on the size of the committee.

Relations to Private Practice

A common problem in the world's salaried medical services is the relationship between the doctor's public and private practices. The doctors usually insist on retaining rights of private practice, since it is profitable. The Ministry of Health or sick funds usually agree in order to please the doctors. Insofar as policymakers think of private practice as a social asset rather than merely a tactical concession to the doctors, they assume that the supply of medical services is elastic: in other words, they assume that the prospect of private fees will cause doctors to work harder, and that heavy consumer demand will be satisfied by an increased volume of medical work beyond salaried hours. Private practice becomes an important safety valve: the doctors would fight more bitterly over the size of their salaries if they could not earn substantial extra income under their own control. Only by conceding rights of private practice could the less affluent countries induce doctors to accept low salaries. The specialists who combine private practice and part-

[24] The various forms of merit pay are described in A. V. Rott and K. M. Pavlenko, *Novaya oplata truda rabotnikov zdravookhraneniya* (Kiev: Zdorovia, 1965), pp. 56, 93, 133. No publications describe the awards procedure.

time salaried appointments as chief-of-service in public hospitals usually earn the highest incomes in the medical profession. If public and private practices were kept separate, no problems would result; but some conflicts of interest do occur, and the supply of medical services is not as elastic as some partisans of private practice hope.

Concessions in Scheduling

In order to please the specialists, Ministries of Health and sick funds often assist their private practices. For example, in the National Health Service of Great Britain, the pay rate for full-time salaried work in the hospitals for many years was lower than the rate for part-time work. Therefore a combination of part-time salaried hospital work and private practice has been considerably more profitable than full-time salaried work. The salaried system itself has contained incentives for part-time instead of full-time work, but critics have succeeded in reducing some of these advantages.

When the National Health Service began, it was widely assumed that considerable private specialty practice would survive, that many specialists would be full-time private practitioners, that special inducements would be necessary to attract distinguished specialists into the hospital service, and that nonteaching hospitals in the provinces would be understaffed without extra rewards. Therefore, the Spens Committee recommended that the part-time consultants be paid at a rate higher than the one corresponding to their proportion of time.

A full-time consultant would work eleven half-days a week, would have no private practice, and would collect a full salary. The Spens Committee recommended that "where x represents the number of half-days per week which the part-time specialist is required to work, his basic remuneration should be $x/11$ of the basic remuneration of whole-time specialists of like status, plus one-quarter of $x/11$ or one-quarter of $(11-x)/11$ of that remuneration, whichever be less." The Committee justified the extra pay on the grounds that doctors working part-time might be expected to see patients treated by their firm or attend committee meetings outside their contracted hours, but the real reason was to induce successful consultants to give some time to the National Health Service.[25]

The subsequent payment system gave to the part-time doctor numerous other advantages that the full-time doctor lacked: in calculating the number of half-days to be paid, a fraction was counted as a full half-day; some of his travel time to and from the hospital was counted in his work time; some

[25] *Remuneration of Consultants and Specialists* (1948) (note 20), pp. 12–13. The scheduling problem and many other aspects of the relationship between private practice and the National Health Service are analyzed in, Saul Mencher, *Private Practice in Britain* (London: G. Bell & Sons, 1967).

of his travel expenses were reimbursed; he was paid for home visits while the full-time physician for many years was paid for none. In addition, the tax laws allowed the part-time doctor to make more deductions of expenses from taxable income than could the full-time doctor.[26] The greatest advantage of part-time appointments was the right of private practice; if a full-time physician took private patients, he violated his contract. In response to these advantages, consultant practice in the hospital service has been basically part-time: three-fourths of the English and Welsh consultants and just over half the Scots have elected to be part-time appointees.

After several years, it became evident that the hospital service could be staffed without special concessions. Spokesmen for full-time hospital consultants criticized the advantages enjoyed by the part-time doctors.[27] Abel-Smith estimated that the extra payments to the part-time doctor made each of his sessions more expensive than those of the full-time doctor's.[28] In addition, part-time doctors were thought to be more expensive to the hospital service because they needed more registrars and house officers. Other critics, including some Labor members of the House of Commons, said that some part-time physicians gave priority to private practice over hospital duties, sometimes put their private patients improperly into free or pay beds, and should not be encouraged by award of an advantageous pay rate.[29]

Since the mid-1950's, the differences between part-time and full-time doctors have been reduced. Since late 1955, full-time doctors have been paid for all home visits, except for the first eight each quarter. The Royal Commission decided that the same salary scales should govern all future recruits to the hospital service. Since consultants, senior hospital officers, and senior registrars already in the service at the time of the Commission report presumably had made career decisions on the presumption that advantageous part-time rates would be paid, the Commission recommended that they could still select weighted rates, but the weighting was considerably reduced and would not be offered to new consultants. Transportation payments will continue to be paid to part-time consultants already receiving them, but they will not be available to new doctors and will probably be abolished for all.[30] Therefore the trend in the English hospital service has

[26] *Report of the Committee of Enquiry into the Cost of the National Health Service* (London: H. M. Stationery Office, Cmnd. 9663, 1956), pp. 141–42; and Royal Commission, *Doctors' and Dentists' Remuneration* (1960) (note 21), pp. 64–68.

[27] "Witnesses for the Whole-Time Consultants' Association," *Minutes of Evidence Taken before the Royal Commission on Doctors' and Dentists' Remuneration* (London: H. M. Stationery Office, 1958), pp. 29–56.

[28] Brian Abel-Smith and Richard M. Titmuss, *The Cost of the National Health Service* (Cambridge: University Press, 1956), pp. 125–26.

[29] E.g., *Parliamentary Debates (Hansard), House of Commons*, vol. 592, no. 153 (30 July 1958), cols. 1404–5, 1453–54.

[30] Royal Commission, *Doctors' and Dentists' Remuneration* (1960) (note 21), pp. 70–72.

been to make the salary scale simpler, more uniform, and without the special concessions favoring private practice. The changes were possible because the consultants were willing. At the same time, in order to appease the general practitioners, capitation was supplemented and thereby made more complicated.

Conflicts of Interest

In the past, public and religious hospitals were designed for the poor. Large numbers of patients resided in open wards and the outpatient departments were crowded and unattractive. Therefore the chief-of-service left the building after his few salaried work hours and saw his private patients elsewhere in town. He treated ambulatory private patients in his office and hospitalized his private patients in single or double rooms in private clinics which he owned, or owned in partnership with other doctors. The public and religious hospitals are now being modernized in northern and western Europe, so the middle and upper classes are more willing to be hospitalized there. But the foregoing contrast between public and private hospitalization remains true in southern Europe and in all underdeveloped countries.

Conflicts of interest beset the specialist when public and private facilities are distinct. If he treats patients in the public hospital's outpatient department, wards, or operating room, he may receive nothing beyond his usual salary. But if he treats that patient in his private office or the operating room of his private clinic, he collects fees either from the patient or from national health insurance. If he hospitalizes the patient in his private clinic, he collects daily inpatient fees from the patient or sick fund.

Seeing the specialist privately has several attractions for the patient. The specialist will give him more time. The chiefs-of-service in the surgical specialties will do the work personally in the private clinic or private office, but otherwise they may delegate it to junior physicians in the public or private hospital. The chief of the obstetrical service will perform the delivery himself in the private clinic, but nurse-midwives continue to handle normal deliveries in most public and religious hospitals in the world.[31]

It is widely believed that a substantial number of hospital specialists decide the conflict of interest in favor of their purse, but firm evidence and figures are lacking. Some of my informants in Latin Europe and in the Eastern Mediterranean believe that some chiefs-of-service and junior special-

[31] Polls of public satisfaction always elicit approval of national health insurance or national health services. But the few surveys that ask about private practice as well usually discover that patients predict even better treatment if they see doctors privately. For example, the Chilean survey in, Salvador Diaz P., "Medicina pública y privada: Las criticas al Servicio Nacional de Salud," *Cuadernos Medico-Sociales*, vol. 6, no. 1 (March 1965), pp. 5–7.

ists with private practices spot potential paying patients in the outpatient departments of public hospitals and divert them into their private practice with assurances of better care. This tactic threatens the attempt by the public hospitals to attract more upper- and middle-class patients, and thereby to alter their traditional image as repositories for the poor. Also, the diversion hurts the public hospital by cutting off income: some older public and religious hospitals have recently installed private rooms that can be rented for extra payments.

Concessions in the Use of Facilities

A trend in northern and western Europe is to induce the chief-of-service to remain in the hospital all day. Younger specialists are showing a greater interest in full-time salaried careers without private practice, but some concessions have been made to their elders. The compromise is to build modern and attractive hospitals, pay high salaries, and offer rights of private practice on the premises. Swedish and German public and religious hospitals have this "geographical full-time" arrangement at present, and it will spread to France and many other countries in the future.

Once senior Swedish doctors left the hospitals around 2 P.M. for their private offices, as in continental Europe today. In order to keep them in the hospitals, their salaries have been raised and they are given private offices virtually free of rent. In return for an office, the assistance of a nurse, and use of the hospital's equipment and materials during private hours, the chief must pay the hospital one krona (i.e., $0.19) per patient-visit. Thus besides paying him a salary, the hospital heavily subsidizes his private practice. In Stockholm, where outpatients are numerous and private fees are uncontrolled, chiefs can earn large private incomes with little overhead. According to the records of a Stockholm hospital that I visited, many chiefs had each taken over five hundred private visits during 1961; in fields where patients make short visits (such as dermatology, orthopedics, and ophthalmology), chiefs each reported from two to three thousand visits.

Despite their nominal full-time appointments, most chiefs in Sweden are really part-time appointees. Their private offices are in the polyclinic part of the building and they are rarely called back to their services during their private hours. In the hospitals I visited, the medical staffs were present five days a week, totaling between thirty-five and forty-five hours. The chiefs devoted four (or occasionally three) afternoons a week exclusively to private practice; the private hours were quite varied and included noon–5 P.M., 2–5 P.M., 10 A.M.–2 P.M., etc. Some of the well-known chiefs in Stockholm occasionally saw a few private patients in the morning, in addition to their regularly scheduled afternoon private office hours; some visited private clinics briefly during the afternoon. (The foregoing summary of time schedules refers to the chiefs rather than the professors of medicine: the latter have no fixed hospital hours and in practice see many private patients at times and places of their own choosing.)

Contact between the Swedish chief and the service during his private hours varies by individual circumstances. Some house staffs in lesser public hospitals are foreign-trained because of the shortage of Swedish-born doctors. Some service chiefs told me they keep in touch with their services by phone or visits during their private hours if they have house men whom they do not fully trust, but they leave the service completely in the hands of their assistants during years of better recruitment. In one of the major Stockholm hospitals, I asked several head nurses whether they had ever contacted a service chief about a problem in the service during his private hours; none ever had, and they considered the chief resident in full authority when the chief was in his private office. Legally, the chiefs are obligated to give their services priority over private practice during their private hours.

Preferential Treatment for Private Patients

Every part-time consultant treats patients both under Britain's National Health Service and privately; any patient may elect private care or completely free care under the Service; to please the consultants during the 1946–48 negotiations, every large hospital has pay beds for private patients as well as National Health Service beds. A patient may choose different types of care at different times: he may visit his general practitioner under the National Health Service and a specialist under a private fee-for-service arrangement; he may make a private office visit to the consultant and enter the hospital under the National Health Service. Scarcities in the Service account for private payments: because of the slow pace of new construction and the shortage of nurses, beds are scarce, waiting lists are long, and the patient can be admitted sooner (particularly for postponable conditions) to a private bed; the patient can see a famous and busy consultant sooner and with greater certainty of personal care in his private office than in the hospital outpatient clinic.

Occupants of "pay beds" must pay all hospitalization costs plus a private fee to the consultant. National Health Service beds are occupied by patients whom the consultants must treat without private fees; the beds in the wards are completely free, but patients must pay the hospital a small extra sum for "amenity beds" located in separate rooms. For some private beds, particularly in London, the consultant may charge any fee, but Ministry of Health regulations impose a maximum fee schedule upon most pay beds. Despite the growth of private hospitalization insurance during the 1950's, the number of pay beds diminished from almost 7,000 to less than 6,000, and now they constitute only one per cent of all beds: waiting lists for National Health Service beds have necessitated conversion of pay beds for public patients; many hospital administrators dislike the idea of pay beds and welcome opportunities to devote them to the hospitals' other needs. Abolition of pay beds has sometimes been demanded by the Labor party.[32]

One alleged problem in the National Health Service is "queue-barging": a patient with a postponable condition that would place him low on the waiting list sees the consultant privately, and the consultant orders his early admission to a National Health Service bed under his firm.[33] Sometimes the occupant of one of the consultant's National Health Service beds allegedly receives his private bill.[34] Some consultants have allegedly admitted private patients to pay beds, charged fees for their services, and transferred the patients to public beds during recuperation, thereby freeing the pay bed for new private patients but delaying persons on the waiting list for public beds. Some hospital administrators suspect that a few consultants see private patients during their outpatient clinic hours at the hospital for public patients; all diagnostic tests for the private patients would be mixed in with the free tests for the other patients.

Abuses like these occur widely in many underdeveloped countries because of frustrating hospital working conditions, very low salaries, and the absence of traditions limiting all-out money-seeking in favor of public service. For example an investigator retained by the government of Ceylon found that many chiefs-of-service used their public hospital beds for private pa-

[32] On pay beds and the controversies surrounding them, see Mencher, *Private Practice* (note 25), chaps. 3 and 4. The available statistics on the utilization of pay and amenity beds are summarized by D. S. Lees and M. H. Cooper, "Amenity and Private Pay Beds," *British Medical Journal* (8 June 1963), pp. 1531–33.

[33] Some critics of part-time consultantships and of pay beds believe these beds enable patients to enter the hospital earlier than more deserving nonpaying patients on the National Health Service waiting list. E.g., *Parliamentary Debates* (*Hansard*), *House of Commons*, vol. 592, no. 153 (30 July 1958), cols. 1405–6, 1454. But this use of *pay beds* by consultant and patient does not violate the law or professional ethics. The violation is preferential admission to a National Health Service bed. In a recent national public opinion poll, half the people had heard, and over one-third believed, the rumor that a private visit to a consultant would result in earlier admission to the hospital. *A Review of the Medical Services in Great Britain* (London: Social Assay, 1962), p. 222. Doctors as well admit this is true. E.g., Ann Cartwright, *Patients and Their Doctors: A Study of General Practice* (London: Routledge & Kegan Paul, 1967), p. 142. Queue-barging is believed to have existed in the prewar voluntary hospitals. Brian Abel-Smith, *The Hospitals 1800–1948* (London: William Heinemann, 1964), pp. 392–93.

[34] Many such violations may be the unintentional result of administrative confusion. The consultant may have assumed that his private patient would be admitted to a pay bed. But the hospital may have converted its pay beds temporarily to public use, or the admitting registrar may have sent the patient automatically to a public bed. (Because of the universal coverage of the National Health Service, every patient may occupy a public bed.) Thus neither consultant nor patient may know that the patient occupies a public bed. Unaware of the intricacies of the system, the patient may not be surprised at receiving a bill from the doctor but no bill from the hospital. For summaries and criticisms of the abuses in the National Health Service arising from specialists' private practices, see David Cargill, *The G.P.: What's Wrong?* (London: Victor Gollancz, 1965), pp. 162–73; and Mencher, *Private Practice* (note 25), chap. 5.

tients, gave priority to public patients paying them secret fees, and shifted their hospital work to assistants. To all this, the Ministry had long acquiesced.[35]

All these violations can be reduced by vigilance and strong action by the hospital group secretary, the admitting registrar, and the chairman of the medical committee of the hospital group. And all abuses can be reduced by the ethical sense of the medical profession. (Ultimately, of course, the best solution is massive hospital construction to eliminate queues.)

To prevent abuses of this sort, Sweden in 1960 abolished the right of public hospital doctors to charge private fees of patients after they were hospitalized. In return, the chiefs' salaries were increased. The Swedish public medical services attempt to differentiate clearly between hospital and ambulatory care: inpatient care is paid for by a combination of public subsidies and patient fees, and doctors' services are covered by the lump sums from the government for hospitalization as a whole; ambulatory care is paid for by the patient on a fee-for-service basis. When the hospital doctors sent bills to their former private patients during periods of hospitalization for inpatient care, some administrators complained that the doctor was being paid twice (by salary and by fee) for the same procedures, and some patients complained they were being charged extra for care covered by their hospital bill. Also, some critics believed that the right to charge inpatients bore the potentialities for abuse found in other countries with under-the-table payments: although everyone in the chief's service was supposed to be treated equally well, the chief might give preference to the patients paying him privately.

Discouraging Private Practice

Few governments have been so dogmatically socialist as to forbid all private medical care. The Stalinist government of Poland attempted to forbid private practice in the hope that the medical profession would work overtime under the salaried national health service. It assumed medical services were inelastic. But it rescinded its policy in 1956, after the doctors refused to extend their salaried hours, thereby causing a lengthening of the queues and a reduction in the amount of medical care. For fear of overburdening the understaffed publicly owned facilities, the Communist government of China for many years has permitted private practice, even when it has dogmatically socialized other sectors of the economy.

Private practice has steadily diminished in the Soviet Union, and therefore few doctors now have any private patients who might benefit from preferential treatment. Private practice is not forbidden, but it is censured publicly and heavily taxed, and therefore ambitious physicians avoid taking

[35] John H. L. Cumpston, *Report of the Medical and Public Health Organizations of Ceylon* (Colombo: Ceylon Government Press, 1950), pp. 27–29, 57–63.

private fees.[36] If a physician sees patients privately, his only attractions are more time and more home visits, since he cannot use state-owned equipment or offices for this care. In other countries, the leading doctors—who are the models in earning and spending for the entire profession—can attain steadily mounting living standards through private practice. But the Soviet Union has always had serious shortages of consumer goods and services, and their salaries already give the leading doctors more money than they can spend.

Some full-time private practitioners can be found in cities or in the Black Sea resorts, and some general practitioners see patients privately after they finish work in their polyclinics. Russia has two other kinds of full-time private practitioners, who have long distressed the Ministry of Health. One is the homeopath, found in considerable numbers in the cities. The other is the *feldsher*, trained by the government and supposed to work in the rural medical services, but who poses as a private doctor in some towns. No-one knows how many *feldshers* do this.

Unnecessary Work

An advantage of salary is that usually it does not encourage the multiplication of procedures not clinically necessary.[37] Payment is made for fixed periods of time and does not increase if the work pace rises. The more common problem is to motivate sufficient effort during the fixed hours. However, some exceptional administrative arrangements make possible the doctor's own control over his work hours and salary, and the multiplication or stretchout of work can become profitable.

Two unusual features of the English hospital service are that the consultant can choose whether to be full-time or part-time, and the consultant and the Regional Hospital Board can bargain over the number of sessions. As I have said, the pay scale in the past has induced most consultants to seek part-time appointments, and the most profitable contracts provide eight or nine sessions weekly. To staff the hospitals and please the doctors, the Boards usually have agreed, although most administrators would prefer full-time doctors. Every hospital group can use a surgeon or internist for at least nine sessions, but the variations arise in using doctors in the narrower specialties, such as dermatology, urology, ophthalmology, otorhinolaryngology, radiology, and others. In many hospital groups, such consultants might complete

[36] Some examples of published criticisms of private practitioners are V. Kopitsyn, "Mir inteligentnovo cheloveka: chastnaya praktika," *Izvestia*, 5 August 1959, p. 6; and M. Derzhavets, "Mesli vracha," *Literaturnaya Gazeta*, 28 June 1950, p. 2.

[37] Therefore, fewer procedures are performed under salary than under fee-for-service, if types of patients and illnesses are held constant. Without further investigation, of course, one cannot assume automatically that all patients are undertreated under the first arrangement and overtreated under the second. Some American comparisons of the effects of the two payment methods under private health insurance are summarized in, Milton I. Roemer, "On Paying the Doctor and the Implications of Different Methods," *Journal of Health and Human Behavior*, vol. 3, no. 1 (Spring 1962), pp. 10–11.

the work load in less than nine sessions. Unlike the usual salaried system, in which the employer or custom fixes the work span, these consultants can govern the period of employment by their own work pace. If they work slowly, multiply optional procedures, and often ask patients to return to the outpatient clinic, they will be needed for many sessions. Some critics—particularly advocates of a completely full-time salaried hospital service—believe that some consultants deliberately work slowly, ask outpatients to return unnecessarily, and increase the waiting lists in their services in order to gain maximum part-time contracts.[38]

The consultant works within a hospital group but signs a contract with the Regional Hospital Board. The Group Committee advises the Board on the number of sessions it needs in each specialty. Many consultants spread their sessions among several hospitals in the group, some work in a few groups in the same region. The fact that the consultants' legal employer (the Regional Board) is different from and is of higher rank than his actual employer (the Group Committee) weakens the latter's control over him. The contractual relationship with the Board instead of with the Committee was one of the concessions made to the consultants during the creation of the National Health Service. Lower ranking doctors have contracts with the Group Committees.

No one knows whether these abuses are exceptional or frequent enough to be a problem. Some potential administrative controls exist: the lay hospital administrator (i.e., the secretary of the Hospital Group Management Committee) is usually the first to hear that the work pace in a service seems unduly slow or artificially inflated; he might then notify the senior administrative medical officer of the Regional Hospital Board or the chairman of the Medical Committee of the Hospital Group; these doctors might then investigate and confer with the offending consultant. But only a strong and confident group secretary initiates such a complaint, since he challenges the clinical policies of a consultant, and since consultants customarily receive much autonomy and respect. A few of my informants—including group secretaries who have confronted these problems—thought that even the boldest lay administrator would hesitate to challenge a consultant's work pace without evidence that the consultant was creating an artificial backlog to induce some outpatients to see him privately. Thus, possibly only the consultant's good faith, the demands of his private practice, and the hospital group's judgment about the reasonable number of sessions for each specialty prevent the unnecessary expansion of work to increase the number of salaried sessions.

Besides the National Health Service, the salaried system of Israeli health insurance may contain features that inadvertently encourage a larger than necessary number of patient-doctor contacts. As I have said, visits to the

[38] For example, *Parliamentary Debates* (*Hansard*), *House of Commons*, vol. 592, no. 153 (30 July 1958), cols. 1476, 1483–84.

doctor occur more frequently in Israel than in any other country. Normally one would expect such a high rate under fee-for-service but not in a salaried system. In many countries the doctor—and particularly the G.P. paid by capitation or salary—prefers to avoid the patient who must make frequent brief visits for injections, checkups, renewals of prescriptions, etc.

But possibly the method of awarding overtime pay to general practitioners in the *Kupat Holim* of *Histadrut*, in the National Sick Fund, and in some other enterprises has been one reason why the doctors have not resisted frequent visits by patients. The collective bargaining sessions between medical employers and the IMA set a normal number of patient contacts for completion during a full day by a salaried doctor, and the physician collects overtime pay if he exceeds the norm. Therefore many doctors have welcomed the short visits by patients needing long-term care, and some of my informants suspected that a few G.P.'s might encourage return visits or might inflate the number of patient-doctor contacts by counting follow-up telephone conversations. As can be seen in the annual *Statistical Abstract of Israel*, the National Sick Fund and the People's Sick Fund have far more return visits (and thus more total patient contacts) than does the *Kupat Holim* of *Histadrut*; a possible reason is that more of the National and People's Sick Fund G.P.'s see their insured patients in their personal offices and can encourage revisits more easily than in the *Kupat Holim* polyclinics, where the patient's visits are influenced by a larger organization. To prevent financial inducements from affecting their doctor's medical actions, some Israeli employers pay all their doctors overtime automatically.

Salaried systems may contain nonsalaried supplements that inadvertently increase work unnecessarily. For example, Italy's public hospital doctors were long paid salaries that they believed were too low for their work. Therefore, for many years the hospital gave the chief-of-service and his assistants part of the daily fee paid by the sick fund for the inpatient care of each insured person. This compensation for work performed motivated specialists to keep their beds filled with frequent admissions and prolonged stays.[39] The funds believed hospitalization costs were unduly high. Another drawback was that the insured person was more remunerative to the doctor than the uninsured patient in the adjoining bed. Consequently, in 1966 representatives of the sick funds, government, and medical societies agreed to raise salaries substantially and to reduce—but not yet abolish entirely—the payment to the specialist for each patient.[40]

39 "Third Conference on Hospital Services in Western Europe," *World Hospitals*, vol. 3, no. 1 (January 1967), p. 55.

40 Carlo Palenzona, "Période de réforme sanitaire, disputes entre médecins, disputes entre ministères," *Concours médical*, vol. 89, no. 7 (18 February 1967), p. 1328; and "Firmato l'accordo interministeriale per i nuovi stipendi ospedalieri," *Quotidiano Minerva Medica*, vol. 16, nos. 61–62 (4 August 1966), p. 975.

Assignment of Tasks

Development of Specialties

Fee-for-service often produces considerable inequalities in the income, status, and size of specialties. But salaried systems are well suited to the full and equal expansion of all specialties. In a hospital or polyclinic, all doctors of the same rank can receive salaries of the same size. Therefore specialties with widely different incomes under fee-for-service—such as surgery, radiology, psychiatry, and preventive medicine—can be paid alike. If their total incomes differ, it is because they earn unequal additional incomes from private practice or from national health insurance using fee-for-service. If there is very little private practice—as in the U.S.S.R.—the salaried system ensures an approximate parity in money and power among all the specialties. In countries where psychiatry, preventive medicine, anesthesiology, and certain other fields lack influence within the committees writing fee schedules and in countries where these specialties have few private patients, the salaried jobs attract enough recruits to ensure the covering of all specialties.

But innovation can be hampered and an unpopular specialty can be neglected if the hospitals are unwilling to create the posts. For example, improved organization and regular payment have yielded many advantages in the National Health Service of Great Britain, but a drawback may be retardation of new specialties. Before the war, a new specialty could be added to a hospital very easily: the medical staff voted to accept the newcomer, he was given a small number of beds, and he found his own patients. Since the newcomer in a voluntary hospital was paid by the patient and not by the hospital, the governing board would risk nothing by allowing entry by a practitioner in a new and perhaps controversial field. But now, a new field may involve an expensive financial risk, and at all levels the hospital service may be cautious. A good example is the role of psychiatry in the general hospital. The visitor to England hears much public debate about the need to improve mental care. If the general hospitals were still organized in their prewar manner, many might invite psychiatrists to conduct outpatient clinics, interdepartmental consultations, and inpatient treatment. But since appointment of psychiatrists now requires a commitment for a specific number of salaried sessions, possibly their inclusion in general hospitals has been retarded and their exclusive identification with mental hospitals has been perpetuated.

Career Lines

In the West, the successful doctor is a practicing specialist who combines hospital work, private practice, and—if possible—teaching in a medical school. In the past, the income structure attracted young doctors into specialty careers, but the salary scales were barriers to many. Specialty credentials required years of postgraduate training in teaching hospitals, but no salaries or low salaries were provided. Therefore, unless a medical student possessed independent means, he had to enter general practice and earn an income. But hospital medical staffs are being organized more extensively in most countries, salaries of junior staff are being raised, and far more young doctors now can afford postgraduate specialty work. Therefore the improved salary scales in hospitals are a principal reason for the widespread trend from general practice to specialty careers: at one time, most medical students in the world planned to enter general practice, but now increasing numbers plan to specialize.[41]

In most of the world, an organizational discontinuity occurs between general practice and specialization. General practitioners work in private offices while specialists alone have hospital privileges; often they are paid by different methods; the successful G.P. is not promoted into specialty practice, but the two are separate career lines depending on educational and financial choices made shortly after the end of medical school.

The Soviet Union is an exception. All the doctors under the jurisdiction of the all-Union Ministry of Health are arranged in a single hierarchy with ranks and salary increments. (The salary scale appears in chapter IV.) After several years of practice and part-time study, a general practitioner can qualify as a specialist. Unlike the West, specialists officially are rated by degrees of skill, according to amounts of postgraduate education. Apparently the rank structure and the salary scale motivate doctors to move out of general practice into specialties and into hospital practice as they grow older. Most G.P.'s are young, and turnover is high.[42]

Usually the clinicians and not the administrators are at the top of salaried scales in medicine throughout the world. But according to the Soviet salary scale in chapter IV, the highest pay is earned by hospital directors and by other administrators. Although we lack survey data about career decisions and career lines, probably this has had the effect of attracting a number of able clinicians into part-time or full-time administration, particularly as they grow older. In contrast, doctors in most other countries lack both the

[41] On the dangers of shortages of general practitioners throughout the world, see *General Practice: Report of a W.H.O. Expert Committee* (Geneva: World Health Organization, 1964), pp. 6–7; Jesse D. Rising, "The General Practitioner in a Changing World," *Canadian Medical Association Journal*, vol. 91, no. 21 (21 November 1964), pp. 1101–5; and Richard M. Titmuss, "The Future of the Family Doctor," *New Society*, no. 96 (30 July 1964), pp. 11–13.

[42] Information from my informants, corroborated by the speech of Minister of Health S. Kurashov, in *Sovetskoe Zdravookhraneniye*, 1960, no. 4, p. 21. The available information about the medical rank structure and career lines appears in, Mark G. Field, *Soviet Socialized Medicine: An Introduction* (New York: The Free Press, 1967), chaps. 5 and 6.

personal interest and pecuniary incentive to become administrators. Soviet doctors wishing to remain in full-time clinical work must take second jobs in medical care, research, or writing in order to earn higher incomes.

Availability of Services

Many countries with salaried national health services are underdeveloped and have very serious shortages of doctors and nurses in rural areas. Salaried pay is the method most easily designed to induce movement into underdoctored areas. If money alone were sufficient to move doctors from one location to another, higher rates could be offered for posts in the villages. For example, in 1937 the Soviet Union extended free medical care to the rural population, and therefore, for the first time it had to induce doctors to practice in the countryside. The salary scale announced in 1942 contained the following regional differentials for physicians in general practice:[43]

Monthly Salary (in Rubles) for Physicians	Number of Years of Experience		
	More than 10	5 to 10	Less than 5
Cities and industrial areas	725	600	500
Rural areas	850	700	550

However, living conditions are so backward in the villages of less developed countries and medicine is so difficult to practice well, that the rural differentials must be much greater to attract doctors. Usually adequate differentials cannot be introduced because a salary structure is based on rank in the clinical and administrative hierarchy. In the Soviet Union, the rural *vrach* would have to be paid a salary at least equal to the service chief of a hospital, but such a deviation from the rank hierarchy is not customary in Soviet salary scales. Since the career structure of urban medicine ultimately is more rewarding than rural medicine, financial reasons reinforce the numerous nonfinancial ones to make rural practice unattractive. The Soviet Ministry of Health attempts to guarantee a minimum number of doctors in rural posts by compulsory assignment during the years just after graduation, but many Medical Institutes allow students to evade these obligations by electing "self-assignment," which is simply the right to look for one's own job without the Institute's assistance. As a result, many urban hospitals and polyclinics are overstaffed, while many rural medical posts are not filled.[44]

[43] Henry E. Sigerist, *Medicine and Health in the Soviet Union* (New York: The Citadel Press, 1947), pp. 313–14.

[44] See the detailed report on the effects of self-assignment in and around Rostov in Vladimir Ponedelnik, "Obshiestvennaya profiesseia," *Izvestia*, 6 July 1960, p. 5. Some statistics on the troublesome problem of turnover in rural areas appear in the Soviet textbook, on personnel planning, I. I. Rozenfel'd, *Planning and Allocation of Medical Personnel in*

Unless the salary system can be modified to include incentives for rural practice, it may unintentionally accentuate rural-urban imbalances. A severe problem in every underdeveloped country is that most of the population is in the countryside while most of the doctors are in the cities. This has been true in Egypt: during the early 1960's, half the country's doctors were in Cairo and Alexandria; the doctor-population ratios were 1:700 in Cairo, 1:1,000 in Alexandria, 1:2,500 for the country as a whole, and 1:15,000 in some rural areas.[45]

The official payment system was one reason for the imbalance. In the absence of any public salaries, all the doctors would concentrate in the cities where the largest numbers of private patients live. Since government salaries were not sufficient to guarantee the living standards sought by Egyptian doctors and since salaries were traditionally only a cushion under a larger *private* practice, the salaries were never large enough to attract enough doctors out of the cities. Since the best paying jobs were offered by urban medical schools and hospitals, the salaried system itself unintentionally attracted the ablest doctors into the cities. For many years, the ambitious program of rural health centers foundered, because few doctors would accept full-time appointments for the low Grade 6 starting salary of EL 240. Five years after the program had begun, only five full-time doctors had been hired, and many centers were staffed only a few hours a week by private practitioners, who drove in from town and collected part-time salaries.[46] Because of the rigidity of the hierarchical salary structure—the rural health officer was considered a G.P. and got a salary lower than the urban hospital specialists—and because of the low budget of the health services, the government was never able to offer large enough differentials to fill these jobs with enough voluntary full-time physicians. Eventually an entirely different system of rural health centers was planned, offering pay outside the rigid civil service salary structure. In addi-

---

Public Health Services (Washington and Jerusalem: National Science Foundation and the Israel Program for Scientific Translations, 1963), p. 134. For other descriptions of the rural-urban imbalance and official denunciations of the behavior of the doctors, see G. Kurzhiiamskii, "Vrach opustil selo," *Meditsinskii Rabotnik*, no. 103 (1961), p. 2; "Dvadsat piatii kongres sanitarno-profylakticheskikh i zdravookhranicheskikh vrachei," *Meditsinskii Rabotnik*, no. 14 (1962), p. 2, and no. 15, pp. 2–3; and Heinz Müller-Dietz, *Medical Education in the Soviet Union* (Berlin: Osteuropa-Institut an der Freien Universität, 1958), pp. 79–80, 95–98. Probably in every country, nonpecuniary motives are far more important for rural doctors than enjoyment of pecuniary advantages, particularly if the differentials are only moderate. See the motivational survey of Chilean physicians reported in, Adela Berdichewsky, "El ejercicio de la medicina en provincia," *Cuadernos Médico-Sociales*, vol. 9, no. 2 (June 1968), pp. 8–11.

[45] Ahmed Kamel Mazen, *Development of the Medical Care Program of the Egyptian Region of the United Arab Republic* (Stanford: dissertation for Ph.D., Stanford University, 1961), p. 104.

[46] Sadek Antonios Bouktou, "Organisation of Medical Care in the Rural Districts of Egypt," *Bulletin of the International Social Security Association*, vol. 7, nos. 1–2 (January–February 1954), pp. 20–21.

tion, it was hoped that a new medical profession could be trained, fired by the Revolution's ideals and willing to serve the countryside instead of seeking financial gain.

The rigid and low civil service salary scales led to such a rural-urban imbalance in Turkey that the government there too had to offer large differentials in favor of rural practice, in order to staff the national health service introduced in 1964.[47] Besides their basic rates on the normally invariant Barem scale, doctors working in the eastern provinces would receive monthly an extra 200 TL, 400 TL, or 600 TL, depending on the degree of underdevelopment of the area. If a doctor had to travel within the province, he received an extra 600 TL a month. In addition, physicians working under contracts forbidding private practice would receive an additional monthly sum of 500 TL, and 800 TL more if they previously had had private practices. An extra 700 TL was paid to specialists. As a result, doctors in the less developed areas of Turkey would earn between 2,300 TL and 3,200 TL monthly, in addition to their basic rates on the Barem scale, which were only a fraction of the regional increments.[48] The government hoped that these unusually high inducements—coupled with controls over emigration—would direct eastward the many doctors who crowded Istanbul.

The conditions under which rural differentials succeed and fail are demonstrated by the experience of Israel. Rural differentials can accomplish a wider spread of medical manpower if the rural doctor is close enough to the big cities to share their culture and to visit on days off, and if the doctor's practice is not technically advanced. In the eyes of the ordinary general practitioner, geographical isolation offsets even the most generous rural subsidies. For any doctor requiring advanced facilities and sophisticated colleagues, working in the city has no alternative.

Because Israel's *Kupat Holim* must staff the medical services of many communal farms and other rural communities affiliated with *Histadrut*, it offers extra pay for rural service. The rural doctor gets between 18 and 38 per cent additional, calculated on basic salary and cost of living allowance together. So that he will be motivated to make a career of rural practice, the doctor

[47] Like Egypt, Turkey has long exhibited the imbalance common to underdeveloped countries with large cities and universities: it graduates far more doctors than can be supported by its private purchasing power, but it has too few doctors for the needs of the population, particularly in the rural areas. In 1960, the numbers of inhabitants per doctor were 635 in Istanbul, 15,400 in Erzurum province, 15,200 in Mus, 23,800 in Agri, 34,800 in Gumusane, and 9,400 in the fifty-one least developed provinces. Ragip Uner and Nusret Fisek, *Saglik Hizmetlerinin Sosyallestirilmesi ve Uygulama Plani Uzerinde Calismalar* (Ankara: T. C. Saglik ve Sosyal Yardim Bakanligi Yayinlarindan, 1961), pp. 144–48.

[48] The new national health service is described in, Alain Vessereau, " 'Socialisation' de la médecine en Turquie," *Concours médical*, vol. 87, no. 25 (19 June 1965), pp. 4337–38, 4341. The payment structure is reported in "Saglik Hizmetleri Sosyallestiriliyor," *Ulus*, 8 March 1963. The basic Barem scale appears in chapter IV, supra. The official exchange rate at present is 1 TL = $0.09.

receives higher supplementary rates each year: 18 per cent for the first year of rural practice, 20 per cent for the second, 22 per cent for the third, 24 per cent for the fourth, then 26, 28, etc. for successive years, and finally 38 per cent after the sixteenth year. Meanwhile, the doctor has probably received several promotions in basic salary grade, besides getting the usual annual seniority increments in each grade, so that his income pyramids steeply. In addition, under the recently established system of lists of regular patients, the rural doctor can collect extra payments for long lists. A doctor responsible for one community collects his basic pay for the first 1,200 people; if he is responsible for two communities, basic pay applies to the first 1,000; for three or more separate communities, basic pay applies to the first 700. For every 100 people above these totals, the rural doctor collects a certain sum monthly; most rural doctors have lists larger than the basic totals and therefore collect the extra payments. After several years of rural service, a doctor would suffer a great decline in income if he returned to urban practice.

The incentives functioned successfully as long as Israel's medical profession consisted predominantly of older immigrants trained in European medical schools. Many had been general practitioners; all were grateful to settle in the new country. Israel had a more urban concentration than its leaders preferred, but still a wider geographical distribution than nearly any other country.[49]

But a new generation was trained in the new medical schools of Jerusalem and Tel Aviv. Young and native-born, they viewed Israel and the rural communities less sentimentally than their elders. The American-oriented medical curricula and postgraduate training in the United States aroused their interest in advanced clinical sciences and led to careers in specialty practice and research. Hardly any entered rural general practice in response to the salary differentials. It appeared as if all would follow their careers in Israeli cities or would emigrate. Therefore the worried government considered passing a law that would oblige young doctors to serve for at least three years in a newly developing region before final certification.[50]

Salaried systems often are devised to affect the distribution of doctors in developed societies, since rural-urban imbalances are present there too. As we saw in chapter IV, Sweden's salaries for each job vary by region: the higher rates are paid not only to compensate for the cost of living but are offered for the regions where recruitment has always lagged. The differentials have not been great enough to solve the regional imbalance, but the situation

[49] H. S. Halevi, "The Demography of the Israel Physicians," *Harofé Haivri: Hebrew Medical Journal*, vol. 1 (1959), pp. 198–200; and Theodor Grushka (editor), *Health Services in Israel 1948–1958* (Jerusalem: The Ministry of Health, 1959), p. 150.

[50] Burton M. Halpern, "New Exodus, Israel's Talent Drain," *Nation*, vol. 200 (10 May 1965), pp. 497–98. A similar regulation was adopted by Greece, after rural differentials had failed to attract medical school graduates into the countryside.

would be worse without them. In Great Britain, the Royal Commission believed that the planned geographical distribution of distinction awards motivated able consultants to work in the provinces, and that without salaries and distinction awards such doctors would have continued to concentrate in London, as they had before creation of the National Health Service.[51]

Position of the Medical Profession

Income

A salaried payment system can place doctors in nearly the highest income group of a society, provided they are free to supplement their rates through their own efforts. If they have rights of private practice or extensive insurance practice, chiefs-of-service in hospitals can earn very high incomes. Individuals in some other occupations—such as industrial executives—may earn more than the best paid specialists, but the specialists as a class may be the country's best paid group.

The specialists who mix salaried and private practice enjoy these advantages consistently in all countries. Table 13 provides an example from Great Britain. In each age group, the consultants are the best paid of all the high-income occupations.[52]

Estimates of total incomes of salaried Swedish doctors in 1965—reproduced in Table 14—demonstrate the importance of the nonsalaried component in lifting physicians into the highest income brackets. The salaries alone would place the hospital doctors near the top of the Swedish income structure: the highest salary paid by the Swedish civil service in 1965 was 101,808 kr. plus a daily cost of living supplement of 31.10 kr., and it was received by only a few men. But the fees earned from national health insurance work and from private practice resulted in totals which *on the average* equaled this, and therefore many chiefs-of-service earned even more.[53]

The advantages of a mixed salaried and private practice appear in the British data: in 1955–56, the full-time salaried consultants earned a median income of £2,914, while the part-time consultants earned a median gross £3,352. This was true in nearly every specialty. Some of the part-time doctors earned very high incomes: 10 per cent earned £5,393 or more, while 10 per cent of the full-time salaried consultants obtained £3,772 or more. Part-time doctors with seven or eight out of the full eleven sessions earned the highest gross incomes.[54]

Earnings rise steadily with age under salaried systems. The doctor is

[51] Royal Commission, *Doctors' and Dentists' Remuneration* (1960) (note 21), p. 82.

[52] Ibid., p. 30. £1 = $2.80 on the free market at the time of the survey, £1 = $2.40 today.

[53] Estimates by the Swedish Medical Association. The free market exchange rate is 1 kr. = $0.19.

[54] Sample survey of 2,095 British consultants by mail. Royal Commission, *Doctors' and Dentists' Remuneration* (1960) (note 21), p. 268.

TABLE 13. MEDIAN INCOMES IN AGE GROUPS, GREAT BRITAIN, FISCAL YEAR 1955–56 (IN POUNDS)

Professions and Occupations	30–34	35–39	40–44	45–54	55–64	30–65
Consultants	2,100	2,460	3,110	3,440	3,600	3,130
General practitioners	1,710	2,120	2,260	2,460	2,180	2,160
Accountants	980	1,250	1,580	1,950	1,900	1,490
Actuaries	1,300	1,660	1,880	2,540	3,010	2,020
Barristers	780	1,310	2,300	2,340	1,990	1,620
Solicitors (England and Wales)	1,120	1,390	1,980	2,290	2,770	1,850
Architects	850	980	1,160	1,380	1,350	1,080
Surveyors	960	1,220	1,770	1,890	1,730	1,360
Engineers	990	1,140	1,280	1,480	1,650	1,210
University teachers	1,060	1,320	1,700	2,000	2,010	1,510
University graduates employed by industry	1,150	1,580	1,900	2,290	2,320	1,570

TABLE 14. INCOMES FROM SALARIES AND OTHER SOURCES EARNED BY SWEDISH DOCTORS IN 1965 (IN KRONOR)

	Salary	Average Total Income, Salary Plus Fees
Hospital doctors:		
Chiefs-of-service	61,000–85,000	110,000
Assistant chiefs-of-service	45,000–69,000	90,000
Assistant physicians	34,000–50,000	65,000
District medical officers:		
County medical officers	61,000	88,000
Rural medical officers	31,000–51,000	85,000
City medical officers	27,000–75,000	85,000
City district medical officers	22,000–28,000	90,000

promoted, acquires automatic seniority increases, and in a few countries receives special merit increases. Salary usually levels off after the late fifties, since seniority increments and promotions rarely continue indefinitely, and because of reductions in hours or in multiple job-holding. The curve for career earnings is quite different from that under fee-for-service, suggested in the last chapter: because a fee system ties the doctor's income so closely to his activities and because he can control his earnings in accordance with his financial needs, income may reach a peak in the middle years under fee-for-service and may level off or drop thereafter.

All statements about career earnings cycles in this book are hypotheses, since we lack studies of individual doctors' life histories under various payment systems. As I said in connection with Table 12, cross-sectional surveys comparing age groups, at the same time may not show the same difference that an individual experiences as he passes through these groups. The apparently lower-paid older persons may have earned even less earlier in life. The middle-aged may earn even more as they grow older.

Since most salaried doctors supplement their salaries with fees, either under private practice or national health insurance, their career earnings curves combine features of the separate curves under salaried and fee-for-service systems. We lack data directly on career earnings, but Table 15 shows the median net incomes of male British consultants in 1955–56 and chiefs-of-service in Swedish hospitals in 1959, classified by age. The British consultants collect private fees in addition to their salaries; the Swedish chiefs receive fees under national health insurance, plus a few private fees. Earnings rise by age groups until the peak is reached in the late fifties. The oldest age group in Britain earns slightly less. The important increments from private or insured practice make the biggest difference in the middle years.[55]

The two flat-rate payment systems—salary and capitation—narrow the dispersion of income within medicine. The market conditions under fee-for-service can produce wide differences in work and in the ability to charge high fees: doctors are unequal in their abilities to attract patients and to impress the other doctors who make referrals. But salary is standardized and varies slightly according to time worked and seniority. Before the National Health Service, the wealthiest consultants in Great Britain earned over ten times the pay of the least successful specialist. In the 1950's, even when distinction awards and earnings from private practice are counted, the minimum pay had been raised and the range had narrowed. Before the Service, the lowest paid specialists included men in all age groups; under the salaried system, earnings depended on career stage, and few specialists failed to rise with age.[56]

Since salaried payment is stable compensation for blocs of work time, it can protect doctors from the fluctuations due to sudden changes in the supply or demand for medical services. For example, the salaried system has been ideally suited to the Israeli medical profession's great problem of assimilating many immigrant doctors in a short time. More than half the country's approximately 5,700 doctors arrived since 1948 as nearly penniless immigrants; all these immigrant doctors are licensed to practice at once. During this period—and particularly during years of heavy immigration from Europe—doctors entered at a greater rate than immigrants generally; therefore the ratio of doctors to people has risen, sometimes in sudden jumps, and now is about 1:430, by far the highest in the world.

In a free market, such a large and rapid influx would depress wages. If it were a competitive market with remuneration by capitation or fee-for-

[55] Sample survey of 2,095 British consultants by mail. Royal Commission, *Doctors' and Dentists' Remuneration* (1960) (note 21), p. 268. Study of tax records of 934 Swedish chiefs-of-service. *Sjukhus och öppen vård: Betänkande av Öhs-Kommittén* (Stockholm: Kungl. Inrikesdepartmentet, Statens Offentliga Utredningar, 1963, Number 21), p. 398.

[56] Compare the Spens Committee report, *Remuneration of Consultants and Specialists* (1948) (note 20), pp. 20–29; and Royal Commission, *Doctors' and Dentists' Remuneration* (1960) (note 21), pp. 30–38, 268–70.

TABLE 15. MEDIAN INCOMES IN AGE GROUPS, BRITISH CONSULTANTS AND SWEDISH CHIEFS-OF-SERVICE

Ages of Doctors	Great Britain (in Pounds), 1955–56	Sweden (in Kronor), 1959
30–34	2,104	
35–39	2,463	
40–44	3,110	
35–44		57,000
45–49	3,380	
50–54	3,511	
45–54		69,000
55–59	3,629	
60 and over	3,303	
55–64		77,000
All	3,122	68,000

service, Israeli medicine would have been particularly vulnerable. Since doctors came from many countries and displayed great variations in professional skill, ability to speak Hebrew, and skill in patient management, competition would have resulted in great initial inequalities in patient loads and incomes, followed by price-cutting by the underemployed. But *Histadrut* and other organizations have organized the entire Israeli labor market so that immigration has not depressed wages: the wages of the employed cannot be cut easily, employees cannot be fired and replaced easily by a new immigrant, and immigrants are hired at the wage scale set for the existing labor force. The same type of labor market is maintained in medicine by the *Histadrut*-influenced employers—*Kupat Holim* and the government—and by the Israel Medical Association and its affiliated medical societies. Immigrant doctors are screened by the employers and hired at the existing salary scales. Medical employers have agreed to combat unemployment by spreading the work: most offer part-time jobs; most offer six-hour and seven-hour work days to senior doctors at full pay, a policy officially designed to fulfill Israel's traditional respect for job seniority, but actually adopted during the late 1950's to spread the work. *Kupat Holim* could have saved much money by adopting different payment methods but, since it is a branch of *Histadrut* and is committed to the parent body's labor policies, it has been willing to spend the extra money to facilitate the adjustment of immigrant doctors.

Parity or Lower Pay for Medicine

In most salaried systems, doctors as a class are among the highest paid in the society, both because the lowest medical category is comparatively high and because the median point for the entire profession is high. Doctors start near the top because most public wage systems in the world fix the beginning point for any occupation in accordance with the amount of preparatory education. Medicine usually is paid more than other professions with comparable amounts of education, on grounds of special knowledge and responsibility.

However, a few countries have wage systems that place medicine parallel to, rather than above, other professional and managerial occupations. In an entirely socialized economy like the U.S.S.R., health was designated one of several economic sectors. Each sector has had its salary scale. The doctors were put only at the top of the health scale and not at the top of the entire national wage system. Pursuant to guidelines adopted by the Central Council of Trade Unions in 1921, doctors were classified among the technical personnel and managers in the field of health, depending on the jobs they occupy. Thus they have been paid more than lower ranks in health and in nonmedical fields, but like the other technical personnel and managers in other fields whose pay scales had similar values in rubles. Since managers and professors in all sectors earn the highest salaries, all managers in industry automatically stand at the top of the industrial salary scales and earn more than the clinicians. Some doctors belong to the high-paid managerial and academic classes by virtue of directorships in medical installations and professorships, but most do not. The spread of the medical profession throughout a salary range parallel to other educated employees is quite different from the concentration of doctors at a level comparable to managers in most other countries.[57]

Doctors may be paid at the same level as all other professions and skilled occupations if their government has imposed austerity on everyone. An example is postwar Poland, which has a very high rate of savings for reconstruction and industrialization. Poland has been able to enforce austerity because much of the economy is owned or managed by the government, including the medical services. Medicine has its own scales but, like other occupations, the differentials by rank are very narrow. According to the basic scale in effect during the early 1950's, the highest basic wage class for doctors with twenty or more years of experience was only double the rate for the newly licensed doctor. First degree specialists with three years of hospital training received an increase of less than 10 per cent over the basic rate; second degree specialists with six years of hospital training received increases of only 15 per cent over the basic rates. Chiefs-of-service, polyclinic directors, and hospital directors obtained extra payments of only between 10 and 25 per cent of the basic rates paid general practitioners. As a result, doctors earned about the same as other professionals, managers, and skilled workers.[58]

[57] The mixture of medicine and other professions and skilled occupations over a considerable pay range is summarized in, Nicholas DeWitt, *Education and Professional Employment in the U.S.S.R.* (Washington: National Science Foundation, 1961), p. 543.

[58] The salary scales for doctors at that time appear in Zwiazek Zawodowy Pracownikow Sluzby Zdrowia P.R.L., *Przepisy Uposazeniowe Sluzby Zdrowia Obowiazujace od Dnia 1 XII 1958* (Warsaw: Panstwowy Zaklad Wydawnictw Lekarskich, 1959), pp. 13–61 passim.

Some payment systems systematically place the medical profession in a less elevated position in the national income structure, and the governments can enforce these priorities. But this is exceptional. The leading examples are the Soviet Union and some of its allies, whose emphasis on industrialization has resulted in giving engineers, architects, planners, designers, other technical professionals, coal miners, and some other industrial time-rate workers higher pay than doctors. At times during the 1930's and 1940's, the basic salary scale for engineers in some parts of the U.S.S.R. was double that of doctors.[59]

The incentive system introduced during the period of rapid industrialization also enabled engineers, industrial managers, and many industrial workers to surpass the medical profession. Managers and engineers could earn production bonuses equal to half or all of their base salaries. Many doctors earned bonuses too, but performance in medicine was less measurable and less prized, the Commissariat of Health was given less bonus money in the annual budgets, and doctors' bonuses were smaller proportions of their base salaries. Since medical performance cannot be rated by productivity measures, doctors were paid by straight-time rates and could not be paid by piece-rates or premium-time rates. Energetic and ambitious factory workers and miners working on piece-rates could surpass the incomes of doctors and indeed could earn more than their own foremen.

However, when emergency conditions eased, laymen ultimately conceded the medical profession a leading position in the Soviet Union as in other countries. Stalin was replaced by a new leadership that had greater respect for the social contributions of medicine. The Medical Workers Union became more active in pressing the wage claims of the doctors before the Ministry of Health and the Central Council of Trade Unions. The wage system was streamlined after Stalin's death, and the industrial occupations were given fewer opportunities to earn bonuses and other extra pay. Medicine acquired almost the same salary scale as engineering, but the latter still had more opportunities for industrial bonuses.[60]

Preserving or Creating Income Differentials between Medicine and Other Occupations

Every profession is convinced of the prime social importance of its work and seeks both the resources and recognition to perform well. Income is a

---

The remarkable similarity among occupations in the distribution of incomes at that time was evident in *Concise Statistical Year Book of the Polish People's Republic* (Warsaw: Glowny Urzad Statystyczny, 1961), pp. 57–59, 77, 117, 126, 135, 144, 158–61.

[59] Compare the salary scale for doctors in 1935 in, Grigory N. Kaminsky, *Okhrana zdorov'ya v sovetskom soyuze* (Moscow: Narodny Komissariat Zdravookhraneniya, 1935), pp. 114–19; with the scale for engineers in, Gregory Bienstock, Solomon M. Schwarz, and Aaron Yugow, *Management in Russian Industry and Agriculture* (New York: Oxford University Press, 1944), p. 93.

[60] B. Sukharevskii, "Razvitii sferi obspuzhivanii i stroitespstvo kommunisma," *Voprosy Ekonomiki*, no. 10 (1964), pp. 10–14.

means for purchasing facilities, a reward for good performance of important tasks, and a symbol of the relative priority given by society to the profession's work. No profession is completely satisfied that society is giving it sufficient means or is obeying the profession's advice urgently enough. Therefore, every profession thinks it is underpaid. Medicine, too, usually protests that its pay is inadequate, even when it is at the top of the society's wage structure. Consequently, official payment systems are continually beset by demands from the medical profession to maintain or to re-establish actual or imagined differentials in relation to other occupations.

Salaried systems in national medical care schemes often arouse discontent, because salary rates usually change only occasionally, and the increases cannot exceed the resources from taxation. Meanwhile, salaries and pay in the private economic sector may be rising, thereby reducing the advantages enjoyed by the doctors. Under a completely salaried system, the physicians cannot increase their incomes substantially through a greater number of procedures, as under fee-for-service.

If a national medical care scheme does not commit itself to guaranteeing preservation of the differentials between the salaried doctors and other occupations, it will antagonize the medical profession. If it bases its remuneration policy on this goal, it runs other risks. The history of salaried pay for consultants in Great Britain illustrates both dangers.

Like the capitation fees for British general practitioners, consultants' salaries remained fixed during the late 1940's and early 1950's, while wages in the rest of the economy rose. When the Danckwerts Award of 1952 produced a large increase that pleased the general practitioners and distressed the Treasury, the consultants also asked for arbitration, but the Minister of Health insisted the issue be settled by bilateral negotiation and by the Whitley Council machinery. The Treasury and the Cabinet were really buying time until they could find money for a new and expensive pay raise. The events bore an undertone of the traditional rivalry between consultant and general practitioner: at the request of the British Medical Association, the Royal Colleges had delayed pressing the consultants' case until the general practitioners' pay had been settled by the Danckwerts Award; the gap between consultants and general practitioners was reduced by Danckwerts, and budgetary limitations postponed a restoration of the old relationship; the leaders of the Royal Colleges asked the Cabinet for a pay increase on the grounds of restoring the pay differential between consultants and G.P.'s, an argument that hardly pleased some of the leaders of the BMA. The Treasury finally agreed to provide enough money to restore the differential between consultants' and general practitioners' pay, and the Medical Whitley Council in 1954 announced the new rates for all hospital doctors.[61]

[61] H. A. Clegg and T. E. Chester, *Wage Policy and the Health Service* (Oxford: Basil Blackwell, 1957), p. 62; and Lord Moran, *Minutes of Evidence* (note 23), p. 196.

Again after 1954, salary scales remained fixed for several years. Meanwhile the economy boomed and pay increased for industrial managers and other salaried personnel in private employment. However, the average total incomes for consultants remained higher than the incomes for all other occupations; rigidities in the salaried system merely narrowed the gap from time to time.[62] Because they were still paid more than anyone else and could earn additional income at their own discretion from private practice, the consultants complained less bitterly about the National Health Service than did the general practitioners.

The Royal Commission and the Review Body during the 1960's adopted the policy that consultants' salaries should preserve pre-existing relationships to the income structure of the rest of the country.[63] Salaries could not be changed frequently, so awards would be made at approximate three-year intervals on the basis of economic forecasts. The Royal Commission and the Review Body estimated the probable increase in the national wage structure and would raise specialists' salaries so that the average over the subsequent period would match the increase of income elsewhere. At the beginning of the award period, the salaries would be high; and at the end of the period, they would be low.

This policy of guaranteeing income parity has proved difficult to administer well and inimical to the national economy. The first problem has been that the award bodies cannot accurately predict movements of incomes in the rest of the country. The salary increases announced in 1960 and 1963 were smaller than the subsequent rises in the rest of the economy. Second, if such an incomes policy were made general throughout the country, every occupation could demand pay rises when any one received an increase; salaries and wages could rise faster than productivity; and a steadily worsening inflation could result. Such a policy is particularly dangerous for a major international trader like Great Britain. Third, the policy has been self-defeating because the other professions would not accept statuses permanently below the consultants. Each profession claims more pay than it is getting, and it points to those who are paid more. The survey data about other professions' salaries and incomes that were published by the Royal Commission had been intended to show the proper differentials between

[62] Royal Commission, *Doctors' and Dentists' Remuneration* (1960) (note 21), pp. 30–31, 39–40, 45–47, 54.

[63] "Now that the vast majority of their earnings come from the state, a monopoly employer for practical purposes, doctors and dentists should have their remuneration settled by external comparison, principally, though not necessarily exclusively, with professional men and others with a university background in other walks of life in Great Britain." Ibid., paragraph 16. The reasoning that led to the Royal Commission's award in 1960 appears in ibid., pp. 4–7, 50–54. The guidelines for the Review Body were stated in ibid., pp. 140–50. Second thoughts about the Royal Commission's data and the difficulties of executing a policy of preserving income differentials are summarized in *Review Body on Doctors' and Dentists' Remuneration: Seventh Report* (London: H. M. Stationery Office, Cmnd. 2992, 1966), chap. 3.

them and the better paid consultants. But several of these professions cited the Royal Commission's report as evidence for successful demands that *they* should be paid more. Finally, a wage policy based on preserving economic differentials ignored other essential criteria, such as the construction of pay grades to regulate recruitment or motivate higher productivity.

In 1966, the consultants and general practitioners sought pay increases that would keep pace with increases in other professions. But the government had been combating inflation, and prices had been moving more slowly. Often, in official payment systems, doctors base pay demands on the need to avoid declines in real income. But in 1966, their requests would have led to temporary gains in real income, while feeding a general wage-price inflationary spiral that the government was combating. Therefore, the Review Body in 1966 stated that its goal would be to optimize recruitment and retention in medicine.

However, fixing pay to regulate recruitment and retention proved equally difficult to administer. Information was not available fast enough and in sufficient volume for planning: very little was known about how the last pay award was affecting recruitment and retention. Projecting the effects of pay awards was very uncertain: any results would be visible only long after the pay awards were made. In 1968, the Review Body resumed its principal emphasis on relativities, on the grounds that current data were sufficient for this basis of decisions, and on the grounds that maintaining existing differentials would protect recruitment and retention.[64]

England illustrates the difficulty of preserving a fixed differential between medical salaries in the *public* sector and the incomes of *privately* employed occupations. Such a policy might be possible in a centrally planned and centrally controlled economy. But even when all occupations are in the public sector, the policy cannot be maintained consistently if pressure groups can gain advantages for one or another group. An example is Israel.[65]

Before Independence, occupations employed by the public organizations among the Jewish population paid nearly the same basic wage, in accordance with the general ideology of brotherhood and self-sacrifice. A standard salary

[64] The issues in 1966 were stated in "Profession's Evidence to Review Body" and "Health Departments' Evidence to Review Body," *British Medical Journal Supplement* (7 May 1966), pp. 127–34. The resumption of the primary emphasis on relativities was explained in *Review Body on Doctors' and Dentists' Remuneration: Ninth Report* (London: H. M. Stationery Office, Cmnd. 3600, 1968); and *Review Body on Doctors' and Dentists' Remuneration: Tenth Report* (London: H. M. Stationery Office, Cmnd. 3884, 1969).

[65] On the turbulent history of Israeli wage policy and the central role of the doctors, see Milton Derber, "Israel's Wage Differential: A Persisting Problem," *Midstream*, vol. 9, no. 1 (March 1963), pp. 60–72; Joseph Ben-David, "Professionals and Unions in Israel," *Industrial Relations*, vol. 5, no. 1 (October 1965), pp. 48–66; and Georges Friedmann, *The End of the Jewish People?* (Garden City, N.Y.: Doubleday Anchor Books, 1968), pp. 107–8. See also Milton Derber, "National Wage Policy in Israel, 1948–1962," *Quarterly Review of Economics and Business*, vol. 3, no. 3 (Autumn 1963), pp. 47–60.

scale with very small increments existed, and the doctors employed by the sick funds and by other Jewish agencies ranked near its top. Since pay was supposed to satisfy people's needs, the important differentials were based on the number of dependents and on seniority.

A steady relationship among occupations might have survived only if the *Histadrut* (the General Federation of Jewish Labor) had retained the central position it occupied before Independence. Since nongovernmental agencies ran the economic and social affairs of the Jewish community under the Arab-oriented British mandate, *Histadrut* was the labor representative of most occupations, a leading entrepreneur, sponsor of the *Kupat Holim* and other social services, and the focus of political activity. After Independence, *Histadrut's* governing body continued to lay down guidelines for pay awards to maintain existing differentials. But the professions—led by the doctors—demanded higher pay than the workers on the basis of their education, skill, and social importance.

Histadrut's guidelines no longer could be enforced effectively, since the professions followed their own leaderships rather than the *Histadrut*. The doctors employed by the government in 1950 struck successfully to force the Ministry of Health and the Government Personnel Committee to bargain with the independent Israel Medical Association and not to set their pay and working conditions in negotiation with the *Histadrut*-affiliated General Association of Government Employees. Thereafter the *Kupat Holim* of *Histadrut* itself—the largest employer of doctors—had to deal with the IMA. Other professional associations broke away from the wage guidelines of the *Histadrut*, even when they nominally remained members of the *Histadrut*. Since they shared a common interest in widening differentials between the professions and other occupations, the professional associations formed a co-ordinating committee with headquarters at the Israel Medical Association.

The self-interested policy on differentials by each occupation has prevented existence of a stable national policy. During the early 1950's, the doctors, followed by the other professions, obtained substantial differentials over the workers for the first time. Then the differentials narrowed, because of pressure by the workers invoking the country's traditional egalitarianism, and because of the equalizing effects of the cost-of-living increases in the salary scales of all occupations. The cycle of wider and narrower differentials in the country continued thereafter in no small part due to the bargaining success—and occasional strikes—of the Israel Medical Association.[66] The

[66] Because other occupations press to catch up with the wage increases granted the first one, Israeli wage differentials remain perhaps the narrowest in the world. Giora Hanoch, *Income Differentials in Israel* (Jerusalem: The Falk Project for Economic Research in Israel, 1961), chap. 1. But the differentials between the liberal professions and other occupations have widened since independence. Ruth Klinov-Malul, *The Profitability of Investment in Education in Israel* (Jerusalem: The Falk Project for Economic Research in Israel, 1966), pp. 15–16, 35–36.

government dared to freeze wages only when war seemed imminent. A Polish-style austerity could not be imposed because the uneasy coalition of political parties that ruled both the government and *Histadrut* feared losses of votes.

Some consequences of the "link-up" practice in Israeli wage administration illustrates a danger of the fixed-differential method of wage policy. The link-up principle means that differentials among certain occupations shall be held constant; when the *Histadrut* and the government in the early 1950's conceded that the professions should earn more than the workers, the professions were linked among themselves. But linking has often boomeranged against wage policy by enabling occupations to gain wage increases before the expiration of their contracts, simply because a linked occupation has secured an increase during *its* bargaining. The situation invites surreptitious encouragement of strategic occupations to which many others are linked, and the medical profession has sometimes done this during periods when its own wage demands were supposed to have been satisfied by a contract. For example, during January 1962 the engineers rejected arbitration awards by two impartial bodies that they had previously agreed to obey, and they called a strike for much higher pay. Resulting from internal politics within the Engineers Union, the strike was one of the most widely criticized in Israeli history. But the country's employed physicians called a half-day sympathy strike. The doctors' sympathy for the engineers was aroused by the link-up practice: if the engineers' pay rose by much, so would the doctors'; the medical profession only four months before had gained a salary increase of its own but could not otherwise obtain more money until the expiration of its contract several years later. Sometimes the bargaining strength of the doctors is increased by assistance of other linked occupations. For example, instead of earning them the united opposition of the country, the doctors' strike in February 1956 was joined by many other professionals and civil servants.[67]

Prestige

It is not surprising that the specialist is widely respected in countries where he receives high salaries and enjoys a lucrative private practice. The chief-of-service of a hospital and the professor in the medical school are among the highest rated occupations in public opinion polls.[68]

But the same high ratings are given the salaried medical profession in countries where the pay is not so generous and where working conditions

[67] Nadav Halevi, "Israel's Wage Dilemma," *Midstream*, vol. 2, no. 4 (Autumn 1956), p. 65.

[68] For example, the Danish public ranked the salaried hospital specialists higher than the fee-earning office practitioners in the survey reported in, Kaare Svalastoga, *Prestige, Class and Mobility* (Copenhagen: Glydendal, 1959), pp. 74–131 passim.

have been difficult. Apparently the value and interest of medical work is not offset in public opinion by limitations on remuneration and facilities. Also, despite the complaints by doctors in such countries, the population thinks they have an admirable life and that its own troubles are worse.

A good example is Poland. The liberal intellectual press in Warsaw frequently reports the medical profession's complaints about pay, working conditions, and an allegedly plunging social status.[69] But the Polish population does not agree. Warsaw inhabitants questioned in 1958 rated doctors ahead of nearly all other occupational groups in social prestige, as a desirable profession for one's child, and even in pay.[70] A sample of Lodz workers interviewed in 1961 believed, on the average, that doctors had retained their prewar financial position and social prestige; many respondents believed that medicine as a profession had risen in esteem and on the financial scale.[71]

Soviet doctors, too, have often complained about their pay.[72] Also, many doctors for years resented that the engineers, who may have seemed to belong to a less "cultured" social class, received more recognition. Nevertheless, Soviet doctors have been paid more than most people, and—since most doctors have been women married to managers and professionals—their family incomes have been high. In response to questionnaires, the postwar Russian escapees said that medicine was more desirable in their eyes than any other occupation and enjoyed the highest regard from the Soviet people. The escapees recognized that doctors received lower material rewards than managers and engineers, but they ranked doctors' living standards ahead of most other occupations. The better paid careers were said to have offsetting disadvantages from political risks and potential demotion for poor performance.[73]

Even in Turkey, where the low pay and slow promotions are said to distress many doctors, medicine is the most highly respected occupation.[74]

[69] E.g., Stefan Baniarz, "Nie Chcę Być Judymem," *Polityka*, vol. 6, no. 25 (23 June 1962), p. 2; Wilhelmina Skulska, "Sluzba Zdrowia I Co Dalej?" *Kultura* (5 December 1965), pp. 5, 9; and Adam Sarapata's opinion polls among doctors, published in *Zycie Warszawy*, late 1959.

[70] Wlodzimierz Wesolowski and Adam Sarapata, "Hierarchie Zawadow i Stanowisk," *Studia Socjologiczne*, no. 2 (1961), pp. 91–124.

[71] Adam Sarapata, "Z Badan nad Przemianami w Hierarchii Zawodow," *Studia Socjologiczne*, no. 1 (1962), pp. 93–112.

[72] Field, *Doctor and Patient* (note 6), pp. 105–7.

[73] Peter H. Rossi and Alex Inkeles, "Multidimensional Ratings of Occupations," *Sociometry*, vol. 20, no. 3 (September 1957), pp. 234–51; and Alex Inkeles and Raymond A. Bauer, *The Soviet Citizen* (Cambridge: Harvard University Press, 1959), pp. 76–78.

[74] George Helling, "Changing Attitudes toward Occupational Status and Prestige in Turkey" (Washington: unpublished paper given at the Fifth World Congress of Sociology, 1962). In Helling's sample of 310 young adults from Western Anatolia, only military careers outranked medicine among rural respondents, while university teaching, engineering and a few high government posts were rated higher than medicine by cosmopolitan city-dwellers. But medicine ranked highest on the average in the entire survey.

One might expect that the salaried and employed segment of the medical profession would enjoy less public respect in countries where most physicians are office practitioners or have high statuses in hospitals. But even they possess the same high prestige as all doctors. For example, a British survey placed the public health doctor—called the Medical Officer of Health—ahead of all twenty-nine other occupations.[75]

Recruitment

Large numbers of students apply to medical schools in all countries, regardless of how doctors are paid. Whether many or few physicians are graduated annually depends upon educational policy rather than upon any inhibiting effects of the payment system. Several countries where much of the profession depends on salaries—Great Britain, Sweden, and Israel—are now graduating too few doctors for their future needs, but the result is due to these countries' preference for small medical schools guaranteeing their students sufficient clinical experience. As a result, these countries' medical schools have far more applicants than places. Another style of medical education—practiced in most of the world, including the Eastern European and underdeveloped countries with salaried national health services—admits and graduates large classes that receive primarily didactic instruction.

If the payment system affects initial recruitment into medicine, it may influence composition rather than number. If other technical and scientific fields seem more competitive, become more challenging, and offer remuneration depending on effort, then medicine may lose the more adventurous and hard-working recruits and may acquire proportionately more students who prefer stable working conditions and predictable careers.

For example, some observers believe that the working and payment conditions in Soviet and Polish medicine during the periods of industrialization resulted in losses of many potential male students to engineering and scientific research, thereby bringing about disproportionately female medical professions. Since they did not expect to be the principal family breadwinners, women were thought to be attracted to a profession that would help relieve human suffering, that would bring no more than a moderate and predictable salary, and that would require no more than fixed working hours in an organized setting. The excessive feminization of medicine began to worry both the Soviet and Polish Ministries of Health during the late 1950's and early 1960's: both countries had always suffered from severe shortages of rural doctors, but a female profession would concentrate in the cities more than ever and would prevent the government from keeping its pledges to

[75] John Hall and D. Caradog Jones, "Social Grading of Occupations," *British Journal of Sociology*, vol. 1 (January 1950), pp. 38–40.

develop rural medical care; women doctors have higher absence rates than men; many women doctors interrupt or terminate their careers to care for children; women doctors change jobs suddenly if their husbands move to other cities.[76] Attracting more men into medicine was an important motive for the governmental and Party leaders' reduction of the salary differentials between engineers and doctors in both countries during the 1960's.

The feminization of Soviet medicine had causes in addition to economics and work organization. A high participation by women in the urban professions has long been a tradition. Because of the killing and wounding of men in wars and purges, women at times have constituted three-fifths of certain age cohorts in the population and a majority of the labor force from these generations. Homemaking careers were made impossible by crowded living conditions and shared kitchen arrangements.[77] The entry of women into salaried medical work may be a worldwide trend. In addition to the advantages of salaried practice mentioned in the text, women doctors in the West may prefer it to private practice because they are relieved of the work and continuing obligations associated with a private office.[78]

Retention and Allocation

Ideally a salary structure should give the holders of each rank the proper balance of incentives and disincentives so that they move through the organizational structure according to the needs of the system. Able persons should be rewarded at a level inducing them to stay in the system, but the next higher level should offer sufficient increments to attract them into positions of more responsibility. Pay should not be so high at intermediate or low ranks that holders become too old or too numerous: instead, economic incentives elsewhere should be attractive enough to induce the less valuable members to leave in sufficient numbers for the nonsalaried opportunities in the profession. Salary is the payment method most susceptible to the rational planning of the allocation and movement of doctors.

The wage that is sufficient to keep persons in a rank varies at different times. Until recently, the lower ranks in hospitals were paid very little and

[76] The debate in Poland broke into the press. E.g., Jerzy Urban, "Medycyna pod Szpilka," *Polityka*, vol. 6, no. 26 (30 June 1962), pp. 1–3.

[77] The predominant numbers of women in Soviet medical schools and medical practice are described in B.-D. Petrov, "Le rôle des femmes dans le service de santé de l'U.R.S.S.," *Concours médical*, vol. 87, no. 11 (13 March 1965), pp. 1899–1900. However, as in the sciences and other technical fields, the principal administrative jobs and professorships in medicine are held by men. De Witt, *Education and Professional Emplyoment* (note 57), p. 522; Galina V. Zarechnak, *Academy of Medical Sciences of the U.S.S.R.* (Washington: Public Health Monograph No. 63, U.S. Department of Health, Education, and Welfare, 1960), pp. 44–48; and John B. Parrish, "Professional Womenpower as a Soviet Resource," *Quarterly Review of Economics and Business*, vol. 4, no. 3 (Autumn 1964), pp. 55–61.

[78] For statistics on the tendency for increasing numbers of women to enter salaried rather than office practice, see Bernard de Fréminville, "Place des femmes médecins dans le monde," *Concours médical*, vol. 88, no. 46 (12 November 1966), pp. 7007–8.

worked hard, but young doctors tolerated the deprivations, in anticipation of future posts as chiefs-of-service, when they too would earn large private incomes and delegate the hospital's work to their assistants. The hope behind the graded salary structures established after the war is that younger doctors will accept lower ranks not in a spirit of current sacrifice in order to achieve future bonanzas, but because they are paid commensurate with their training and work and because they hope to progress in an orderly sequence toward higher responsibilities. But countries differ in how far their financial capacities permit realization of these reforms. Substantial discrepancies among countries have existed, while the medical profession has become more mobile and multilingual.

One result of these cross-national differences in the salaries and working conditions of intermediate ranks has been complaint. Because some have studied in the more generously endowed countries and others have heard idealized reports, younger doctors in hospitals, on medical school staffs, in research institutes, and other organizations in many countries have called for improvements in their own systems. They have criticized not only pay but the excessive authority of the chiefs-of-service and professors, excessively pyramidal structures due to the limited numbers of chiefs and professorships, shortages of research funds and facilities, and the limited professional freedom of the junior staff.[79] Younger doctors have been a principal force behind reform.

An example is the enthusiastic support by the younger doctors of the establishment in France of a full-time salaried medical service, in both teaching and nonteaching hospitals. Until the 1960's, France had the traditional system of low pay, with chiefs finally recouping after their appointments for the many years of deprivation. The reform was favored by some of the older chiefs who had passed the years of most profitable private practice; but it was opposed by the intermediate group who were becoming chiefs during the 1960's, since they still needed to make up for the years of low income. The new system is being introduced gradually. Young doctors entering the hospital service will be full-time and salaried throughout their careers. The doctors who were already chiefs during the early 1960's can choose to be part-time with the customary remunerative private practice or to be full-time at the new salaries. As the part-time doctors retire, all ranks will be full-time and salaried, without an outside private practice.[80]

[79] For example, the criticisms of European hospital staff structure after their study in America by Renzo Tomatis, *Il laboratorio* (Turin: Giulio Einaudi, 1965); and Urs Peter Haemmerli, "Principes d'organisation dans un hôpital d'enseignement Américain," *Médecine et Hygiène* (Geneva), vol. 17 (30 January 1959), pp. 38–39.

[80] The basic decrees adopted during 1958 through 1960 are summarized in, Paul Comet, *L'hôpital public* (Paris: Berger-Levrault, 1960). The administrative plans are in, Jean-Jacques Ribas and Michel Rougevin-Baville, "Les centres hospitaliers et universitaires et la réforme médicale," *Droit social*, vol. 25, nos. 9–10 (September–October 1962),

The alternative to reform is migration, and postwar medicine has seen a movement of younger salaried doctors to hospitals and research institutes in countries offering more pay and better working conditions. In general, the movement has been from underdeveloped countries to the more developed; from Southern Europe northward; and from many European and non-European countries to the United States and Canada. As a result, many countries have lost promising young specialists that they needed; but their public medical services lack the money to raise salaries and to provide the research facilities that seem so attractive in the United States. Some countries, such as Great Britain, lose young hospital doctors to more attractive systems (such as the United States, Canada, Australia, and New Zealand) and attract replacements from less affluent countries (such as Pakistan, the West Indies, and Cyprus).[81]

If a salaried medical service is ruled by officials with data about personnel flows and with power to manipulate pay rates, they can raise or lower salaries in the light of needs. For example, data in the 1960's showed that British hospitals had too few registrars, a number of registrars and house officers had emigrated, and remuneration was one of their complaints about the National Health Service.[82] Therefore the Review Body recommended that the registrars receive a higher position in the salary scale, in order to motivate more to stay.[83]

Combinations of pecuniary and organizational changes were made to correct numerical imbalances in the British hospital services in earlier years too. Administrative modifications are needed to achieve a desired effect,

---

pp. 488–99. The first CHU's are described in, Marilise Pascaud, "Tour de France des C.H.U.," *Concours médical*, vol. 88, no. 15 (9 April 1966), pp. 2631–37; and A. Lemaire, G. Baldassini, and R. Goutières, "Le secteur Saint-Antoine du Centre Hospitalier et Universitaire de Paris," *Presse médicale*, vol. 73, no. 44 (23 October 1965).

[81] On the migration of doctors generally and the possible role of income differentials, see "Outflow of Trained Personnel from Developing Countries: Report of the Secretary General" (New York: United Nations General Assembly, 23rd Session, 5 November 1968, A/7294), pp. 35–40; and studies cited in, Stevan Dedijer and L. Svenningson, *Brain Drain and Brain Gain: A Bibliography on Migration of Scientists, Engineers, Doctors and Students* (Lund: Research Policy Program, 1967). On the loss of doctors to the United States because of higher salaries and other advantages, see *Migration of Health Personnel, Scientists, and Engineers from Latin America* (Washington: Pan American Health Organization, 1966), passim, esp. chaps. 4 and 5; Carl E. Taylor et al., *Health Manpower Planning in Turkey* (Baltimore: The Johns Hopkins Press, 1968), pp. 39, 60–62; and Burton M. Halpern, "New Exodus: Israel's Talent Drain," *Nation*, vol. 200 (10 May 1965), pp. 497–99. On the costs to the developed countries who also suffer losses, see "Minister Addresses Young Doctors," *British Medical Journal Supplement* (24 September 1966), pp. 134–35.

[82] Brian Abel-Smith and Kathleen Gales, *British Doctors at Home and Abroad* (Welwyn: The Codicote Press, 1964), chap. 4; Minister of Health Kenneth Robinson's statement during question time in the House of Commons, summarized in *Lancet* (29 October 1966), pp. 974–75; and John R. Seale, *The Supply of Doctors and the Future of the British Medical Profession* (London: Fellowship for Freedom in Medicine, 1962).

[83] Review Body's seventh report, *Doctors' and Dentists' Remuneration* (note 63), pp. 33–37, 82.

since changes in remuneration are limited in size to preserve the general form of the salary scale and because nonpecuniary motives often have countervailing effects, particularly in medicine. For example, during the 1950's there developed a surplus of senior registrars (since there were not enough consultantships to allow promotion for all) and a shortage of registrars (since the surplus of senior registrars discouraged many doctors from entering hospital careers). To stimulate recruitment of registrars, the Royal Commission recommended a pay raise but avoided making it so high as to encourage them to remain too long instead of entering general practice.[84] Classical economic theory would have dictated a pay cut for the senior registrars, but this was impossible, since their salary would no longer have matched the hierarchical structure of the medical staff. The senior registrars got a pay raise too, but a smaller one than the registrars'.[85] Another committee recommended administrative measures to reduce the number of senior registrars, such as more frequent revision of the number of posts and more thorough screening of candidates.[86]

Conclusion: The Effects of Salary

Salaried payment is part of an organized medical service. Therefore the possible advantages and weaknesses of salary payment depend on the traditions and medical organization of the country: salaries can be associated with excellence or with weakness. Hasty care, few home visits, excessive referrals, and other defects occur in some countries but not in others. Certain desirable results—such as nonmercenary attitudes, close colleague relations, interest in personal professional growth, economical care, etc.—are certainly not universal in all countries with salaried medicine, but cross-national variations exist as a result of tradition, the attitudes of the medical association, the organization of the system, the ratio of doctors to resources, and so on. The mixture of part-time salaried practice and part-time private fee-for-service practice can generate serious administrative and ethical problems that would not exist under any payment system covering the full working day. Probably all salaried practice has the virtue of greater administrative simplicity than fee-for-service and capitation systems. As a general rule, salaried systems do not encourage unnecessary treatment or medically unjustified multiplication of procedures, but the latter is possible in a few systems where doctors can earn overtime or can select the amount of salaried work time.

Since salaries are fixed and publicly known, they invite invidious com-

[84] Royal Commission, *Doctors' and Dentists' Remuneration* (1960) (note 21), pp. 92–93.
[85] Ibid., pp. 91–92.
[86] *Medical Staffing Structure in the Hospital Service: Report of the Joint Working Party* (London: H. M. Stationery Office, 1961), pp. 19–26.

parisons between medicine and other occupations, and doctors' pay may become controversial: doctors may press to equal or surpass other salaried occupations; lower ranking doctors may grumble about the better paid; other salaried occupations may complain that their common employer (such as the hospital or the government) favors doctors unduly. Salaried systems easily become targets for discontent, even when the basic problem is a limited national income: under fee-for-service, a low-paid doctor in such a country could not point to a specific scapegoat; in an equally unrewarding salaried system, it is easy to blame the government. Since medicine is a high-status profession and doctors are aware of foreign trends, even a high income by domestic standards may not be fully satisfying, if the country's doctors select as their reference group a better paid foreign medical profession. Despite controversies, the salaries paid doctors are usually very high by a country's income standards, and specialists can earn even more through supplementary private practice. In nearly all countries, the most prized medical careers combine salaried specialty work and private practice.

Since an extensive salaried system is part of an organized medical service, the latter may be part of a larger public service. Thus many decisions about doctors' pay are part of larger economic plans. Doctors may believe themselves badly treated if the government's economic policies give priority to other occupations. Sometimes the medical profession may do relatively well, but by means of pressure group action that upsets the régime's plans. The outcome results from the comparative power of the planners and of the medical association, and it is affected by the prestige of medicine in public opinion.

Some salary structures are delicately attuned to encourage movements of doctors into certain jobs and regions, and to discourage other career choices. These incentives succeed if they coincide with other rewards and professional values. By themselves, the monetary incentives may not be enough to compensate for undesirable features of jobs and regions. In practice, very large differentials usually are not provided to attract doctors into less popular assignments, because of the need to preserve a rank hierarchy in pay. For example, most countries are short of doctors in rural areas, because few salaried systems violate the rank principle to the extent of placing rural general practitioners higher than most specialists.

X

EFFECTS OF CAPITATION

Capitation shares many of the attractions of salaried payment, since both are flat-rate methods. Many administrators prefer capitation since financing is predictable: costs do not fluctuate or rise excessively because of the work of doctors and the illnesses of patients. Billing for procedures is not a part of the plan, and therefore administration is simpler than under fee-for-service.[1]

Those who favor capitation also believe that it fosters good medicine. The doctor has a continuing relationship with a patient on his list. Unlike many salaried systems, the doctor—and not an organization—has the direct contact with the patient. Compared to fee-for-service, the turnover of patients should be lower and the doctor-patient relationship should persist in both sickness and health. The doctor should be motivated to practice preventive medicine: he gains no added income from treatments, and a desire to conserve effort should induce him to keep his patients healthy.[2]

[1] The British general practitioners interviewed by a visiting American doctor said that the elimination of collections and the reduction of paper work were among the greatest merits of the National Health Service. Paul F. Gemmill, *Britain's Search for Health* (Philadelphia: University of Pennsylvania Press, 1960), pp. 123–25. In Montague's survey of doctors in three countries, the English had more complaints than the Americans about pay, facilities, and the organization of medical services, but fewer complained about clerical work. Joel B. Montague, Jr., "Professionalism among American, Australian, and English Physicians," *Journal of Health and Human Behavior*, vol. 7 (Winter 1966), pp. 286–87. Capitation has more administrative overhead than salaried systems, because it must incorporate checks against inclusion of a patient on more than one list, so that different doctors do not earn several capitation fees from the same patient. The British investigating procedures are described in *Report of the Committee of Enquiry Into the Cost of the National Health Service* (London: H. M. Stationery Office, 1956), pp. 169–72.

[2] For such clinical arguments on behalf of capitation by an administrator of Spain's insurance programs, see Enrique Serrano Guirado, *El Seguro de Enfermedad y sus problemas* (Madrid: Instituto de Estudios Politicos, 1950), pp. 313–14. During the negotiations to harmonize national health insurance in all the Common Market countries, some officials of sick funds and trade unions favored extending the Dutch capitation system throughout European general practice for some of the reasons given in the text. Jean Mignon, "Vers

Encouraging Good Medicine

Proper Referral

One of the potential weaknesses of capitation payments is neglect. Since income increases with length of list, the doctor is motivated to enroll many regular patients. But since the doctor earns the same capitation fee regardless of the amount of care, he may be motivated to minimize time and work for each patient. The longer his list, the greater the need to economize on time. Therefore, despite its expected advantages, some policymakers have decided that capitation will not work well enough in practice.

The Commission that investigated German social security during the 1960's searched for any reform that would combat the venal multiplication of procedures long thought endemic in German health insurance. At first inspection, capitation seemed superior. But the belief that the capitation system produces neglect—thereby creating worse problems than overuse under fee-for-service—led the Commission to recommend retention of Germany's existing system.[3]

Professional ethics usually are too strong to lead any doctor to neglect completely a time-consuming or troublesome patient. Rather, referrals may be made more often than is justified by ideal medical policy. A widespread impression among many hospital directors and others acquainted with medical affairs in Great Britain and Holland is that undue numbers of troublesome and time-consuming patients are referred by general practitioners to the outpatient departments of hospitals.[4] G.P.'s themselves can give the necessary long courses of treatments to patients suffering from chronic diseases like diabetes, arthritis, hypothyroid, and pernicious anemia; but many hospitals find that busy G.P.'s send these time-consuming patients to them. Some G.P.'s may send patients with puzzling symptoms to the hospital for diagnostic examination at once, without taking time for a thorough examination. The G.P. loses nothing, since he continues to receive his capitation fee; hospital doctors get more work without more income, since they are paid by salary. Of course, referral by general practitioners to hospitals is a growing trend throughout the world and is beneficial when the patient receives care the G.P. cannot provide, but my British and Dutch

---

l'harmonisation européenne des régimes de sécurité sociale," *Concours médical*, vol. 85, no. 1 (5 January 1963), p. 94; and Mignon, "La rémunération à l'acte en question?" ibid., vol. 85, no. 7 (16 February 1963), p. 1085.

[3] Sozialenquête-Kommission, *Soziale Sicherung in der Bundesrepublik Deutschland* (Stuttgart: W. Kohlhammer GMBH, 1966), pp. 230–31.

[4] If capitation leads to over-referral, not all general practitioners react in the same way. Wide individual variations in the propensity to refer patients to outpatient departments of hospitals appear in the data summarized in William P. D. Logan, *General Practitioners' Records* (London: H. M. Stationery Office, 1953), pp. 34–35.

informants believed that some referrals are unnecessary and are even undesirable, since the patient is sent to a stranger by the doctor who knows him best.

Excessive referral by the general practitioner to the hospital was believed one of the weaknesses of the capitation system under Britain's National Health Insurance,[5] and the National Health Service has not solved the problem. Fry estimates that 40 per cent of the referrals to the casualty department in a southeast London hospital were unnecessary and could have been treated by G.P.'s.[6] Priest estimated that 16 per cent of the patients referred to him in a hospital's outpatient department had nothing more than psychoneurotic problems that their G.P.'s should have managed.[7] In surveys by the Central Office for Public Health Care, specialists in Amsterdam hospitals reported not only unnecessary referrals but also insufficient diagnostic reports and medical histories from the general practitioners who sent patients for good medical reasons.[8] Inadequate medical education, no continuing postgraduate education, and the absence of incentive pay, therefore, may result in the worst combination: many general practitioners performing insufficient diagnostic work either by themselves or with the aid of laboratories, and too many patients transferred to the hospital outpatient departments for complete investigations.[9]

If straight capitation produces excessive referrals, one solution might be a monetary inducement: a general practitioner would be paid extra for each time-consuming person on his list, such as an elderly person or a baby. Under unweighted capitation, equal lists earn equal fees but may create unequal work, if one list contains more older patients and babies. Weighted capitation fees were favored by the Spens Committee but were long opposed

[5] Hermann Levy, *National Health Insurance* (Cambridge: University Press, 1944), pp. 128–29; and Richard M. Titmuss, *Essays on the Welfare State* (London: George Allen & Unwin, 1958), p. 212.

[6] Lionel Fry, "Casualties and Casuals," *Lancet* (16 January 1960), p. 166. Excessive referrals are reported also by Gordon Forsyth and Robert F. L. Logan, *The Demand for Medical Care: A Study of the Case-Load in the Barrow and Furness Group of Hospitals* (London: Oxford University Press, 1960), p.105; and by Ann Cartwright, *Patients and Their Doc ors—A Study of General Practice* (London: Routledge & Kegan Paul, 1967), pp. 122–36 passim.

[7] Many of the patients whom Priest believed could have been treated by the general practitioners complained that their G.P.'s never gave them enough time. General practitioners vary greatly in their referral rates. The precise policy and appropriate means for allocating patients between the general practitioners and the hospital are still unsettled: if the G.P. is expected to avoid unnecessary referrals to consultants, he should have more facilities for examination and treatment. W. M. Priest, "A Thousand Outpatients," *Lancet* (17 November 1962), pp. 1043–47.

[8] Arie Querido, *The Efficiency of Medical Care* (Leiden: H. E. Stenfert Kroese N.V., 1963), pp. 54–56. Perhaps the Dutch specialist is less irritated by over-referral than his British counterpart: he earns extra fees, but the latter is salaried.

[9] The poor quality of diagnostic work in British general practice and the resultant volume of undetected illnesses in the patients whom the G.P.'s see are described in, Gordon Forsyth, *Doctors and State Medicine* (London: Pitman Medical Publishing Co., 1966), chap. 5.

by the British Medical Association.[10] Until the Central Pool system for calculating fees was modified, extra payments for time-consuming patients would reduce the basic capitation fee and would shift incomes from doctors with long lists to doctors with difficult lists. General practitioners with high incomes from long lists have carried much weight within the BMA.

However, British doctors during the 1960's increasingly insisted that extra pay be furnished for extra work. Finally, as part of the general reforms during the mid-1960's, a higher capitation fee was awarded for one type of time-consuming patient: for the ordinary patient, in 1969, the annual fee was £1–1–6, but for the patient aged sixty-five and over it was £1–10–0.[11] The Central Pool was abolished, and therefore the extra payments for older patients did not reduce the basic capitation fee and did not reduce the incomes of G.P.'s with lists comprised of younger persons. The weighted capitation fee was an additional payment by the Treasury.

Another method for discouraging over-referral combines statistical detection and administrative regulation. Like such measures against abuse in specialty practice, this procedure is used in the national health insurance system of Holland. Dutch general practitioners now are paid by unweighted capitation. Statistics on referral are regularly computed for each G.P. Lists of referral rates are kept for all doctors. Local lists are mailed periodically to all doctors in many communities; names of doctors are omitted, but each can recognize his own referral rate and see how it compares with others. Such public knowledge places pressure on the individual doctor to reduce his own rate, if it is excessive. If several doctors seem to be chronically out of line or if the community average seems out of line with those of other communities, the subject may be discussed in meetings of the local chapter of the medical association. The medical community itself is directly interested in preventing a deviant from over-referring: this tactic raises costs and thus absorbs money available for raising the capitation fee next year; the doctor who economizes on his time with health insurance patients has a competitive advantage over other doctors when seeking and treating private patients. If the statistics show excessive referral in the community, officials of the sick funds—who are interested in curbing costs—may complain to the local

[10] Compare *Report of the Inter-Departmental Committee on Remuneration of General Practitioners* (London: H. M. Stationery Office, Cmnd. 6810, 1946), pp. 10–11; with "Proceedings of the Annual Representative Meeting," *British Medical Journal Supplement* (20 July 1957), pp. 41–42; and "Witnesses for the British Medical Association," *Minutes of Evidence Taken before the Royal Commission on Doctors' and Dentists' Remuneration* (London: H. M. Stationery Office, 1958), pp. 264–65.

[11] The reasoning behind the "modified capitation system" appears in "Second Report of Joint Discussions between General-Practitioner Representatives and the Minister of Health," *British Medical Journal Supplement* (16 October 1965), pp. 154–55. The report concluded that "all the available evidence confirms that on average patients over the age of 65 make heavier demands on their doctors than do younger patients," but that there was insufficient evidence to justify special rates for other classes of patients.

chapter of the medical association. The role of the local medical society is formalized in Amsterdam: a committee of seven doctors investigates cases of over-referral and has power to reprimand, fine, or suspend miscreants from insurance practice.

Dutch sick funds employ "control doctors" who represent the funds within the medical profession. They deal with individual doctors who may refer too many patients, overperform specialist procedures, overprescribe drugs, and otherwise exceed professional norms. They perform other medical-administrative tasks, such as approving hospitalization of patients. For every geographical unit of about 100,000 insured people, there is one full-time salaried control doctor, employed by one or more sick funds. If a G.P. has consistently been referring to specialists far more patients than the local norm—e.g., 50 out of 100 patients when the statistical average is 30 out of 100—the control doctor is supposed to confer with him. Most of the control doctors are former general practitioners and can speak from personal experience.

These controls check deviations from the norm but not the norm itself. However, by restraining deviations among communities and among individual doctors within the same community, the Dutch system probably checks rapid increases in the norm.

Italy's principal national health insurance scheme pays the general practitioners either by capitation or fee-for-service. The financial structure and administrative controls have been designed to discourage excessive referrals by doctors paid by capitation, but neither measure has been sufficiently effective. During the early 1960's, INAM (Istituto Nazionale per l'Assicurazione contro le Malattie) had three basic annual capitation fees according to the type of patient: L 2,310 for each farm worker and each dependent; L 2,870 for each urban worker (in industry, commerce, financial businesses, and domestic service) and each dependent; L 3,990 for each pensioner and each dependent. (At that time, the free market exchange rate was 100 lire = $0.16.) The weighting was supposed to compensate for differences in the doctor's work: pensioners give doctors more work than urban employees, while the farm population visits the doctor less often. Nevertheless, since extra work did not give the general practitioner extra income (except for additional fees for visits), many informants believed that G.P.'s referred too many patients to the polyclinics for work the G.P.'s could do themselves. Thus the G.P. conserves his time for his private practice, while losing little or none of his INAM income. But the result has been a large patient load at the polyclinic and pressure upon INAM to increase the salaried hours for the specialists and general practitioners—the latter often doing in the polyclinic what they and their colleagues might have done in their office practices.

Provincial offices of INAM keep statistics on referral, sick leaves, prescribing, and certain other work of the general practitioners. As in Holland

and many other countries, the provincial medical officer of INAM is supposed to judge when a G.P.'s referral rate is out of line with the statistical average of the community, and this control doctor then asks the G.P. to reduce his rate. But this is not done often in cases of over-referral to the polyclinic. INAM treats its doctors gingerly, particularly during the recurring strikes of the 1960's, for fear that excessive controls over clinical judgment might create new rebellions. The control doctors have concentrated recently on the problem of prescribing drugs, which has grown rapidly and is INAM's largest operating expense, and they often hesitate to harass doctors with additional charges of over-referral. High referral rates seem to have the sanction of tradition: general practitioners in the past have done only the simplest work, they have been expected to refer any complex work to specialists, and INAM until recently assumed that its G.P.'s would do the same. More office practice would require higher fees and incentives to purchase modern equipment.

Adequate Care

Do general practitioners paid by capitation fail to give patients minimum physical care when clearly no one but they can give it? My informants in England and Holland did not believe this a problem. Although the quality of care varies according to the G.P.'s skill and facilities, gross neglect in order to economize on time is believed rare. Care may be too rapid for comprehensive treatment and emotional support, but many patients come not to expect them under the official medical scheme. However, they might expect something more if they were paying privately.

A survey by Amsterdam's Central Office for Public Health in 1950 and 1951 estimated that the G.P. with a large practice saw forty-seven patients daily in his office and spent about three minutes on each patient. The rest of his time was devoted to home visits under national health insurance, private office visits, and private home visits. Some general practitioners had shorter lists under health insurance, but managed these patients at the same tempo. Work pressures have eased slightly in Amsterdam since this survey was conducted, and they have always been lower in the provinces. The average British general practitioner in the 1960's had a shorter list than the physician in Amsterdam, less private practice, and an average of about thirty-three patient contacts per day. The average British G.P. spent between four and seven minutes on each office visit and between twelve and twenty minutes on each home visit.[12]

---

[12] The Dutch survey is in, Querido, *Efficiency of Medical Care* (note 8), p. 37. The British data are reported in, College of General Practitioners, *Reports from General Practice: Present State and Future Needs* (London: College of General Practitioners, 1965), pp. 9, 20–23; and David Mechanic, "General Practice in England and Wales: Results from a Survey of a National Sample of General Practitioners," *Medical Care*, vol. 6, no. 3 (May–June 1968), pp. 249–51. Most British patients would prefer more time and more psychosocial care from the G.P., but they blame his speed on the National Health Service rather than on him. Cartwright, *Patients* (note 6), pp. 7–8, 30–31, 35, 112–16.

Neglect is uncommon, judging from polls of public satisfaction. In Great Britain, most patients are satisfied with their general practitioners: of a national sample of the British population in the late 1950's, 86 per cent approved the work of their present G.P., only 15 per cent had ever changed general practitioners out of dissatisfaction, and 72 per cent of the families had no family members who had ever changed general practitioners out of dissatisfaction.[13] In a national sample survey in 1965, 86 per cent of the British population said the general practitioner was "good at his job" and only 3 percent said he was not.[14] A few British patients report delays in making home visits and not enough personal attention, and they suspect they would be treated more thoroughly in private practice.[15]

Public opinion polls conducted in Holland reveal little discontent. For example, more than half the residents of Sassenheim get their medical care under national health insurance; nearly all the respondents approved the medical services and commended the doctors.[16] Querido's numerous surveys of the population of Amsterdam reveal little complaint.[17]

Basic reasons for the adequacy of minimum physical care include the high standard of ethics of the English and Dutch medical professions and the work habits of individual doctors. Instead of the capitation fee causing a standardized and low rate of work, Lees' British data show that the consultation rate varies widely among doctors with similar lists, apparently according to their consciences and habits. Doctors do not respond identically to the monetary incentives, but many other variables affect their performance.[18] Another reason why deliberate neglect does not seem a widespread problem is the freedom of the patient to select a new general practitioner if he believes his present one is not sufficiently attentive. If the G.P. is obviously negligent, he risks losing capitation fees.

[13] Political and Economic Planning, *Family Needs and the Social Services* (London: George Allen & Unwin, 1961).

[14] *Gallup Political Index*, no. 64 (August 1965), p. 121, published by Social Surveys (Gallup Poll) of London.

[15] Enid Hutchinson, *General Practice: A Consumer Commentary* (London: Research Institute for Consumer Affairs, 1963), pp. 10–11; and Cartwright, *Patients* (note 6), passim. The cross-national study of the utilization of medical care in England, Yugoslavia, and America found that large majorities of British patients reported their G.P.'s "unhurried" and prepared to "listen" and "explain." But the proportions were even higher in American private practice. Kerr L. White et al., "International Comparisons of Medical Care Utilization: Feasibility Study," *New England Journal of Medicine*, vol. 277 (September 7, 1967), p. 520.

[16] Ivan Gadourek, *A Dutch Community* (Leiden: H. E. Stenfert Kroese N.V., 1956), pp. 147, 251.

[17] Querido, *Efficiency of Medical Care* (note 8), p. 43. Winkler Prins' survey of four Dutch communities—including Amsterdam—also reported high satisfaction and great personal reliance on general practitioners. J. Winkler Prins, *Huisarts en Patient* (Amsterdam: J. A. Boom en Zoon, 1966), chap. 6 and appendix 2.

[18] D. S. Lees and M. H. Cooper, "The Capitation Fee," *Lancet* (20 April 1963), pp. 880–82.

Another reason for the adequacy of care under capitation in both England and Holland is the disciplinary machinery. Regulations in both countries specify the doctor's minimum obligations. Neglecting a patient in Great Britain, for example, may result in his complaint to the local Executive Council, with the resultant humiliation of an investigation, a possible reprimand, or a possible fine. Considerable newspaper publicity is now given to the rare instances of disciplinary action and it is believed that English patients have become increasingly sensitive in protection of their rights.[19]

In Great Britain, the "Terms of Service for Practitioners" in effect at the time of writing are *The National Health Service (General Medical and Pharmaceutical Services) Regulations 1966*, Statutory Instrument No. 1210. Because of the danger of neglect under a flat-rate payment system, the Terms of Service specify many minimum duties of the G.P. in such diverse areas as the number of office hours, the number of weeks at work, speed of response to emergency calls, availability for night calls and weekend calls, and so on. The existence of the Terms of Service is one of the numerous sources of resentment among G.P.'s concerning the collectivization of practice and the erosion of the model of the independent physician. All general practitioners are bound by the Terms, but no individual has a voice in the creation or application of its details; at best the individual doctor can refuse to adhere by taking the prohibitive financial risk of not participating in the National Health Service. The Terms are written by collective negotiations between the medical societies and the Ministry of Health.

Even in Spain—where the national health insurance system has been beset by insufficient money and by a load that has outstripped facilities and personnel—patients commend their doctors. A survey of insured persons during the early 1960's registered many complaints about hasty and superficial treatment and the absence of free choice of a doctor. But the respondents blamed the *system* and not the doctors: although half had complaints about medical care, over two-thirds commended the physicians and thought the doctors were doing as well as could be expected under difficult circumstances.[20] Another national survey of the Spanish public in 1965 also elicited high commendation of the doctors and widespread criticism of the administrative organization of SOE (Seguro Obligatorio de Enfermedad).[21]

One problem in countries with insufficient income to pay the doctor high fees for long working hours is the temptation to divert public patients

[19] Some results of the disciplinary procedure are summarized in *A Review of the Medical Services in Great Britain* (London: Social Assay, 1962), pp. 38–39. The G.P.'s surveyed by Cartwright were aware of and resentful of these strict obligations. *Patients* (note 6), pp. 55–58.

[20] Manuel Gomez-Reino, "El Seguro de Enfermedad visto por sus personales," in, Enrique Martin Lopez et al., *Estudio sociologico sobre el Seguro de Enfermedad* (Madrid: Ministerio de Trabajo, Secretaría General Técnica, 1964), 4: 93, 99–106, 116–20, 129–32. Complaints about the excessive patient load are echoed by the doctors. Ibid., pp. 199–202, 290–95.

[21] Amando de Miguel Rodriguez et al., *Informe sociológico sobre la situación social de España* (Madrid: Fundación FOESSA, 1966), pp. 141–46.

into private practice: if the sick fund can pay only low fees, it can demand only short hours; if he is paid little for this limited time, the doctor will not voluntarily give extra time for work that overflows his fixed hours; if the rest of his work day is more lucrative, the doctor may accept a public patient during his private hours only if the patient will pay the customary private fee. It is believed that some Spanish and Italian general practitioners give private care to patients on their official insurance lists outside the hours reserved for that practice; if a G.P. has a long list and rushed office hours, a private fee is the best way for a patient to get enough of his time for thorough care. As in other countries with capitation systems, it is illegal to charge a private fee for a patient on one's national health insurance list, and SOE and INAM doctors thereby risk suspension or expulsion. As in Holland and other countries with national health insurance and national health services, SOE and INAM employ regional control doctors whose numerous duties include the investigation of violations. Disciplinary tribunals hear charges and are empowered to penalize doctors, but have few cases. Partly because of this situation, SOE and INAM attempted to narrow the differentials between insured and private fees during the 1960's.

Styles in Medical Treatment

One would expect a capitation system to produce fewer optional diagnostic and therapeutic procedures than a fee-for-service system. The small amount of comparable data supports this hypothesis. For example, doctors paid under capitation under INAM in Italy write fewer pharmaceutical prescriptions per insured person than doctors paid by fee-for-service, and this difference is true within all provinces.[22]

The conservative effects of capitation may strengthen a clinical conservatism common to countries using this form of payment. For example, my informants believed that English and Dutch patients receive fewer diagnostic tests and fewer treatments than (for example) the American patient, but that the explanation was not confined to the capitation system. Traditionally these physicians have not relied on laboratory tests and diagnostic equipment as much as (for example) Americans and Germans, but they have preferred to use interviews, observation, and personal intuition. Similarly, they have followed traditions of caution in giving injections, drugs, and other therapies. As the fashions of scientific medicine spread, underinvestigation and therapeutic caution will probably diminish. Another nonpecuniary reason for the limited use of diagnostic aids and mechanical therapies by many general practitioners, paid under foreign capitation systems is their limited office equipment, which I shall mention again below.

[22] *Alcuni dati nazionali e provinciali sull'assistenza medicogenerica e farmaceutica distinti secondo il sistema di compenso al medico* (Rome: Istituto Nazionale per l'Assicurazione contro le Malattie, 1966), pp. 39–58.

Home Visits

Since they are not rewarded under capitation, one might expect a drastic decline in home visits. As we have seen in other chapters, home visits seem to have diminished either absolutely or proportionately even under payment systems that specifically reward them.

But more than monetary incentives affect the clinical habits of doctors. National tradition and administrative sanctions may prevent the trends in England and Holland from assuming the expected magnitude. Home visits have always been considered essential parts of general practice in both countries and the G.P. is still supposed to include them in his daily schedule. Refusal to make a home visit by day or night is very risky in England: the patient or his family may complain to the Executive Council, and members of the Council and of the Local Medical Committee consider such refusals to be very serious violations of the G.P.'s contract with the National Health Service. Occasionally general practitioners have been expelled from the National Health Service or have been forced to resign because of refusal to pay an emergency home visit. Publicity in the newspapers and in medical journals reminds both patients and doctors of these sanctions.[23]

For a considerable period after the start of the National Health Service, home visiting remained as common as before the war: between one-quarter and one-third of contacts were in the patient's home.[24] During the late 1950's and early 1960's, the rate may have declined in England and Wales. But in Scotland—where general practitioners also were paid by capitation—half of all contacts continued to be made in the home, and the rate did not diminish.[25]

Doctors in several countries have pressed for the replacement of capitation by fee-for-service systems that would pay the doctor for his work.[26] Some public medical schemes succeeded in preserving capitation recently by supplementing it by such fundamentally different methods as flat payments for all doctors or fees for individual procedures. These concessions were made in Italy. INAM previously had allowed general practitioners to

[23] Almont Lindsey, *Socialized Medicine in England and Wales* (Chapel Hill: The University of North Carolina Press, 1962), pp. 221–22; and Cartwright, *Patients* (note 6), pp. 68–76.

[24] Lindsey, *Socialized Medicine* (note 23), pp. 213–14.

[25] College of General Practitioners, *General Practice* (note 12), pp. 18–21. One-fifth of the English general practitioners in the studies summarized by Lees and Cooper ("Capitation Fee," note 18) still conducted more than half their patient contacts in homes, and half the doctors performed more than 30 per cent of their contacts in homes. Some of Mechanic's respondents still did considerable home visiting. "General Practice" (note 12), pp. 250–51.

[26] The declining use of capitation in Germany, Denmark, and Norway during the twentieth century is described in I. G. Gibbon, *Medical Benefit: A Study of the Experience of Germany and Denmark* (London: P. S. King & Son, 1912), chap. 8 and pp. 64–68, 227–30, 236–76 passim; Barbara N. Armstrong, *The Health Insurance Doctor: His Role in Great Britain, Denmark, and France* (Princeton: Princeton University Press, 1939), pp. 139–42; and James Hogarth, *The Payment of the General Practitioner* (Oxford: Pergamon Press, 1963), p. 104.

choose between straight capitation or a simple fee-for-service that paid for office and home visits. The doctors paid by capitation complained they were not getting enough money for the effort expected, particularly for home visits in the rural areas where capitation was most common. Consequently, it was suspected that home visits were not made often enough. Therefore the 1966 national agreement between the medical associations and INAM created a third system of payment that the local offices of the doctors and sick funds could elect: the general practitioner would collect an annual capitation fee for all persons on his list, and it would cover all office visits; but each home visit would yield an additional fee on an item-of-service principle.

The fees in lire are:

	Region 1	*Region 2*	*Region 3*
Capitation fees for all office visits annually:			
Farmers	2,300	2,000	1,800
Other occupations	2,600	2,300	2,000
Children under six	2,900	2,550	2,200
Pensioners	3,200	2,800	2,400
Fee for each home visit	1,030	990	950

The regions of Italy are classified by cost of living. In general, Region 1 is the north, Region 2 is the center, and Region 3 is the south. In addition to capitation fees, each practitioner under this system receives an additional loading of L 500 or less for each person. He earns lower loadings per insured person if his list is longer.[27]

Night and Weekend Visits

A fundamental issue in a capitation system is whether a doctor is responsible for the patient at all times. A fee-for-service system might assume that a physician can freely decide when he is available, but monetary incentives would extend his working hours: the greater his available time, the more fees he can collect, and visits at inconvenient times usually are paid for at higher rates. Salaried systems are commonly parts of organized medical care with fixed working hours, and services are always available, since the organization retains another doctor to work when one's hours of availability end.

In theory, this is not always true: in much of the world the salaried chiefs-of-service in hospitals and Britain's consultants are on call at any time. But in practice, their responsibility is limited. Since the organization hires other salaried doctors when they are away, they are rarely called during their hours of private practice and rest.

But capitation systems usually assume the total dependence of a patient on his doctor and the total responsibility of the physician. Nevertheless, the

[27] "Conclusa la vertenza Medici-Mutue," *INAM Informazioni*, vol. 13, no. 8 (August 1966), pp. 1, 2, 4.

doctor's capitation fees remain the same if a patient makes frequent demands at inconvenient hours. Normally doctors paid by capitation either make night and weekend visits themselves, hire substitutes for standby duty, form partnerships and rotate the standby duty, or subscribe to "duty rotas," by which the G.P.'s in a community assign one of their number in rotation to take all the local off-hours calls. None of these methods offsets the economic disincentive against performing night or weekend work inherent in capitation.

This problem was one of the numerous sources of tension surrounding the payment of general practitioners in the National Health Service. The doctors wished to have some option about availability, complained about unreasonable demands by patients at inconvenient times, and grumbled about the expense of hiring standby physicians during nights, weekends, and vacations. Night calls are not as common as doctors believe, but night calls evoke their hostility and seem very salient, since the doctors cannot control their own lives and must obey rather than direct the patients.[28]

The profession's representatives and the Ministry of Health negotiated an agreement in 1965 and 1966 designed to mollify the doctors by giving them financial rewards for burdensome calls. The general practitioners' official Terms of Service were clarified so that the typical work schedule was defined as five and a half "reasonable" working days forty-six weeks a year. The general practitioner could agree in his contract with the Executive Council whether to be available during evenings, on Saturday afternoon, and on Sunday. If he agreed, he would receive a £200 supplementary practice allowance, a 2s. 0d. supplementary capitation fee for each patient in excess of 1,000 on his list, and a £1 fee for each night visit between midnight and 7 A.M. Therefore, to remove the disincentives from capitation, devices more akin to salary and fee-for-service were added. Doctors could perform the off-hours work themselves or could hire standby physicians.[29]

Emergency night and weekend calls declined during the early years of the National Health Service. The disincentives of the capitation system of payment were not the only reasons. Another cause was earlier referral of women and children to general practitioners. Not covered by the prewar

[28] Max B. Clyne, *Night Calls: A Study in General Practice* (London: Travistock Publications, 1961), pp. 4–6, 10, 12, 76–77, 80, 95–96, 164–65; and Cartwright, *Patients* (note 6), pp. 40–41, 75.

[29] "Second Report of Joint Discussions Between General-Practitioner Representatives and the Minister of Health," *British Medical Journal Supplement* (16 October 1965), pp. 154–55; and *Review Body on Doctors' and Dentists' Remuneration: Seventh Report* (London: H. M. Stationery Office, Cmnd. 2992, 1966), pp. 53, 63–64, 69. Duty rotas are described by Lindsey, *Socialized Medicine* (note 23), pp. 181–82. The various methods used by G.P.'s to cope with night and weekend calls on the eve of the new payment system are reported in the survey conducted by Ann Cartwright, "General Practice in 1963: Its Conditions, Contents and Satisfactions," *Medical Care*, vol. 3, no. 2 (April–June 1965), pp. 73–75. A substantial minority of the doctors in Cartwright's survey felt oppressed by round-the-clock obligations.

National Health Insurance and reluctant to pay fees, many women and children previously had delayed consulting doctors.[30] For this reason, some general practitioners told Hadfield, the demand for home visits in their practices had increased, but the demand for night visits was smaller than before the National Health Service.[31]

Modernization of Practice

Ideally a payment system should induce doctors to develop their facilities and staff. As we saw in chapters VII and VIII, some fee schedules under national health insurance motivate doctors to buy and use the newest diagnostic and therapeutic devices, since the fee schedules make them profitable as well as a source of professional pride. A drawback of straight capitation is that it provides only an uncertain incentive: the G.P. risks losing fees only if patients can recognize that one of his competitors has a more modern practice. But it is important that general practitioners paid by capitation modernize their offices, since reasons will be fewer to make unnecessary referrals to hospitals or polyclinics. Doctors often resist proposals to condition pay awards on modernization of facilities, on the grounds of undue interference by the public authorities.

The dilemma of how to motivate modernization of facilities under capitation is apparent in the experiences of countries that try to make the fee sufficient for voluntary purchases and in other countries that attempt to supplement the basic fee. Holland illustrates the limited success of the first tactic; England demonstrates the difficulties in administering the second. The Dutch capitation fee is fixed by the negotiating committee on the assumption that some of the money will be used for equipment, journals, and other costs. But only personal ambition governs the amount of money invested in self-improvement. Observational studies by Amsterdam's Central Office for Public Health during the 1950's concluded that too few general practitioners had equipped their offices adequately.[32]

For many years the National Health Service of Great Britain encouraged the purchase of new equipment, ancillary staff, journals, and other modern aids more directly by paying each G.P. an expense allowance from the Central Pool. But he got cash instead of materials; he was paid regardless

[30] Gemmill, *Search for Health* (note 1), pp. 128–31.

[31] Stephen J. Hadfield, "A Field Survey of General Practice 1951–52," *British Medical Journal* (26 September 1953), pp. 683–706.

[32] Querido, *Efficiency of Medical Care* (note 8), pp. 36–39. The Royal Dutch Medical Association subsequently tried to persuade general practitioners to improve their practices by sponsoring demonstrations and by negotiating with municipalities for better office accommodations.

of whether he purchased anything, and expense allowances varied by length of list. Thus in practice the expense allowance was simply an extra capitation fee. If anything, the system encouraged underspending for office expenses, since the doctor was free to keep the balance. Besides the capitation fees themselves, the practice expenses were another incentive for long lists: as lists increase in length, the unit costs of the practice decrease and net profits rise.

After it became evident that many doctors did not spend the expense allowance for its ostensible purpose, one of the fundamental controversies in the history of the National Health Service developed. Some critics recommended reimbursement for actual expenses rather than automatic cash payments, but the BMA defended the automatic payments on the grounds that every doctor has an approximately equal tendency to underspend his allowance at certain career stages and overspend at other stages.[33] Meanwhile, some observers believed that too many general practices were backward.[34] The National Health Service in 1964 tried to make an award for practice expenses conditional upon its actual use for the purpose: two-thirds of doctors' spending for secretarial and other expenses would be reimbursed, and the entire pay award for 1964 would be devoted to that purpose.[35]

The BMA and the leaders of the Executive Councils had not been averse to some obligation that doctors use certain practice expenses for the intended purpose, but the Review Body's decision seemed too sweeping. At first no money was given for increasing G.P.'s net incomes, and it appeared as if the Review Body and the National Health Service might regularly influence medical practice by means of the payment system. The more militant group representing the G.P.'s—the General Practitioners Association—opposed the terms of the award on principle, and the BMA joined it. Their argument emphasized the freedom of the doctor as a professional and

[33] Compare "Witnesses for the Medical Practitioners' Union," *Minutes of Evidence Taken before the Royal Commission on Doctors' and Dentists' Remuneration* (London: H. M. Stationery Office, 1958), pp. 106, 112–14, 126–29; with "Witnesses for the British Medical Association" (note 10), pp. 282–89, 1285–86.

[34] The primitive offices of many of England's impecunious prewar solo G.P.'s are described in, Joseph S. Collings, "General Practice in England Today," *Lancet* (25 March 1950), pp. 555–85. Many offices visited by Hadfield in 1951 and 1952 were deficient. "Field Survey" (note 31), pp. 700–1. That many premises remain inadequate is evident from Cartwright's survey conducted just before introduction of the new method for bestowing expense allowances. *Patients* (note 29), pp. 75–76. Patients' judgments may not be sufficiently informed to exercise adequate control over their G.P.'s. A national sample of the public was considerably more generous than the reformers: 70 per cent thought their G.P. was "efficient in organising his work," 68 per cent thought the offices were "well equipped," and few were critical. *Gallup Political Index*, no. 64 (August 1965), pp. 121–22, published by Social Surveys (Gallup Poll) of London.

[35] *Review Body on Doctors' and Dentists' Remuneration: Third, Fourth and Fifth Reports* (London: H. M. Stationery Office, Cmnd. 2585, 1965), pp. 12–13, 22.

as an "independent contractor": how the doctor used his expense money was entirely a matter for his own judgment, and the laymen in the Review Body had no authority to influence his decisions by making conditional pay awards.[36]

The dispute over practice expenses was the first in a series over the system of paying doctors under the Central Pool method during 1964 and 1965. The Ministry of Health released the pay award of 1964 without conditioning it on the actual spending for ancillary staff, but controversy continued over this and other issues. A strike of general practitioners was threatened in 1965.

Finally, as I said in chapter V, the Central Pool method of deriving fees was abandoned, and a new capitation system was adopted. Because the Central Pool was abolished, increases in practice expenses no longer would cause corresponding decreases in capitation fees and net income. A basic practice allowance was given every G.P. with a list of at least 1,000 patients, without a showing that he had purchased equipment or publications. (The basic practice allowance no longer was a fixed sum for each person on the G.P.'s list: the old method was believed to have given doctors with short lists too little money for expenses and to have given G.P.'s a monetary incentive to amass very long lists at the same time that the Service tried to discourage long lists by loadings on capitation fees.) The principle of reimbursement was introduced for hiring assistants and for rentals, but a compromise in administration preserved the independence of the doctor from government supervision. In an agreement with the profession's representatives, the Minister of Health disclaimed any interest in fixing standards of staffing, inspecting doctors' practices, judging the qualifications of ancillary staff, and deciding that sufficient staff was hired at the proper rates. The agreement placed the doctor's pecuniary self-interest in control of his staffing decisions: the National Health Service would not reimburse him for all salaries but would pay 70 per cent of the first £500 and 50 per cent of additional spending. Full direct reimbursement for rent had been recommended in the profession's own "Charter for the Family Doctor Service," and the Ministry agreed, with the understanding that the two sides could negotiate standards of "reasonable" rental.[37] The principal burden for the improvement of practices was shifted from the payment system to a General Practice Finance Corporation created by Parliament in 1966. The G.P. need not justify his spending for new construction and equipment to administrators in the Ministry of Health; he would borrow money on banking principles

[36] Editorial, "The Review Body's Award," *British Medical Journal* (13 February 1965), pp. 397–99.

[37] "Family Doctor Service: Joint Report on Discussions between General Practitioner Representatives and the Minister of Health," *British Medical Journal Supplement* (5 June 1965), pp. 239–40.

from an independent public corporation, and therefore he would preserve his self-image as an "independent contractor."[38]

The difficulty of modernizing office practices under capitation in less wealthy countries is illustrated by the experience of INAM in Italy. For many years, wages were low, the revenues of INAM were limited, and therefore payments to general practitioners were low. (As I said earlier, capitation is used in many rural districts and small towns, while an abbreviated fee-for-service system is used in cities.) In 1953 the annual fee for all INAM patients covered by capitation was only L 550; as recently as 1961, the fees ranged between L 1,500 for farm workers and L 2,550 for pensioners. Lists have always been short, since doctors are numerous, the medical associations press INAM to spread the work, and loadings that decrease with length of list discourage the accumulation of too many patients. Therefore the general practitioner maintained a primitive office, made many home visits, and referred patients requiring more complex care.[39] INAM built polyclinics where salaried specialists and general practitioners gave the ambulatory care that the office practitioner lacked the facilities to provide. By the large increase in fees during the 1960's, INAM hoped that general practitioners finally would have enough money to modernize their offices and make fewer unnecessary referrals.[40]

One-third of the general practitioners paid by capitation have lists of under one thousand patients; three-fifths have lists of under 1500 patients. The list system is used by all general practitioners. Those paid by fee-for-service have even shorter lists. For many years the fees were also low under the fee-for-service option of medical pay: in 1953, the office visit was only L 183 everywhere in the country, and the home visit was only L 367; as late as 1961, the office visit ranged between L 300 and L 270, the home visit between L 600 and L 540. (The free market exchange rate has been approximately L 100 = $0.16.)

Organization of Practice

As in other countries, the British G.P. was traditionally an independent small businessman. Some had salaried young assistants who hoped to become heirs or junior partners; some had full partnership agreements. But most

[38] The purposes and administration of the Corporation were discussed in the debate on the "National Health Service Bill," *Parliamentary Debates* (*Hansard*), *House of Commons*, vol. 723, no. 40 (3 February 1966), cols. 1372–1432. The Minister describes the profession's preference for loans rather than grants at col. 1424.

[39] *Alcuni dati nazionali e provinciali sull'assistenza medico-generica e farmaceutica distinti secondo il sistema di compenso al medico*: *Anno 1965* (Rome: Istituto Nazionale per l'Assicurazione contro le Malattie, 1966), p. 6.

[40] Even when they earned enough money, many G.P.'s kept it instead of investing it in their practices. For example, the prosperous doctor in a Southern town described in, Edward C. Banfield, *The Moral Basis of a Backward Society* (Glencoe: The Free Press, 1958), pp. 92, 99.

worked alone; underfinancing of facilities and ignorance of the newest clinical developments inevitably resulted.

The National Health Service has tried to motivate collaborative arrangements to pool resources, share facilities and knowledge, and spread the work by efficient division of labor. The Service and the local health authorities have created health centers with central services and with offices for general practitioners working either as individuals, partnerships, or groups.[41]

The Service at various times used the method of paying doctors to encourage the formation of partnerships and groups. For many years the loadings on the capitation fees for partners were calculated so that patients were allotted among the partners in the most profitable way: extra capitation payments were paid every G.P. for every patient over 500 but not exceeding 1,500 on his list, under a payment policy to discourage very long and very short lists; but a partner with a very long list and a partner with a short list were allowed to report that their two lists consisted of the average number of patients. Therefore the partners' total income was higher than if they practiced independently.

But these advantages were reduced during the 1960's for several reasons. Many partnerships were organized not to improve practice but for monopolistic purposes: if a G.P.'s list became so long that a competitor might be tempted to open a practice nearby, the G.P. might take on junior partners in order to increase his list. Many partnerships were not truly collegial but were dominated by a principal, who made most of the decisions and obtained most of the income, regardless of how the work and patient lists were distributed. The incentives in the payment system led to some sham agreements designed merely to gain the advantages: two G.P.'s might continue to practice separately but sign a nominal partnership agreement so they could average their lists and gain a higher income by means of the better distribution of the loadings.[42]

Many reformers favored the medical group over the partnership, which was the organization preferred by the most influential practitioners. The group was more egalitarian, its terms usually precluded exploitation of other members by a principal, more doctors were involved than in partnerships, the members could not practice in separate places as in the sham partnership agreements, and it was more likely to acquire sufficient facilities and ancillary staff. One of the supplements in the modified capitation system initiated in 1966 was a £200 annual addition to the basic practice allowance of any

[41] The enthusiastic promotion of health centers and their limited acceptance by general practitioners is summarized by Lindsey, *Socialized Medicine* (note 23), pp. 169–74.

[42] The characteristics and weaknesses of partnerships are summarized in ibid., pp. 164–67; and David Cargill, *The G.P.: What's Wrong?* (London: Victor Gollancz, 1965), pp. 137–38. The reduction of the special advantages for partnerships was announced in the *Report of the Royal Commission on Doctors' and Dentists' Remuneration* (London: H. M. Stationery Office, Cmnd. 939, 1960), pp. 105, 118–19.

G.P. practicing in a group.[43] The special payment was designed to accelerate the gradual growth of group practice. Deep-seated customs must change before group practice becomes as common as in the United States, but the younger general practitioners clearly seem more interested than their elders.

Preventive Medicine

One of the principal arguments for capitation is motivation for more preventive medicine: since they gain nothing additional from treatments but instead must work harder, doctors should attempt to prevent persons on their lists from getting sick.

The modest growth of a preventive viewpoint has been one of the disappointments of England's National Health Service, and it is now realized that changing the compensation method is insufficient to overcome powerful clinical traditions. Medical education, the content of journals, professional shoptalk, and public expectations still lead the general practitioner to define his task as therapeutic care of patients who come to him with problems, rather than as preventive medical investigation of all the persons on his list.[44] Preventive medicine takes time, and the average G.P.'s day is fully occupied with the sick people who come to his office or who request home visits.

British general practitioners have been interested in administering preventive inoculations and special preventive examinations—such as tests for cervical cancer—because they were rewarded individually on an item-for-service basis. But these extra procedures did not arise out of capitation; they were compensated on different principles and actually undermined the capitation system. Until 1966 these fees were paid from the Central Pool before the Pool was divided into capitation fees, and therefore they were a competing way of earning money. The smallpox epidemic of 1962 led to so many vaccinations that the Central Pool was noticeably diminished, doctors received lower capitation fees and smaller incomes than expected, and doctors paid entirely by capitation grumbled that some brethren might be giving unnecessary inoculations. This experience was a principal reason for the abolition of the Central Pool after 1965.

Dutch general practitioners do not perform much preventive medicine in return for their capitation fees but—like their British counterparts—they

[43] The earlier encouragement of group practice is described by Lindsey, *Socialized Medicine* (note 23), pp. 167–68. The new supplement is explained in the Review Body's *Seventh Report* (note 29), pp. 66, 70.

[44] Hadfield, "Field Survey" (note 31), p. 687. Of the general practitioners interviewed by Cartwright in 1963 only one-third favored routine checks on middle-aged women and only 15 per cent favored routine checks on middle-aged men. "General Practice" (note 29), p. 80. Cartwright's survey in 1964 revealed limited preventive work. *Patients* (note 6), pp. 79–99.

do some of this work for extra fees. Dutch national health insurance is considered a vehicle entirely for curative medicine. The Cross Associations and other organizations are expected to do all the preventive medicine in the country, such as health examinations, chest X-rays, immunization, health teaching, and sanitary inspections. Most general practitioners perform these tasks on their regular insured and private patients on behalf of the Cross Associations and municipalities. They earn extra income by collecting fees on an item-of-service basis.[45]

Continuity of Care

Capitation fees should be ideally suited to fostering continuity of care. The individual registers with a doctor, and the G.P. receives a fee periodically for being responsible for that individual. Changing of general practitioners is not believed common in England and Holland, in large part because of the payment system and the administrative effort of switching. Perhaps even stronger reasons are the English and Dutch national traditions emphasizing the need for each person to have regular relations with a particular general practitioner.[46]

But discontinuity occurs when the patient enters a hospital. Almost always, whenever they are used to pay part of the medical profession, capitation fees cover only ambulatory general care. If the general practitioner continues to treat the patient in the hospital, usually he collects fees on an item-of-service basis, as he did in many prewar British hospitals. More commonly in the world, the general practitioner—however he is paid—must transfer control of the hospitalized patient to a closed staff of specialists paid by salary or fee-for-service.

The division has widened in Great Britain since the National Health Service filled nearly all hospitals with closed salaried staffs. Now a steadily diminishing number of general practitioners controls beds in hospitals, much of this care is restricted to obstetrics, and much of it is in smaller communities.[47] Separation from the hospital is one of the British general practitioners' principal complaints against the National Health Service.[48] The average

[45] Querido, *Efficiency of Medical Care* (note 8), p. 37.

[46] Large proportions of the British public keep their G.P.'s for many years. Cartwright, *Patients* (note 6), pp. 100–1.

[47] Ibid., pp. 17, 137–40.

[48] The exclusion of some G.P.'s and their grievances are summarized in, Rosemary Stevens, *Medical Practice in Modern England* (New Haven: Yale University Press, 1966), pp. 85–86, 100–5, 158–68, 361–65. The National Health Service now tries to increase the G.P.'s exposure to hospital medicine by making the paid part-time jobs of "clinical assistant" more attractive and by enabling the G.P. to use the hospital's diagnostic facilities on behalf of his own patients. See the Review Body's *Fifth Report* (note 40), p. 21; and "Third Report of Negotiations on Family Doctor Service," *British Medical Journal Supplement* (7 May 1966), pp. 139, 143–44.

G.P. rarely visits his patient in the hospital.[49] His diagnosis often is ignored by the house staff, which makes its own investigation from its supposedly more sophisticated viewpoint. Some general practitioners complain that they cannot regain control over their patients after referral to the hospital. The consultants—and particularly the younger ones—were said not to trust the G.P.'s competence and insisted on giving the patient regular care in the outpatient department, instead of referring him back to the G.P.[50] However, most English patients, who have come to accept the division between the specialist and the G.P., are no more satisfied with inpatient treatment by their regular G.P.'s, and do not expect to be visited by them while in the hospital.[51]

An increasing minority of G.P.'s earn extra fees working as part-time "clinical assistants." But they are not responsible for their own patients, and they are clearly subordinate to the consultant. Besides the disadvantage of this status, the work as clinical assistant once was controversial because its payment came out of the Central Pool, thereby diminishing the average G.P.'s basic compensation from capitation.[52]

Rewarding Superior Performance

Ideally, any differentials should favor the better doctor. But, as in the case of motivating the modernization of practices, simple payment formulae may have the opposite effect, and earmarking specific sums arouses protests about undue influence by the public authorities in professional spheres.

As we saw in the last chapter, eminent salaried consultants have had extra "distinction awards" since the inception of Britain's National Health Service. The Spens Committee hoped that the payment system for general practitioners could incorporate differentials for quality of performance,[53] but in practice incomes have depended primarily on the market structure: the highest pay has been earned by G.P.'s who located in underdoctored areas and amassed the longest lists. Spokesmen for the BMA once claimed that length of list roughly correlates with quality in the sense that only a doctor who satisfies his patients can keep so many, but others have contended that length and quality were independent. The Royal Commission hoped that merit awards might be worked out by negotiations between the Ministry

[49] Ann Cartwright, *Human Relations and Hospital Care* (London: Routledge & Kegan Paul, 1964), chap. 10 and pp. 191–92.

[50] Hadfield, "Field Survey" (note 31), pp. 697–98; and Cartwright, *Patients* (note 6), p. 144.

[51] Cartwright, *Human Relations* (note 49), pp. 120–22, 125.

[52] Stevens, *Medical Practice* (note 48), pp. 160–61.

[53] *Remuneration of General Practitioners* (note 10), p. 8.

of Health and the BMA,[54] but the subsequent conversations were fruitless. It is very difficult to modify a capitation system to reward quality as well as quantity.[55] Also it is very difficult to measure quality differences among general practitioners, and few persons are acquainted with enough G.P.'s to make nationwide judgments.[56] But the fact that consultants had distinction awards rankled, and the apparent decline in the morale and recruitment of general practitioners required a remedy.

Therefore the proposed reforms in 1965 and 1966 included a new set of basic payments to reward general practitioners by status. The doctors' representatives preferred seniority payments that would be applied automatically and that would create no invidious comparisons within general practice; the representatives of the National Health Service favored distinction awards for general practitioners. The compromise agreement between the medical societies and the Ministry adopted both seniority payments and distinction awards. Without merit awards, the senior doctors and the general practitioners with the longest lists would be earning more than the ablest doctors who gave time-consuming care, and general practice would continue to be unattractive to the best young doctors. About 30 per cent of all G.P.'s would be eligible for extra annual payments for "special experience and service to general practice," but only a select few would receive the highest awards. The Review Board in 1966 recommended two grades: the smaller sum was lower than the *C* distinction awards for consultants but the higher payment exceeded a *B* distinction award for consultants. 2,500 G.P.'s would receive £750 annually in addition to their other income, while 100 would receive £2,500 annually. For a G.P., the higher award was a very substantial increment and—it was hoped—would be an effective incentive to stimulate good work and keep able doctors from becoming specialists or from emigrating.[57] Since they were parts of the basic practice allowances, the merit awards were not an intrinsic part of a capitation system of payment; indeed, they were designed to offset the effects of capitation resulting from the incentive to amass long lists.

A committee representing the general practitioners drafted criteria and procedures. Because the issue had been so controversial and because favoritism was feared, the criteria and mechanics were more formalized than the system for giving distinction awards to hospital consultants. The criteria for

[54] *Report of the Royal Commission on Doctors' and Dentists' Remuneration* (London: H. M. Stationery Office, Cmnd. 939, 1960), pp. 120–22. The recommendation was echoed by the Review Body in its *Fifth Report* (note 35), pp. 27–29.

[55] "Evidence of H. M. Treasury, Ministry of Health, and Department of Health for Scotland," *Minutes of Evidence Taken before the Royal Commission on Doctors' and Dentists' Remuneration* (London: H. M. Stationery Office, 1958), pp. 831–33, 837.

[56] "Witnesses for the British Medical Association," ibid., pp. 274, 1282–83.

[57] "Second Report of Joint Discussions . . ." (note 11), p. 158; and the Review Body's *Seventh Report* (note 29), pp. 65, 95.

inclusion on the special list for French doctors had been confined purposely to the fewest and least controversial attributes, but the proposed British criteria included many of the distinctions that had been used by research investigators. Besides the amount of postgraduate and continuing medical education, the general practitioner could earn points by renting special premises, keeping an appointment system, maintaining good records, conducting special preventive clinics besides his usual office hours, using advanced screening and diagnostic clinics, working in hospitals, and participating in research. Regional panels would obtain information from every general practitioner by questionnaire, they could use informants, and they would recommend awards. Final decisions would be made by a Central Selection Body drawn from the leadership of general practice. In order to prevent merit awards from affecting the flow of patients, the lists would be confidential; but to prevent favoritism, general practitioners could inspect the lists for their region.[58]

The report was the most careful plan for introducing merit pay into any official payment system, but it became no more than a model for future policymakers. The general practitioners were asked to vote on "the principle of payments for special experience and service to general practice," and over 75 per cent disapproved.[59] Therefore the G.P.'s ended by obtaining what they had originally demanded: seniority payments and stratification of the profession by seniority and length of list, but no distinction by merit.

Economizing on Use of the Doctor's Time

One of the potential weaknesses of any service benefits scheme is excessive demands by patients who are not genuinely ill, thereby leaving doctors too little time to care for sick people adequately. The need to deter unnecessary demands upon physicians is a motive for the proposals for cost-sharing and cash benefits described in previous chapters. Unnecessary demands are particularly irritating under salaried or capitation systems, since they bring no added income to the doctor. The problem has been much publicized in Great Britain, because average lists have been longer than in other countries using capitation, the National Health Service has encouraged people to seek medical care, and the general practitioners have been chronically discontented about their pay and working conditions.

58 "Report of the Working Party on Additional Allowances for Special Experience and Service to General Practice," *British Medical Journal Supplement* (11 February 1967), pp. 39–42. Since the working party consisted of doctors active in medical societies, their criteria for merit included holding offices and serving on committees. Another criterion was designed to commit the National Health Service to expand the much-debated right of general practitioners to have their own beds in hospitals, which some critics thought was essential to high quality medicine: a G.P. could earn points by having such beds.

59 "Merit Awards Ballot," ibid. (29 April 1967), p. 25.

For many years, the National Health Service tried to discourage long lists and spread the work by the "loadings" mentioned earlier. For example, during the early 1960's, the basic annual capitation fee was 19s. 6d. and the loading was an additional 14s. 0d. for each patient from 401 to 1,600 on a single practitioner's list. Loadings were abandoned after 1966 in Great Britain, but they are still used in Holland.

The loadings and the administrative ceilings on length of lists deal only with the number of patients: neither they nor any financial device in modern capitation systems can discourage individual patients from making clinically unnecessary and time-consuming demands. Surveys of general practitioners in Great Britain reported many complaints that a few patients took excessive time with unnecessary home and office visits.[60] This issue was one reason for the vote of the Annual Representative Meeting of the British Medical Association in 1965 to consider shifting general practice to fee-for-service: as in private practice, the doctor would be paid every time he was called unnecessarily.[61]

The Ministry of Health opposed such a fundamental change in the payment system. The outcomes of sweeping changes cannot be predicted. The Ministry believed that G.P.'s should educate patients not to use medical services unnecessarily; but fee-for-service might have the opposite effect, since the doctor would profit from many visits.[62]

It seemed impossible to introduce a deterrent into the payment system without discouraging legitimate visits by patients whose uncertain conditions deserved investigation and without violating the National Health Service's touchstone of free medical care. The Beveridge Report that inspired creation of the National Health Service had stated: "It is proposed accordingly that, in the contributions suggested as part of the Plan for Social Security, there shall be included a payment in virtue of which every citizen will be able to

[60] *Abuse and Misuse: A Critical Problem in the Family Doctor Service* (London: General Practitioners' Association, 1965), pp. 13–20, 59–65, and the many studies summarized therein at pp. 21–31; Mechanic, "General Practice" (note 12), pp. 247–49; and Cartwright, *Patients* (note 6), pp. 15, 40–41, 44–52, 162. On the other hand, when asked to keep a diary and rate each case as it came up, G.P.'s estimated fewer unnecessary visits than the numbers they gave in surveys. Cartwright, *Patients* (note 6), p. 48. Many admirers of the Service have conceded that unnecessary visits are an important problem, such as Cargill, *The G.P.* (note 42), pp. 17–18, 52–62, 174–76.

[61] "British Medical Association: Annual Representative Meeting, Swansea 1965," *British Medical Journal Supplement* (17 July 1965), pp. 67–68. Before the barrage of complaints in the 1960's, the profession had seemed satisfied with capitation, although it would have preferred supplements to compensate for burdensome work. E.g., surveys of doctors, such as John H. F. Brotherston, Ann Cartwright, and Fred M. Martin, "The Attitudes of General Practitioners towards Alternative Systems of Remuneration," *British Medical Journal Supplement* (17 October 1959), pp. 119–23, and reports of committees of the profession, such as *A Review of the Medical Services in Great Britain* (London: Social Assay, 1962), pp. 54–57.

[62] "Second Report of Joint Discussions . . ." (note 11), p. 159.

obtain whatever treatment his care requires, at home or in an institution, medical, dental or subsidiary, without a treatment charge."[63] Opposition to cost-sharing has remained an article of faith of the Labor party since the inception of the National Health Service. The introduction of charges precipitated Aneurin Bevan's resignation from the Cabinet.

Therefore, the Ministry launched a national publicity campaign to "Help Your Doctor" by not bothering him with unnecessary requests.[64] The Minister of Pensions and National Insurance changed the rules for national insurance certification, so that fewer office and home visits were necessary to certify the patient's disability.[65]

Position of the Medical Profession

Income

No controlled experiments have estimated the economic consequences of different payment systems, when they are applied to comparable patient loads. But it is widely assumed that a doctor would earn more under fee-for-service than under capitation, since he would be motivated to do more work. For this reason, medical associations usually press to abandon capitation while administrators in sick funds and governments prefer that it be kept.[66]

In all countries, general practitioners earn less than specialists but more than most other wage-earners. The gap between specialists and G.P.'s narrows in countries where both are paid by fee-for-service and where the official medical schemes allow the general practitioners to perform advanced procedures. In contrast, capitation places general practitioners substantially below the income levels of specialists. This can be seen by comparing Table 5

[63] *Social Insurance and Allied Services* (London: H. M. Stationery Office, Cmnd. 6404, 1942), p. 162.

[64] *Annual Report of the Ministry of Health for the Year 1965* (London: H. M. Stationery Office, Cmnd. 3039, 1966), p. 12. The profession's representatives and the National Health Service also agreed to encourage the use of efficient appointments systems. Arnold France, "Limiting Unnecessary Demands on Family Doctors: Letter, August 23rd, from the Permanent Secretary of the Ministry of Health," *The G.M.S. Voice*, 6 September 1966, pp. 3–4. As in most countries, appointment schedules have been used by only a minority of British general practitioners. Cartwright, *Patients* (note 6), pp. 16, 155–59; and Cartwright, "General Practice" (note 29), p. 72.

[65] "Family Doctor Service" (note 37), p. 240. Doctors had long complained about the number of office and home visits solely for the purpose of signing certificates. As in the case of night visits, research on the work loads of average practice showed that such contacts were only a small fraction, but they seemed salient and annoying to doctors. E.g., Teviot S. Eimerl, "Patterns of Illness in a Family Practice," *World Medical Journal*, vol. 12, no. 2 (1965), pp. 44–45; and Cartwright, *Patients* (note 6), pp. 28–29, 42, 45–47.

[66] For example, the division of views in Great Britain, cited in "Second Report of Joint Discussions . . ." (note 11), p. 159.

(wherein both German G.P.'s and specialists were paid by fees and can perform many of the same procedures) and Table 13 (wherein British G.P.'s were paid by capitation and consultants were paid by a combination of public salary and private fees.)

Table 13 showed the median incomes in the mid-1950's for general practitioners, consultants, and other well-paid occupations in Great Britain. In each age group, the general practitioners earned more than all or most nonmedical occupations. The G.P.'s fell behind significantly only after the age of fifty-five, when G.P.'s contracted their practices, but a few other occupations attained their peak incomes because of promotions, seniority salary increments, or attainment of senior positions in partnerships.

But the British general practitioners in Table 13 earned consistently less than the consultants, and the differential widened with age, as consultants acquired seniority increases, distinction awards, and more lucrative private practices. The differential was even wider before World War II, when proportionately less of the G.P.'s practice was covered by capitation fees from national insurance, when he also collected item-of-service fees from a low-income population, and when he had serious collection problems.[67]

Capitation may operate less advantageously for general practitioners in Holland than in Great Britain, according to the Dutch data in Table 6. Contrary to the British situation, the Dutch G.P.'s earn less than other well-paid occupations.

Although capitation may be associated with incomes that are lower than the very highest and that inspire noisy campaigns for improvement, the results may satisfy most individual doctors. For example, in Curwen's survey of motives for entering general practice in Great Britain, many decided they could earn an adequate livelihood, while the more challenging and more remunerative consultant's career required too much study and work.[68]

Among both G.P.'s and consultants, according to Table 16, the middle-aged earn more than the younger or older, but the range by age is narrower for G.P.'s.[69] Capitation rates remain the same, and age variations in length of list may not be large enough to offset the changes in consultants' salary over time, resulting from salary increments and distinction awards. In the higher income brackets, the rise in consultants' pay is obviously much sharper

[67] The average annual incomes of British general practitioners in 1936, 1937, and 1938 are estimated in the two Spens Committee reports: the report on general practitioners, *Remuneration of General Practitioners* (note 10), pp. 4, 22–24; and *Report of the Inter-Departmental Committee on the Remuneration of Consultants and Specialists* (London: H. M. Stationery Office, Cmnd. 7420, 1948), Tables 4 and 6.

[68] M. Curwen, " 'Lord Moran's Ladder'—A Study of Motivation in the Choice of General Practice as a Career," *Journal of the College of General Practitioners*, vol. 7, no. 42 (January 1964), pp. 45–52.

[69] The data are drawn from Royal Commission, *Doctors' and Dentists' Remuneration* (note 42), pp. 261, 268. The free market exchange rate was £1 = $2.80 at that time, but £1 = $2.40 today.

TABLE 16. INCOMES IN AGE GROUPS, GREAT BRITAIN, FISCAL YEAR 1955–56 (IN POUNDS)

Age	Average	Lower Quartile	Median	Upper Quartile	Highest Decile
General practitioners:					
Under 35	1,704	1,213	1,650	2,104	2,571
35–39	2,139	1,648	2,116	2,613	2,994
40–44	2,256	1,784	2,263	2,734	3,183
45–54	2,449	1,900	2,455	2,955	3,442
55–64	2,203	1,602	2,184	2,732	3,241
65 and over	1,736	1,070	1,675	2,330	2,933
All	2,145	1,574	2,107	2,677	3,165
Consultants:					
30–34	2,131	1,888	2,104	2,287	2,586
35–39	2,569	2,187	2,463	2,824	3,461
40–44	3,290	2,714	3,110	3,671	4,498
45–49	3,635	2,835	3,380	4,178	5,158
50–54	3,890	2,995	3,511	4,501	5,700
55–59	4,095	3,050	3,629	4,791	6,024
60 and over	3,693	2,932	3,303	4,485	5,663
All	3,393	2,558	3,122	3,816	5,007

than the rise in general practitioners' pay, but much variation among these consultants arises from private practice. Consultants reach their peak incomes at a later age than general practitioners. This too results partly from the difference between salary and capitation and partly from the consultants' greater opportunity for private practice. The income range within each age group (resulting from a comparison of upper and lower quartiles) also differs according to the payment system. The inter-quartile range remains remarkably stable for the G.P.'s paid by capitation but rises steeply with age for the consultants, as distinction awards and private fees raise their upper income bracket. Among the young doctors, the range is smaller for consultants than among general practitioners: the younger consultants rely on straight salary, but variations in length of list cause the capitation system to produce a wider range of incomes.

The Royal Commission polled assistant general practitioners too. Their annual pay was lower than the salaries of senior registrars and similar to the salaries of registrars. The biggest jump in a G.P.'s pay occurs during the step from assistant to principal. If the lowest hospital ranks are included, the specialist salary scales have a wider range than the average G.P. is likely to experience during his career.[70]

Straight capitation probably produces a career cycle in earnings quite different from that of other well-paid occupations. As I said in previous

[70] Ibid., pp. 264–67.

chapters, data comparing age groups at the same time—see Table 16—are not the same as direct reports about individuals' earnings at successive ages. However, cross-sectional surveys can support more accurate speculations about career earnings cycles. Under straight capitation, British general practitioners reached their peak earnings between the ages of forty-five and fifty-four, according to Table 16. But, according to Table 13, other leading occupations in Britain showed higher, the same, or only slightly lower levels in the older age groups. Although the incomes of individual general practitioners may have steadily risen during their careers under straight capitation, probably the gross incomes of many dropped as they aged. Meanwhile, the incomes in the other occupations probably rose steadily until retirement. This hypothesized difference in career earnings cycles was a principal reason why the leaders of British general practice during the 1960's pressed for a reduced reliance on capitation and for the introduction of larger basic practice allowances and seniority increments. The Review Body also attempted to add distinction awards that would enable many G.P.'s to maintain high incomes during later stages of their careers and that would give very high incomes to a few. The new payment structure was expected to produce a new career earnings cycle without the downturn or leveling-off believed to exist before.[71]

The capitation system has the virtue of enabling the individual and the Treasury to predict the doctor's income for the year, an important argument in countries that are attentive to the dangers of budgetary deficits. If the individual doctor wishes to expand his income suddenly, he cannot do so within the framework of his current practice but must seek new patients (not always easy) or must obtain an additional part-time job from a local health authority, a private business firm, or a private insurance firm. If a significant proportion of the country's population—particularly the wealthy —is not covered by the official scheme, the doctor can expand his income through private practice. Private practice is an important supplement to the income earned by capitation fees in Holland and Spain, where medical care is given through national health insurance that is not universal. But one of the grievances of British general practitioners is that private practice has virtually disappeared for them: all inhabitants of Great Britain are covered under the National Health Service, nearly all come to the general practitioner under the official scheme, and patients see doctors privately only for specialty care.

[71] The Chairman of the General Medical Services Committee said of the proposed system, "There could be an incentive to young doctors to enter general practice—by virtue of a good career structure in general practice, which offers prospects at all stages comparable with those of any other branch of medicine, even right to the top." J. C. Cameron, "Advice to Family Doctors," *The G.M.S. Voice*, 9 May 1966, p. 1.

Numerous English general practitioners have taken part-time government or private jobs to overcome the rigidity of the capitation system in their National Health Service practice. The Royal Commission found that one-third of all general practitioners spent part or most of their time outside panel practice; they earned annual incomes higher than G.P.'s who practiced full-time in the National Health Service.[72]

Private general practice patients in Great Britain total fewer than 4 per cent of the population. Of the general practitioners, about 3 per cent are full-time private practitioners, about 10 per cent have a predominantly private practice mixed with National Health Service work, and 25 per cent have a subsidiary private practice, according to the Royal Commission's information.[73] However, much of this work may refer to private jobs rather than private office practice. It is widely believed that private general practice is declining; statistics show that it is done predominantly by older doctors and will diminish with retirements. The National Health Service caused private general practice to disappear far more precipitously than anyone expected.[74] During disputes over pay, some general practitioners threaten to create private schemes outside the National Health Service and some critics recommend replacement of the entire structure by private health insurance, but enough doctors and patients remain dedicated to the existing system to scotch these revolts.[75]

Capitation has the virtue of stabilizing the doctor's income during the year. Medicine is a seasonal field, and fee-for-service causes income to fluctuate.[76] Some of Hadfield's and Gemmill's respondents in Great Britain said that formerly their incomes had been higher during the first and fourth quarters and much lower during the second and third, but that the National Health Service had given them greater stability in personal budgeting.[77]

Does a straight capitation system produce less economic inequality among general practitioners than fee-for-service? As yet we do not have statistics about income distribution in enough countries. The Royal Commission reported income distribution by age for general practitioners in England, the United States, and Canada, and the range of variation within the profession seems not too different. Possibly the decline in income in later years

[72] Royal Commission, *Doctors' and Dentists' Remuneration* (note 42), pp. 116, 260.

[73] Ibid., p. 116; and Royal Commission, *Supplement to Report: Further Statistical Appendix* (London: H. M. Stationery Office, Cmnd. 1064, 1960), Table 102.

[74] D. S. Lees, "Private General Practice and the National Health Service," *Sociological Review Monograph Number 5* (July 1962), pp. 33–36; and Cartwright, *Patients* (note 6), pp. 10–15.

[75] E.g., Samuel Mencher, *Private Practice in Britain* (London: G. Bell & Sons, 1967), chap. 5.

[76] The annual cycle varies in shape, depending on the weather and the occurrence of epidemics. In France, for example, doctors normally send the largest numbers of bills during the autumn and late winter, while the summer is slack. Edouard Garbe, "Le travail du médecin praticien—Étude statistique," *Cahiers de sociologie et de démographie médicales*, vol. 5, no. 2 (April–June 1965), p. 70.

[77] Hadfield, "Field Survey" (note 31), pp. 691–92; and Gemmill, *Search for Health* (note 1), p. 125.

is smaller in England than in America, partly as a result of the minimum guaranteed by a list under the capitation system.[78]

The Planning of Income Differentials

In most countries, the decisionmakers try to preserve existing differentials among general practice, specialty practice, and other well-paid occupations. It is very difficult to achieve planned income targets for an entire profession under fee-for-service, and therefore the decisionmakers usually increase the fees from time to time in accordance with increases in the cost of living, under the assumption that other occupations have risen a like amount. The decisionmakers are under less pressure by the doctors to bring about an average target income for the profession under fee-for-service, since the individual has a better chance to enhance his own pay through his own efforts. But a flat rate payment method is usually designed to bring about a target income, the profession is fully aware of the resulting differentials, and the individual physician usually can expand his revenue only by seeking outside sources rather than by working harder under the official payment scheme.

Relativities in pay will not become controversial under capitation if the general practitioners accept the existing differentials and if the economy remains stable. For many years, Dutch general practitioners adjusted to capitation satisfactorily for these reasons. But if the economy is in flux and the cost of living rises quickly, the doctors can easily become disenchanted with capitation. During the mid-1960's incomes and living costs rose suddenly in Holland, the annual review procedure did not raise capitation as fast as the G.P.'s wished, they felt that they were falling behind other occupations, and some of their criticisms of the administration of capitation extended to the flat-rate system of payment itself.

General practitioners' pay has been so turbulent in Great Britain in large part because they want improvements in the existing differentials. At first, this was the policy of the National Health Service. As I explained in chapters V and VI, the Spens Committee in 1946 recommended that English general practitioners be raised *above* their prewar position in the economy, an unusual policy directive for a nationalized industry. Payment procedures and funds are more flexible in prosperous private occupations, and usually great improvements in an occupation's relative position occur only in private

[78] Royal Commission, *Doctors' and Dentists' Remuneration* (note 42), pp. 261, 326. Comparisons were possible only with the United States and Canada. I suspect that in countries with too many general practitioners for full employment, a fee-for-service system (along with other causes) produces greater economic inequalities among G.P.'s than does capitation.

employment. In the postwar economic boom in Europe, it has been privately employed industrial and white collar workers who have improved their positions most, and pay lags in the nationalized industries have been a widespread problem.

The Spens Committee did not realize it was proposing an exception to subsequent history: because of higher prices, higher income taxes, and higher pay among workers, the relative economic position of the European middle classes has declined since World War II,[79] but acceptance of the Spens Report committed the National Health Service to guarantee a *higher* position for the general practitioner. Since the price level and wages in the English economy were rapidly rising, the target was rising; because Treasury budget ceilings limited the expansion of the Central Pool, and since the Pool had to pay for a steady increase in the numbers of doctors and patients, the financial means lagged behind the target. An additional problem was the ambiguity of the target. The Spens Report had committed the National Health Service to "improve" the economic status of the G.P., but no one could be certain what level of pay would constitute a sufficient improvement. The purpose of the expert commission was to produce unambiguous policy guidelines, but the apparently logical and factual report had contained unanticipated weaknesses. The BMA was convinced that the government's formulas fell short of the commitments both had accepted, the BMA charged the government with betrayal and bad faith, and there seemed no way of resolving this debate through bilateral negotiation. Thus the Spens criteria generated rather than resolved conflict.

The controversy also demonstrated the problems arising from a failure to fit means to ends. The Spens Report's recommendations concerning the optimum distribution of income among G.P.'s, the levels of income at different career stages, and other topics could be achieved most efficiently by a carefully constructed salary system. But the BMA wished to avoid salaried general practice at all costs, since it wished G.P.'s to retain the status of "independent contractors." The BMA was passionately committed to the Spens goals, while just as passionately opposed to the most efficacious means of attaining them.[80] Unless supplemented by special payments resembling salaries or unless altered by special formulae that destroy its advantageous administrative simplicity, capitation produces income inequalities according to the length of the practitioner's list and not according to merit or career stage. Thus, contrary to the aims of the Spens Committee, straight capitation

[79] On the decline of professionals relative to workers, see Tibor Scitovsky, "An International Comparison of the Trend of Professional Earnings," *American Economic Review*, vol. 56, no. 1 (March 1966), pp. 25–42.

[80] Harry Eckstein, *Pressure Group Politics* (London: George Allen & Unwin, 1960), pp. 98–100 and chap. 6 passim.

resulted in giving the highest incomes to those G.P.'s who practice in densely populated but unpopular districts, such as industrial cities.[81]

British general practitioners have tried to improve their financial position, not only relative to lay occupations but also relative to the consultants. But the consultants have been just as determined to preserve their differentials over the G.P.'s. At times the consultants succeeded by inducing governments to grant the same increases as those obtained by the G.P.'s. For example, the last chapter summarized events in the early 1950's, when the consultants supported an increase for the G.P.'s and then obtained a comparable increase later, on the stated grounds of re-establishing a normal differential. The Royal Commission and Review Body during the 1960's tried to avoid becoming enmeshed in this competition by deciding the consultants' and general practitioners' pay together and by insisting that any unilateral claim by one group be approved by the other.

Preserving the differential by identical awards proved very difficult, because consultants and general practitioners were paid by different methods. For example, the Review Body in 1963, predicting that the nation's wages would rise by 14 per cent during the subsequent three years, decided to raise all physicians' net incomes by 14 per cent, and therefore increased both hospital doctors' salaries and part of the general practitioners' Central Pool by this figure. However, the system operated to widen the differential: the specialists received a 14 per cent increase in salaries; but much of the increase in the Central Pool was absorbed by a deficit from the previous period, by increased payments for work outside of panel practice, and by other charges. Consequently, the obscure operations of the Central Pool left the average G.P. with a much smaller net increase than the consultants received. An impasse resulted when the G.P.'s claimed they were underpaid relative to other occupations, and the Review Body responded that they were not. These experiences led to the general practitioners' attacks on the payment system, ultimately resulting in the government's abolition of the Central Pool.[82]

[81] How the capitation mechanism and the Central Pool system inevitably caused the Ministry of Health to follow procedures and distribute incomes in ways deviating from the Spens Committee's planned differentials is described in "Witnesses for the Ministry of Health," *Minutes of Evidence Taken before the Royal Commission on Doctors' and Dentists' Remuneration* (London: H. M. Stationery Office, 1958), pp. 790–91, 844–45.

[82] The prolonged controversy over the differentials between the general practitioners and the consultants is summarized in Stevens, *Medical Practice* (note 48), chaps. 9, 20, 21. The argument by general practitioners for a narrowing of the differentials on grounds of increasing similarity in skills and responsibility appears in *The G.P.A. Report—Part Two: Doctors' Remuneration* (London: General Practitioners' Association, 1965), pp. 47–51. The Review Body's rejection of the G.P.'s claims of underpayment appears in its *Fifth Report* (note 35), pp. 23–25. The Review Body's temporary abandonment of differentials as criteria for making payment decisions is summarized in its *Seventh Report* (note 29), chap. 3.

Prestige

Since the public's respect for the medical profession does not depend on the payment system, it is neither magnified nor diminished by the use of capitation in a national medical scheme. As in nearly all countries, medicine ranks at the top of public surveys of occupational prestige in The Netherlands.[83]

Spain is one of the few countries where medicine is not among the most respected occupations.[84] Although Spain's SOE pays doctors by capitation, this fact seems to have no relation to the position of medicine. Rather, according to Kenny, doctors are not highly respected in Spain because of the persistence of a folk-religious attitude toward the causes and cures of illness.[85] Before the modern organization of medical practice, medicine was not one of the highest ranking occupations.[86]

Recruitment

Capitation by itself makes medical careers neither more nor less attractive. Recruitment has flourished in some countries with capitation, but it has lagged in others. Many other factors operate besides the mere existence of a flat-rate system of payment. Even a much criticized type of capitation fee may seem tolerable in the light of a country's total opportunity structure.

Both Holland and Spain have recruited enough doctors for their needs. Despite the use of a method of payment that most doctors in the world oppose, Dutch general practice seems to have suffered less from the rising popularity of specialization than has general practice elsewhere. And despite the complaints by SOE's doctors against low pay and an excessively bureaucratized system,[87] Spanish medical schools continue to attract very large numbers of students and SOE can pick its general practitioners from long waiting lists or from crowded competitions.[88] For example, when SOE in

[83] Cartwright, *Patients* (note 6), p. 52; F. van Heek et al., *Sociale Stijging en Daling in Nederland* (Leiden: H. E. Stenfert Kroese N.V., 1958), 1: 25–26; and Gerrit Kuiper, *Mobiliteit in de Sociale en Beroepshierarchie* (Utrecht: van Gorcum and Co., 1954), p. 49.

[84] Unpublished surveys of the Spanish population by Data S. A. of Madrid and by other polling organizations.

[85] Michael Kenny, "Social Values and Health in Spain: Some Preliminary Considerations," *Human Organization*, vol. 21, no. 4 (Winter 1962–63), p. 285.

[86] F. Polo y Fiayo, *El médico gobernante* (Madrid: Javier Morata, 1930), pp. 11–34.

[87] Salustiano del Campo Urbano, *Problemas de la profesión médica española* (Madrid: Comision Nacional Española del Instituto Internacional de Estudios de Clases Medias, 1964), pp. 52–54; and Gomez-Reino, "Seguro de Erfermedad" (note 20), pp. 241–53, 263–71.

[88] During the decades since the creation of SOE the number of students in medical faculties has steadily risen, and the proportion of university students in medicine has increased. *Estadistica de la enseñanza superior en España, curso 1963–64* (Madrid: Instituto Nacional de Estadistica, 1966), pp. 8–9.

1967 announced an open competition for 372 places in general practice and for 305 specialty posts, 3,800 G.P.'s and 3,200 specialists entered.

Although applications for medical schools in Great Britain have continued to exceed the available enrollment, retention of young general practitioners became a problem during the 1960's. Several hundred emigrated each year. Primarily they complained about the organization of general practice—contacts with hospitals were too few, some could not set up independent practices or become partners, and so on—but a minority added remuneration to their other objections. The Review Body became concerned, since the ratio of general practitioners to population was deteriorating, and medical progress was increasing the work load per patient. Therefore, in order to raise general practitioners' morale and to improve recruitment and discourage emigration, the Review Body in 1966 raised general practitioners' pay.[89] But other nonmonetary reforms were also needed.[90]

Conclusion: The Effects of Capitation

Apparently gross neglect of patients does not occur in any of the countries that have used capitation systems. Certain important countervailing forces protect the patient, such as the individual doctor's ethical conscience, the medical profession's group opinion condemning dereliction of duty, and the danger of official complaints and lawsuits. But capitation results in excessive transfers to services outside the G.P.'s panel practice. For example, the G.P. may refer the time-consuming patient to another organization, particularly the outpatient department of the hospital, unless effective administrative deterrents exist.

Because of their standardized character, simple capitation fees provide no pecuniary motives for more effort or for work of better quality. If professional conscience is supplemented by monetary incentives, capitation must be modified in ways that rob it of its administrative simplicity. Higher capitation fees can be offered for the types of patients who will likely be more burdensome; basic payments can be offered the most capable doctors in order to reward superior performance or more time-consuming work; a minimum income can be guaranteed doctors with short lists; fees on an item-of-service basis can be offered for more onerous tasks; practice expenses can be reimbursed. Under pressure from the medical profession, some national schemes have incorporated these supplements to stimulate better

[89] Review Body's *Seventh Report* (note 29), chap. 4. For the government's concern about recruitment and retention see the summary of question time in the House of Commons in *Lancet* (29 October 1966), pp. 974–75.

[90] An eloquent statement of the need to improve working conditions in order to raise the performance and retention of doctors appears in the Review Body's *Seventh Report* (note 29), pp. 29–30.

work or to mollify the discontented, but such revisions illustrate the worldwide trend away from simple capitation.

Capitation cannot reorient styles of medical practices, but it can support traditional approaches. Probably it reinforces a conservative approach to the patient, and unnecessary or drastic medical procedures are not encouraged. If medical care and medical education traditionally emphasize therapy, more than a capitation system is necessary to instill a preventive viewpoint. The method of lists under capitation can foster greater continuity of care than general practice under fee-for-service, but it cannot counteract a country's customary division between general practice and specialty work.

Capitation tends to reinforce the distinction between G.P. and specialist by depriving each of the financial motives to perform the other's procedures. It survives best where the evolution of medical practice and the aspirations of doctors do not blur the difference. This has long been true in the two countries with the most firmly based capitation traditions, England and Holland: general practitioners were based in private offices and specialists did most of their work in hospitals; general practitioners gave basic care and specialists did advanced tasks; there was little overlap in work sites, tasks, and class status. However, general practitioners in the world have been rising in skills and aspirations, have attempted to share the specialists' professional opportunities and position, and have either pressed to abandon capitation (as in Germany) or obtained revisions of capitation that resembled features of specialists' payment methods (as in England).

XI

DESIGNING EFFECTIVE PAYMENT SYSTEMS

To the public, money often seems the medical profession's principal interest. Claims about money and facilities are the only occasions when laymen and doctors converse about the same topics with a common vocabulary.[1] Probably in all countries, the principal newspaper coverage of medicine concerns disputes over doctors' pay and over the inadequacies of hospitals.[2]

But of course doctors are at least as deeply concerned with the substantive content of their work: that employment should yield more than instrumental returns is one of the essential characteristics of a profession. Even during the most bitter payment disputes with sick funds and governments, the average practicing doctor works as always, is preoccupied with the technical aspects of his duties, and is a spectator (albeit an interested and irritated one) to the remuneration controversy. Because of the customary professional autonomy over the substance of the job and because of its supposedly esoteric nature, doctors make little effort to communicate knowledge to the laity about the other things that interest and motivate them, and the medical administrators and press hardly bother to learn and publicize these matters.

[1] One of Britain's former Ministers of Health recalls: "The unnerving discovery every Minister of Health makes at or near the outset of his term of office is that the only subject he is ever destined to discuss with the medical profession is money.

"Cynically, but unjustly, he may be tempted to assume that this is because money is the only thing the medical profession cares about. It is not so. What has happened is that the nationalised service makes money the sole terminology of intercourse between profession and government. If, for instance, legal advice and representation were nationalised on principles similar to those of medical care, the lawyers would no doubt be found on the same terms with the administration." Enoch Powell, *A New Look at Medicine and Politics* (London: Pitman Medical Publishing Co., 1966), p. 14.

[2] This is true even in countries where the government discourages publicity about trouble and where the press is co-operative. For example, a recent content analysis of Spanish newspaper coverage revealed far more articles about payment disputes than about any other topic in national health insurance. Diego Ignacio Mateo del Peral, "El Seguro de Enfermedad a través de la prensa de Madrid," in, Enrique Martin Lopez et al., *Estudio sociologico sobre el Seguro de Enfermedad* (Madrid: Ministerio de Trabajo, Secretaría General Técnica, 1964), 3: 121.

The fact that pay is not the only preoccupation of the medical profession has important consequences for remuneration policy. The procedures for determining and distributing pay are symbolically significant, and the doctors consider them at least as important as the amount of money. Procedures must satisfy any profession's distinctive concern with sharing in all managerial decisions and reserving all clinical decisions to itself. Unless pay is adequate for a satisfactory living standard and for buying some facilities, recruitment may suffer and practitioners will be overworked.[3] Adequate financial rewards, of course, must be combined with satisfying technical working conditions and with the personal appreciation of patients.[4] Therefore, once the procedures and levels of pay suffice, and if the nonpecuniary rewards are protected, doctors will adjust to any system of compensation. In practice, the most familiar system usually arouses the least protest.

Like any profession, doctors as a group expect to be consulted in public decisions about their pay and other aspects of their work. Many disputes have revolved about the administrative setup of a payment system: if the government and sick funds have full power to fix doctors' pay, or if the government and funds negotiate but can and do make unilateral decisions afterward, the system will be upset by strikes and protests. Doctors prefer either payment systems that they control completely or—since hopes for total power are unrealistic—true bargaining situations that yield pay rates promulgated by agreement. If the law or custom requires that the announcement of the pay rates and of the administrative rules be decrees of the government or sick funds, medical associations are not disturbed, provided the enactment is *pro forma* and automatically promulgates the negotiated agreement. The recent trend in Europe—and probably the future trend in the rest of the world—is replacement of unilateral public payment announcements by bargaining for contracts.[5] The State retains an irrevocable right

[3] If rates from any clinical job are low and if private practice is limited, doctors must hold several jobs in addition to whatever office practice they can attract. Many will be tired and give hasty care. Almost none will have the time and energy for continuing their education. For example, the difficulties of many Turkish and Greek doctors, described by Carl E. Taylor et al., *Health Manpower Planning in Turkey* (Baltimore: The Johns Hopkins Press, 1968), pp. 50–51; and by Richard H. Blum and Eva Blum, *Health and Healing in Rural Greece* (Stanford: Stanford University Press, 1965), p. 224.

[4] The nonmonetary gains in general practice can be rewarding even during bitter disputes over pay, as exemplified by Peter Manngian, *Goodbye, Doctor, Goodbye* (London: Abelard-Schuman, 1963), pp. 151–55. Usually complaints about their pay are merely part of a more general dissatisfaction by hospital doctors over underfinanced working conditions. E.g., " 'Charter' for Hospital Doctors," *British Medical Journal Supplement* (29 October 1966), pp. 171–74.

[5] On the harmonious transformation of French medical decisionmaking during the 1960's, see Jean Mignon, "La réforme du régime conventionnel par le décret du 7 janvier 1966," *Droit social*, vol. 28, nos. 7–8 (July–August 1966), pp. 434–38. Even before the reforms of 1966, the officially authoritarian payment system was administered in an increasingly collaborative manner. François Sellier, "La situation sociale," ibid., vol. 27, no. 4 (April 1965), pp. 254–56. The absence of a bargaining mechanism and the retention of sole authority over fees by the sick funds and government angered German doctors for

to reduce or postpone pay awards during national economic crises, but the doctors do not protest this power when it is used with manifest reason.[6]

Professions usually believe they are underpaid and make ceaseless demands for better pay, more social recognition, and better facilities. Partly this results from the belief of each profession that the problems it specializes in solving are particularly threatening to society, and that society *must* be eager for salvation at any cost. Partly the scope of these demands results from a belief that the government could easily raise all the necessary money by its taxing powers and by budgetary reallocations.[7]

Certain administrative remedies might moderate these demands. First, the medical profession needs to be informed better about where it actually stands in the nation's income and prestige structure. As we have seen throughout the book, medicine ranks very high in salary and prestige in all countries; where its living standards fall below those of doctors in other countries, the reason is poverty in the home country, but doctors usually rank much higher than their fellow citizens. Doctors think they earn less than they do.[8]

A second remedy is to reorganize the confrontation system. At present in most countries, the doctors bargain only with the Ministry of Health or sick funds and rarely see the men from the Treasury who recommend the tax rates and write the budgets. Nor do the doctors debate with the rival claimants to the government's limited money, such as the other government Ministries or the other occupations that seek higher pay. In practice, the persons whom the doctors see are not true adversaries but usually favor the doctors' interests openly or covertly. Sometimes the Ministry of Health or the sick funds become the doctors' advocates in the periodic battles of the budget in the government.[9] Since the doctors do not debate with their true

---

decades. This power of the sick funds remains an unresolved irritant in Italian national health insurance today despite raises in pay. Carlo Palenzona, "Période de réforme sanitaire, disputes entre médecins, disputes entre ministères," *Concours médical*, vol. 89, no. 7 (18 February 1967), pp. 1328, 1331.

[6] For example, no sooner had Britain's general practitioners won the award that ended the prolonged crisis over pay in 1966, than the government proclaimed the Incomes Standstill and postponed the increase. After getting full explanations from the Prime Minister and Minister of Health, the leaders of the medical societies recommended that the profession co-operate. An essential condition was that austerity should apply to all. However, when loopholes exist in wage policy, medicine is more successful than other occupations in extracting special concessions from the government. For example, the pay awards to British general practitioners earlier during the 1960's summarized by Rosemary Stevens, *Medical Practice in Modern England* (New Haven: Yale University Press, 1966), p. 301.

[7] Powell, *Medicine and Politics* (note 1), pp. 20–25.

[8] This discrepancy has been true for many years. For example, American doctors during the early 1930's thought they were underpaid, but their relative position was very high. Harold F. Clark et al., *Life Earnings in Selected Occupations in the United States* (New York: Harper & Brother, 1937), pp. 15–16, 23–25, 70–79, 257–68.

[9] A common phenomenon in government is that even the bodies that regulate a private interest come to sympathize with that group. Samuel P. Huntington, "Groups, Agencies, and Clientelism" (Cambridge: unpublished paper from the Department of Government,

critics and competitors, and since they bargain with friendly agencies, they easily acquire the habit of making ambitious demands for pay and facilities without regard to social priorities.

So many occupations now depend on public pay or public facilities in every country that national forums might be created with profit. The demands for large pay increases or facilities for one group might be discussed in the intergroup forum, and periodic recommendations about priorities and distribution might be issued. A pay demand that could withstand such scrutiny would clearly be supported by a social consensus lacking under the present system of unilateral pressures upon the public authorities. The doctors would have the novel experience of learning about the economic needs of other sectors of the society and would see how allocations for their pay and facilities fit into society's total set of priorities. In its clinical work, the medical profession has clear-cut institutions for meeting its social responsibilities; but mechanisms are needed to make it socially responsible economically as well.

The medical profession should be induced not only to participate in decisions about the relation between its pay and the rest of the economy, but also in decisions about the allocation of national resources for medical care. A serious problem in some countries—such as Britain and France—is the lag in spending for hospital buildings and nurses' pay while the doctors press successfully to keep their own pay ahead of other leading occupations. All participants in medical services should meet in forums to debate whether such priorities in allocation of limited resources are generally accepted. Doubtless these groups will find common ground in a collective appeal to the Treasury for more money for medical care, but the problem of allocating what they get will always exist.

Encouraging Good Medicine

No method of payment is simple and produces easily predictable consequences.[10] The success of any remuneration procedure depends on many other variables, such as the ethics of the medical profession, the co-operation of the medical association, the amount of money available, the facilities for practice, the expectations of the population, and so on.[11] Every payment

Harvard University, 1951). Britain's Review Body was supposed to price doctors' pay awards within the financial capabilities of the government, but within a few years it was practicing the generosity characteristic of special purpose agencies. Its award in 1966 exceeded the government's resources and was scaled down by the Cabinet. Therefore, some mechanisms are needed to achieve a more unified conception of the public interest not only for the private groups but also for their individual regulatory agencies.

[10] The next paragraphs summarize the effects of payment systems on the performance and position of doctors. For some able remarks on the administrative advantages and disadvantages of each payment system, see James Hogarth, *The Payment of the General Practitioner* (Oxford: Pergamon Press, 1963), chaps. 13 and 14.

[11] The results of every payment system in every occupation depend on the total complex of institutional determinants and personal motives. This is well stated in Marriott's

system carries potentialities for neglect and abuse as well as motivations for good work. Every payment system has mixed success in practice, because so many other variables affect doctors' performance and because its own inherent potentialities are mixed. Any change in an existing system will agitate those who decline in relative position within the medical profession, and financial concessions to mollify their complaints will destroy the "fine tuning" essential to a theoretically ideal payment structure. Therefore planning commissions often begin searches for the ideal payment system optimistically, but they usually end by noting the drawbacks of every known procedure, by foreseeing the difficulties of achieving rational reform at home, and by unenthusiastically agreeing to continue the familiar payment system of their own country, with some modifications to appease the doctors and discourage abuse.[12]

Remuneration to reward superior work presents dilemmas. The best incentive system must be individualized: since every person has a slightly different set of motives and responses, payment should be designed especially for him. But the trend in the modern world is to collectivize labor agreements and to standardize pay rates for all workers in a particular category: incentive systems tend to disappear and individuals receive the same rates despite personal differences in motives and performance.[13] In completely private practice—within limits of the market and of local professional custom—doctors can fix their own fees idiosyncratically, in ways that may not relate to quality of work. The trend in national health insurance and national health services is to adopt standardized nationwide fees or salaries. Disputes lead to further standardization, in order to minimize controversy. Consequently, work of different quality often begets like reward, and nonpecuniary professional motives must be the factors that produce superior medical care. If the standard rates reward quantity of work (as in fee-for-service) or do not reward extra effort (as in salary or capitation), there is the danger of unintentionally discouraging the superior work that takes time.

---

analysis of the effects of pay on the performance of industrial workers. R. Marriott, *Incentive Payment Systems* (London: Staples Press, 1957), esp. chaps. 7 and 8.

[12] For example, the report by a committee of the British medical societies endorsing capitation because the alternatives were even more unacceptable. *A Review of the Medical Services in Great Britain* (London: Social Assay, 1962), pp. 54–57. By the same negative reasoning, an official German advisory committee endorsed its traditional service-benefits fee-for-service method over capitation and cash benefits. Sozialenquête-Kommission, *Soziale Sicherung in der Bundesrepublik Deutschland* (Stuttgart: W. Kohlhammer GMBH, 1966), pp. 220–31, and esp. p. 231.

[13] These trends are common in nonmedical pay in many countries. For example, see *Managerial Compensation* (Ann Arbor: Foundation for Research on Human Behavior, 1965), pp. 2–4, 39–40, 43–46; David W. Belcher, *Wage and Salary Administration* (Englewood Cliffs, N.J.: Prentice-Hall, Inc., 2d ed., 1962), pp. 545–51; and Burkart Lutz and Alfred Willener, *Niveau de mécanisation et mode de rémunération* (Luxembourg: Communauté Européenne du Charbon et de l'Acier, 1960), part 2.

Some payment systems have experimented with special rewards for doctors who are judged superior, in contrast to the attempt to reward specific *procedures* of high quality. One method is to raise basic pay, such as the distinction awards to British specialists; another method is to allow some physicians to collect higher fees from patients willing to pay them, as in France. Ideally such rewards—whether of doctors or for procedures themselves—should be individualized. But in practice in merit pay administration in other occupations, the unions usually press for obvious criteria and automatic application, while management often decides that bureaucratized procedures are less controversial. Similarly in medicine, merit pay may succumb to standardized methods, thereby losing its effectiveness upon quality of performance. For example, after several years of fruitless discussion over the method of designating superior doctors, the solution in France was to so classify doctors automatically if they held certain hospital posts or had taken postgraduate training. Once the simple criterion is achieved by many doctors—e.g., when many have taken postgraduate courses—the connection has attenuated between the award and quality of work. Since the medical profession is as unenthusiastic collectively about merit pay for a few as is any large class of workers, probably few countries will include such rewards in the official payment system. The British general practitioners' success in resisting merit payment and in obtaining automatic seniority increments may be typical. For the moment, British specialists receive distinction awards upon the recommendation of investigators and committees who deliberate secretly about the qualities of specific individuals; but the method is often criticized, and more standardized criteria and automatic procedures can be expected.

Inclusion of practice expenses in pay to guarantee superior facilities is another matter that should be individualized but in practice is standardized throughout the profession, regardless of need. Like the members of any other group, many doctors would claim such subsidies when the public authorities believed they were not needed or had not been earned. The medical profession is particularly sensitive to the discretionary power of public authorities over professional practice. Therefore the trend is to omit practice expenses from the system of paying doctors under public medical schemes. Separate government programs may help groups or single practitioners obtain facilities, and therefore the sufficiently troubled remuneration system for work is not complicated further. More commonly, especially outside the most affluent Western countries, the trend is to remove the facilities for public medical care from the doctors' ownership and control: ambulatory and hospital treatment are given to insured patients in buildings and with equipment owned by the sick funds and the government, and the doctor is paid only for his work. If they obtain enough income and clinical autonomy in hospitals, polyclinics, and other organized establishments, most doctors in the world seem happier without the expense and trouble of equipping and managing their own enterprises.

The quality of work can be promoted through a public remuneration scheme by confining payment for particular procedures to holders of specialty credentials in those fields. Therefore surgery cannot be performed by general practitioners or by specialists in other fields, and obstetrics can be performed only by obstetricians and general practitioners who are trained and certified by the licensing body in that field.[14] Besides confining complicated work to those with advanced training, the practice has the probably beneficial result of reducing competition for patients, since each specialty has a monopoly in its field. One of the few ways that a payment system can directly regulate the quality of care, this rule has the drawbacks of dividing the medical profession and depressing the skill and status of general practice. The specialists—and particularly the surgeons—become much wealthier and more powerful than the doctors in the medical specialties and in general practice. Unless they are persuaded of the value of family care, general practitioners may be chronically discontented.

A payment system must coincide with the total organization of medical practice. Incentives to practice good medicine will have no effect except to produce irritation if the doctor cannot follow through. For example, any policy to encourage preventive examinations by office practitioners through special payments presupposes access to a sufficient number of laboratories or hospital outpatient departments. The parlous state of French hospitals has limited the number of full-time salaried appointments for the many young doctors aspiring to careers in clinical science and research. Only after the construction of many new hospitals with adequate laboratories, examination rooms, and libraries can the recent reforms be implemented in the organization and remuneration of hospital practice. If a flat-rate payment system is not to produce over-referrals to hospitals, the general practitioners must have sufficient access to full diagnostic and therapeutic facilities, as experience shows in Great Britain and Holland.

Good medical services should have no administrative barriers to the seeking of care when it is needed. Cash benefits schemes are criticized because they lead to some delays and some complete failures in obtaining medical care, although they are often defended as effective deterrents to abuse.[15]

[14] The unrestricted collection of fees for any procedure under private practice and the open staff structure of most hospitals have allowed American general practitioners to perform surgery and obstetrics for some time, often with debatable results. "Physicians Who Perform Surgery," *Progress in Health Services: Health Information Foundation*, vol. 10, no. 6 (June 1961), pp. 1–6; Richard Carter, *The Doctor Business* (Garden City, N.Y.: Doubleday & Co., 1958), pp. 125–26, 184, 187, 193–95, 230; *Prepayment for Medical and Dental Care in New York State* (New York: School of Public Health and Administrative Medicine, Columbia University, 1962), pp. 199–248 passim. As national health insurance spreads in the United States, a decision will have to be made about this increasingly disputed issue.

[15] Cash benefits schemes and cost-sharing by the patient are based on the classical economic assumption that medical services are typical consumer goods that will be pur-

However, making the payment system easier for the patient will not assure prompt use of medical services. Apathy and the obligations of work and family may be even greater deterrents than money.

Ideally a payment system should encourage the right distribution of specialties in a country, so that referrals can be made to fully qualified persons. The payment system should be designed in the light of its allocation effects as well as its income effects: its rewards to certain deserving specialties should not attract so many doctors that shortages result in other needed skills.

However, the experience in some countries shows that internal politics within the medical profession can result in the underevaluation and underpayment of certain specialties. The leading victims are usually psychiatry, preventive medicine, and dentistry. In addition, some specialties may not develop because other specialists find it profitable to take over their procedures or to delegate the work to persons under their supervision, such as nurses. The victims of this manipulation of the payment schedule and rules include anesthesiology, radiology, internal medicine, and pediatrics. On the other hand, fee schedules usually itemize the procedures of the surgical specialties at length and work to the financial advantage of their practitioners. As in so many other areas of remuneration policy, a well-organized and equitably paid profession can be created under a public medical scheme only if the various factions are committed to the success of the system and to the reasonable prosperity of each other. A salary structure can guarantee more equal income and status among the specialties than can fee-for-service. Since all but the shortest fee schedules may inherently benefit the surgical specialties most and may encourage the medical specialties to undertake an undue amount of mechanized treatment, perhaps they should always include case payments for the supportive specialties, generous enough to reward time-consuming interviews, emotional support, and other work not easily itemized.

If a public medical care system seeks to guarantee superior care, it must include machinery for expert review of work. The patients may be satisfied—as they usually are in public opinion polls on medical care—but they may not be qualified to judge the quality of the treatments they receive.[16]

chased very wastefully if they are cheap or free. James M. Buchanan, *The Inconsistencies of the National Health Service* (London: Institute of Economic Affairs, 1965), pp. 5–7, 12–13. But critics deny that the demand for medical care is on a par with the demand for other goods and services: usually it is sought only when necessary. Eveline M. Burns, "Policy Decisions Facing the United States in Financing and Organizing Health Care," *Public Health Reports*, vol. 81, no. 8 (August 1966), p. 676. On the differences between markets for medical care and other markets characterized by greater consumer power, see Kenneth J. Arrow, "Uncertainty and the Welfare Economics of Medical Care," *American Economic Review*, vol. 53, no. 5 (December 1963); and Richard M. Bailey, "An Economist's View of Health Services Industry," *Inquiry*, vol. 6, no. 1 (March 1969), esp. pp. 11–13.

16 Research in the United States showed that samples of hospital inpatients were highly satisfied with treatments judged of low quality by observers qualified in medicine. *Prepayment for Medical Care and Dental Care in New York State* (New York: School of Public Health

Preventing Abuse

Certain desirable procedures can be encouraged by special fees. However, a dilemma is to prevent the fees from motivating unnecessary and excessive performance. For example, procedures that do not harm the patient—like preventive examinations and home visits—can be done excessively for fees that were merely supposed to motivate performance when necessary. No system has devised payment formulae or administrative procedures that strike the perfect balance. And the nature of the "perfect balance" is not certain: the "right number" of home visits is disputed, and "too many" preventive examinations might even be good. More serious problems are, unnecessary and financially motivated procedures that harm the patient.

A proper combination of financial formulae and controls can diminish abuses. Many countries should study the variable charges in Dutch fee-for-service and case payments: numerous delicately attuned and frequently updated formulae reduce the rewards of excessive repetitions of work without discouraging long-term care in individual cases. Administrative controls over cases of deviation are effective when they are accepted by the profession, but often they arouse so much resistance they are not adequately enforced. Evaluation of the doctor's work by a lay administrative organization seems to strike at the profession's insistence on autonomy. A promising solution is the new French plan to develop control committees and consultations that bring together doctors representing the sick funds and medical association.[17]

One of the unusual features of doctors' pay is that medicine is among the few occupations in the public sector that can determine its own earnings: particularly under fee-for-service, physicians have considerable discretion in prescribing the number and type of procedures that will bring them money. An argument for salaries is less opportunity for the venal multiplication of procedures, but that danger is replaced by the risk of neglect. Administrators prefer salaries instead of payment systems allowing the expansion of work and earnings by the doctor's own discretion, since the work and expenditures of medical services are more predictable.[18]

---

and Administrative Medicine, Columbia University, 1962), chap. 7, part D; and *A Study of the Quality of Hospital Care Secured by a Sample of Teamster Family Members in New York City* (New York: School of Public Health and Administrative Medicine, Columbia University, 1964). The British patients surveyed by Cartwright did not believe their G.P.'s referred them too often to hospital outpatient departments, but more expert judges thought the doctors did. Ann Cartwright, *Patients and Their Doctors* (London: Routledge & Kegan Paul, 1967), p. 125.

[17] "Rapport du Haut Comité Médical de la Sécurité Sociale sur le fonctionnement et l'organisation du contrôle médical," *Notes et études documentaires*, no. 3088 (9 May 1964), pp. 10–28.

[18] Former British Minister of Health Powell recalls the essential administrative differences between the sectors of the National Health Service that paid doctors by salary and the Executive Councils that paid general practitioners by capitation and dentists by

Ultimately, abuse is discouraged by the conscience of the medical profession, and standards are observed more widely if the profession is adequately paid, if it is not overcrowded and competitive, and if the leaders of the medical societies are committed to the success of the public medical care scheme. In the past, codes of medical ethics were individualistic and were enforced accordingly: they condemned offenses against the patient and against fellow doctors. Venal acts against the sick funds or government were not specifically covered; medical associations in most countries did not feel responsible for enforcing the sick funds' or government's payment rules; and often medical associations sided with the individual doctors against the control procedures. But as better consultative mechanisms and mutual confidence develop between medical associations and public medical care schemes, codes of medical ethics may expand to include violations of regulations, and the medical associations feel responsible for protecting the funds.[19]

One of the numerous dilemmas in administering medical pay is opportunity for private practice by physicians receiving most of their income from the public medical care scheme. Doctors press for the right of private practice, since they earn considerable extra income thereby and also enjoy a freedom that seems symbolically prized. Medical administrators concede the right, since the official payment system need not bear the burden of determining doctors' entire income. One reason why the general practitioners have been more satisfied with health insurance in Holland than in Great Britain is the greater opportunity to supplement capitation income by one's own private practice in The Netherlands. As a result, the private patient receives more attentive diagnoses, more emotional support, more convenient appointments, and more home calls. Given their successful history in bargaining with sick funds and governments, doctors are not likely to give up rights of private practice. Instead, some countries with high personal incomes and powerful medical professions—such as Switzerland today and possibly the United States in the future—may incorporate rights of private practice into the official scheme itself, by means of a cash benefits system, a sliding scale of charges to the patient, and a fixed schedule of reimbursements by the funds.

---

fee-for-service. In the first two, the Ministry can budget; in the third, at best it can merely make estimates of the probable costs it will be required to pay. *Medicine and Politics* (note 1), p. 30. In order to make capitation and fee-for-service predictable, administrators in Britain and Germany developed the method of central pools. The public authorities provided lump sums and the doctors were paid fees calculated by dividing the pools by the numbers of patients or services. But doctors press—usually successfully—to abandon these methods when the resultant payments are disappointing.

[19] Such an expansion of the traditionally individualistic French medical ethics is suggested in, Jean-Robert Debray, *Le malade et son médecin* (*Déontologie médicale*) (Paris: Éditions Médicales Flammarion, 1965), pp. 137–42, 158–64. Articles 30 and 48 of the Code of Medical Ethics decreed by the French government already state that coverage by a third party payer should not induce physicians to perform more procedures than are clinically necessary.

In service benefits schemes, perhaps the only foreseeable solution is to pay doctors enough under the official rates so that the insured patients are not treated materially worse than the private patients. Here too, the policies of the medical association can be a powerful influence in minimizing discrimination. Ideally, private practice should become a method of buying amenities rather than better physical treatment, but the distinction is not clear in practice.

Discouraging Neglect

Professional ethics guarantee that doctors will not neglect patients who seriously need physical care, no matter how objectionable the remuneration under the public medical scheme. Under completely private practice, the profession donates considerable work, and the public system has the advantage of ensuring some payment. But a drawback of flat-rate payment systems is that, if a hospital outpatient department or polyclinic is available, the doctor may refer time-consuming and unprofitable patients that he ought to treat himself. The patient is neglected in lacking continuity and thoroughness of care.

Over-referral can be discouraged by extra fees for time-consuming patients, as in the modified capitation system instituted in England in 1966. Also it can be discouraged by the vigilance of the medical association. Sometimes the profession can be persuaded to donate the extra time, as it often does under the sliding scales of private practice. An example is Holland. Before 1956, the general practitioner collected a higher capitation fee for older persons. But the sick funds confronted a familiar dilemma: the persons who were the greatest burden on medical services—the chronically ill and elderly—contributed the least to their own support in current payroll taxes. To economize, the extra capitation payment for the elderly was abolished, and the Treasury and the doctors agreed to donate support: the Treasury would supplement the elderly persons' low insurance premiums, and the general practitioner agreed to give full care in return for the same capitation fees applying to everyone. Nevertheless, as we reported in chapter X, some over-referrals occur.

Professional statesmanship to discourage neglect is more difficult to promote in underdeveloped countries. There the public hospital doctor and polyclinic doctor receive low salaries and in return are confronted with large numbers of patients with poor prognoses. Facilities usually are inadequate and overcrowded. Compared to the West, patients are usually far below the doctor's cultural level. Often the society has a tradition of duty to one's own family, rather than to the public welfare, and unselfish service to the poor is rare in the upper class. The medical association usually is weak and inactive. The visitor sees examples of poor communication, rudeness, and neglect by many of the salaried doctors. Improvement would require not merely more pay but a restructuring of the society.

Recruitment and Allocation of Doctors

Despite the publicized disputes between medical associations and public medical authorities, recruitment does not seem affected in any country. Students enter medical schools in larger numbers than ever because of the prestige of medical careers, the intrinsic interest of the work, and the relatively high incomes that can be earned under all payment systems. Perhaps the expansion of competing career opportunities in the natural sciences has changed the composition of medicine's new recruits, but the numbers continue to grow.

Although a country's payment system may not discourage recruitment, it may encourage emigration. Although a doctor earns more than most of his countrymen, he may obtain an even better income in another country without the need to hold several jobs or to maintain a rapid consultation schedule. A serious problem has been the permanent emigration of doctors from the less developed countries to the more developed, and from some developed countries to the United States. Dissatisfaction with the total organization of practice seems at least as important as pay alone. Some young doctors emigrate because at home they must wait too long for promotions in the hospitals; others are attracted by funds and facilities for research, particularly in the United States. Therefore improvements require a reorganization and expansion of opportunities going beyond remuneration alone.

Remuneration has not succeeded in curbing the internal migration of doctors. At a time when the spread of national health services and national health insurance commits public authorities to provide full benefits in the countryside, the severe rural-urban imbalance of the medical profession remains in underdeveloped countries and the imbalance in favor of the cities may be increasing in the developed countries. No one knows whether pay ever can equalize the distribution: no country (except for Turkey, currently) has been able to violate the rank structure by offering rural doctors enormous differentials, and smaller differentials cannot attract doctors away from the facilities, personal amenities, and supplementary private practice in the cities.

Probably neither high pay nor ideal facilities can attract doctors into country towns and rural areas in sufficient number. For example, the hospitals and offices in the northern and rural areas of Scandinavia can hardly be improved upon as settings for practice, but still they are seriously understaffed and rely on temporary appointees from abroad. Probably the public authorities must rely in the future on persons other than doctors who are recruited from these areas and are trained in many of the skills of general medicine. For example, in northern Sweden much of this work must be done by female public health nurses, aided by efficient emergency transportation for the more serious cases. In many underdeveloped countries, male medical assistants can be trained for rural practice.[20]

Further remedies aside from pay are needed to repair the imbalance in location of services within the cities: probably more home visits should be made than are made at present, in the light of current thinking about comprehensive patient care, but the trend is toward fewer home visits by doctors. The present differentials in fees for home visits in most official schemes are not enough to increase the number, and flat-rate payment systems probably contain disincentives that can be offset only by strong professional traditions in favor of home visiting. Except in a few countries, most home visits are made only in clinical emergencies, and probably little home visiting is done with enough frequency and thoroughness to learn about the patient's total environment. If the trends continue toward increasing specialization and reliance on profitable and advanced equipment in offices, another form of medical organization, rather than futile efforts to manipulate fees, probably will be necessary for adequate medical service in the home. One solution is close collaboration between general practitioners and public health nurses: they would share lists of patients, and the nurses would perform the routine home visits and teach the preventive medicine.[21]

The Collectivization of Medical Care

The development of payment systems that will encourage good medicine, will be economical, and will be harmoniously accepted by everyone is part of the larger task of improving the organization of medical care on a national

[20] For many years the training and use of assistant doctors was considered a stopgap until underdeveloped countries trained enough physicians. Self-serving by many medical assistants led to disillusionment and plans to phase out their training. For example, see Edwin F. Rosinski and Frederick J. Spencer, *The Assistant Medical Officer* (Chapel Hill: The University of North Carolina Press, 1965); Clement C. Chesterman, "The Training and Employment of Auxiliary Personnel in Medical and Health Services in Tropical Africa," *Journal of Tropical Medicine and Hygiene*, vol. 56 (June 1953), pp. 123–34; and J. D. Cottrell, "Auxiliary Health Workers in the Eastern Mediterranean Region," *Journal of the American Medical Women's Association*, vol. 10, no. 7 (July 1955), pp. 237–42. However, even if these countries could train enough doctors to increase the ratio to the population, the rural imbalance will remain. Therefore an effective system for training and regulating medical assistants will be necessary, such as the recommendations in, Maurice King (editor), *Medical Care in Developing Countries* (Nairobi: Oxford University Press, 1966), chaps. 1, 3, and 7.

[21] For a recommendation that public health nurses undertake much of the general practitioner's less complex work, see *Reports from General Practice: Present State and Future Needs* (London: College of General Practitioners, 1965), pp. 31, 42–43, 49–52. On the possible reorganization of medical practice to transfer lesser medical tasks to auxiliaries, see Rashi Fein, *The Doctor Shortage: An Economic Diagnosis* (Washington: The Brookings Institution, 1967), pp. 111–29.

scale. The public presses for adequate facilities that can be used by anyone in need, and therefore government and collaborating private organizations in all countries develop nationwide institutions for the education of professional staff, hospitals, ambulatory treatment, preventive services, financing of demand, and so on.[22] To achieve efficiency, economy, and safety, government directly—or by means of *qua si* public agencies created under law—imposes rules upon all the medical services or organizes its own services in more standardized and co-ordinated ways. Such rationalization and planning occur in many other sectors of modern society. The standardization of doctors' pay follows the trend toward uniform wage rates in national labor markets in all other economic sectors.

The Adjustment to Standardized Procedures

When their interests benefit, workers and employees press for standardized wage rates and regularized procedures for wage determination. Like any other group, the medical profession in many countries has pressed for changes that have introduced standardized payments and flat rates in place of the more individualized charges characteristic of a completely private market. Because collecting through a third-party enables doctors to collect minimum fees for all their patients, doctors use sliding scales less often and narrow the range of charges. Whether under private or insured practice, medical societies often prefer standardized rates in order to reduce competition and acrimony within the profession.[23] Doctors favor a rate structure according to the work load only if the results are favorable. As recent events in British and Spanish general practice show, they may press for equal basic practice allowances that guarantee minimum incomes, seniority payments that reward long service, and retirement programs that guarantee security—all of which introduce salaried elements and depart fundamentally from the image of independent contractors who depend entirely on their market position.[24]

[22] The various contributions by government and by mixed public-private efforts in providing and regulating medical services in the world are summarized in, Eveline M. Burns, "The Role of Government in Health Services," *Bulletin of the New York Academy of Medicine*, 2d series, vol. 41, no. 7 (July 1965), pp. 754–94.

[23] On the American trend toward standardized fees that differentiate payment only according to the time and nature of the procedure, see Herman Miles Somers and Anne Ramsay Somers, *Doctors, Patients, and Health Insurance* (Washington: The Brookings Institution, 1961), pp. 53–54; and Herbert E. Klarman, *The Economics of Health* (New York: Columbia University Press, 1965), pp. 22–23. Average fees vary among regions, but the differences may be narrower than is generally assumed. See *Medical Care Financing and Utilization* (Washington: Health Economics Branch, Division of Community Health Services, Public Health Service, U.S. Department of Health, Education, and Welfare, 1962), p. 67.

[24] The disadvantages of the British general practitioners' status of independent contractor paid under the old capitation system and the advantages of the salaried systems enjoyed by civil servants and consultants are compared by Powell, *Medicine and Politics* (note 1), pp. 33–34.

Throughout the world, professionals are increasingly subject to public regulations, or to rules that are conditions for participation in extensive public programs, and increasing numbers of professionals work in organizations. Doctors, like all other professionals encountering these trends, need to reconcile their customary self-image of total autonomy with the new requirements of organizational and social responsibility; their need for discretion must be combined with the organizations' needs for stability and predictability; collaborative decisionmaking and amicable relations must be created with lay administrators; new habits must be learned, such as remembering rules, filling out forms conscientiously, and following orderly time schedules.[25] More generally, new adjustments must be made as the profession becomes a public agency:

> when a society offers monopolistic privileges to a group, it has the right to expect the group to discipline itself with regard to the public interest and to avoid exploitation of the public. No group is entitled to a monopolistic grant of power from the state, including the power to control entrance into a profession, unless it assumes a reciprocal obligation to use that power in the public interest. But it is not easy for government officials to develop the expertise required to judge and to control the actions of a professional group. The answers must be found between the two limits of trying to get a profession to exercise control over itself and shifting the task of controlling a profession to government officials.[26]

The rhetoric of some spokesmen of the medical profession and the occasional bitter outbreaks over pay should not mislead one into believing that doctors are not capable of quick adjustment to a more "socialized" system of providing and paying for medical care. In some countries, gradual adaptations have been occurring for some time; elsewhere enactment of innovations had been long resisted but often was quickly implemented when passage finally occurred. In no country was the organization and ideology of private office practice more firmly established than in France, but since the 1960's the profession has been adapting with remarkable harmony to the controlled system of fees, the spread of full-time salaried hospital staffs, and even the first glimmerings of private and public group practice.[27] Medical associations

[25] The mutual adjustment problems of professionals and organizations are summarized in, W. Richard Scott, "Professionals in Bureaucracies—Areas of Conflict," in, Howard M. Vollmer and Donald L. Mills (editors), *Professionalization* (Englewood Cliffs, N.J.: Prentice-Hall, Inc., 1966), pp. 265–75. The consequential transformation of all the liberal professions in all countries is predicted in, Jean Savatier, "Qu'est-ce qu'une profession libérale?", *Projet*, New series, no. 4 (April 1966), pp. 451–64.

[26] Eli Ginzberg, "The Political Economy of Health," *Bulletin of the New York Academy of Medicine*, 2d series, vol. 41, no. 10 (October 1965), p. 1032.

[27] The collision between the requirements of national health insurance and the traditional individualism, autonomy, and secretiveness of French medicine are described in, Henri Hatzfeld, *Le grand tournant de la médecine libérale* (Paris: Les Éditions Ouvrières, 1963). Subsequent adaptations by the doctors are summarized in, Michel Carré, *Quelle médecine voulez-vous?* (Paris: Éditions Laffont, 1964). Suggestions for modernizing the profession's

and practitioners can adjust to modern methods of organization and remuneration—like any occupation—if the doctors are paid well enough and if they participate regularly in all decisions. As in other sectors of society in most countries recently, if an interest group has a satisfactory status—an important qualification—bargaining for economic benefits within established institutions replaces the former ideological attacks on the legitimacy of the public authorities.[28] The younger doctors in all countries seem more willing to adjust readily to the new conditions of social security, salaried jobs, and group practice.[29]

Besides standing consultation mechanisms, other administrative provisions are necessary for the harmonious conduct of a public mechanism dispensing professional services. One principle that doctors adamantly defend is the freedom to join or to leave a public program. A common solution is a policy of individual adhesions: the system is created by statute, and any doctor is free to join or stay out. A more cumbersome solution is one arising from a corporative tradition of social organization, as in France: the medical association in an area can join the system on behalf of all its members, but in districts where the dissenters are too numerous to support a collective decision, individuals can join. The drawback of this method is collective control: the individual dissenter is bound by the majority's decision to sign a contract.[30] Although closed panels can survive in private health insurance, their use in large public programs cannot long resist the attacks of the medical profession, since they jeopardize doctors' incomes and their freedom to appeal to the entire public. The standards of medical education and licensing should be high enough so that free entry does not reduce the quality of care.

---

ideology appear throughout, Debray, *Malade et son médecin* (note 19). The surprisingly rapid spread of group practice in a country where the medical associations had long opposed it on principle is described in, M. Thiercelin, "Le développement de la médecine de groupe et le régissant la coopération médicale," *Concours médical*, vol. 87, no. 11 (13 March 1965), pp. 1869–70, 1873. These changes correspond to the spread of formal organization, planning, and standardization of procedures and services throughout French society. The nation-wide trends are summarized in, Jean-Daniel Reynaud (editor), *Tendances et volontés de la sociéte française* (Paris: Futuribles S.É.D.É.I.S., 1966).

28 These developments in intergroup relations in other economic sectors of Europe are described in, Seymour Martin Lipset, "The Changing Class Structure and Contemporary European Politics," *Daedalus* (Winter 1964), pp. 280–86.

29 E.g., Jean Bui-Dang-Ha-Doan, "Les anciens internes des Hôpitaux de Paris et leur devenir," *Cahiers de sociologie et de démographie médicales*, vol. 4, no. 3 (July–September 1964), pp. 103–8; and Martin S. Weinberg and Elina Haavio-Mannila, "The Medical Profession in Finland," *Journal of Health and Social Behavior*, vol. 8, no. 1 (September 1967), pp. 229–32.

30 Some observers recommend the replacement of this method by the more common rules allowing any doctor to join or secede from the public program at his discretion. The program would take effect upon passage of laws, not upon the signing of contracts between the public authorities and the medical association. Jean Mignon, "Adhésion individuelle ou engagement individuel?", *Concours médical*, vol. 87, no. 22 (29 May 1965), pp. 3821–24; and "Les options fondamentales de la Confédération des Syndicats Médicaux Français," ibid., vol. 88, no. 12 (19 March 1966), pp. 2089–90, 2093–94.

Participation in the decisions of public medical schemes and commitment to the success of these programs will not cause the doctors and the medical association to abandon self-interest. Like every occupation in the public service, they seek higher pay and better working conditions and argue that the nation will benefit through better recruitment and improved performance. As the profession becomes more involved in the management of the public system, the leadership of the medical association changes: the demagogic leaders of a self-centered interest group are replaced by men more skilled in planning and committee work. But when the profession feels it is not paid or appreciated enough, these leaders will again assume the roles of militant and sometimes vitriolic spokesmen for a pressure group. If they do not, they will be beset by internal rebellions within the medical association and by breakaway societies.[31] These occasional outbreaks do not mean the doctors are more self-centered or irreconcilable than other occupations in the public service: their demands and threats are merely more publicized, and they are more successful in getting what they want.

Planning Medical Pay

Modern society not only is becoming more organized it is becoming more planned. Governments try to estimate the future needs and expenditures for medical care as for other public services. In practice, predictable budgeting is difficult, because utilization often exceeds expectations. Certain types of medical payment present greater planning problems than others: in particular, one cannot estimate accurately the total budget for medical services rendered by fee-for-service, because procedures may increase greatly in number; and if the planners predict only moderate increases in fees, the doctors may successfully obtain large increases that keep pace with the cost of living and other economic indicators.[32] For such reasons, administrators and planners prefer salaried systems.

[31] Both the British Medical Association and the French *Confédération* passed through these stages. As they become more integrated in decisionmaking, the leaderships were transformed. But during the 1960's, more militant general practitioners accused the leaders of excessive collaboration with the public authorities at the expense of the doctors' pecuniary interests and professional freedom. Schismatic groups arose and pressed the BMA and the *Confédération* to remain aggressive during payment negotiations. On factionalism in British general practice, see David Mechanic and Ronald G. Faich, "Doctors in Revolt: The Crisis in the British Nationalized Health Service," in, Ian Weinberg (editor), *English Society* (New York: Atherton Press, forthcoming), and Samuel Mencher, *Private Practice in Britain* (London: G. Bell & Sons, 1967), chap. 5. The French events are summarized in part in Carré, *Quelle médecine?* (note 27); and in the articles by Roland Mane and Jean-Jacques Dupeyroux in *Droit social*, vol. 25, nos. 9–10 (September–October 1962), pp. 516–29.

[32] Incomes of doctors rise much faster than fees because of increases in productivity. For example, greater productivity—not higher fees—has been the principal reason for the spectacular growth in American physicians' incomes in recent decades, according to

Planning requires explicit decisions about the location of medicine in the total system: an amount of money must be allocated for medicine in comparison to the amounts for other economic sectors, and targets for medical incomes must be established in comparison with other occupations. Planners have long been accustomed to estimating society's needs, priorities, and allocations in industry, transportation, education, and some other sectors. But until now—except possibly in some Eastern European countries—planners have not yet developed adequate criteria for determining the proper place for medical care in the total economy and for the medical profession in total distribution of income. Spending on hospitalization, treatments, and drugs has rapidly mounted at the discretion of doctors and hospitals because of the absence of planned goals and because consumer interests have not been well represented in medical markets. Medical care now absorbs a large percentage of the public revenues and national incomes of some countries where a different order of priorities might be better, like Italy and Israel.

Criteria for Determining Medical Pay

No public medical scheme can function—particularly if it affects most doctors—without decisions concerning the relative position of the medical profession in the country's distribution of personal income. Controversies over criteria might persuade policymakers that the safest method is to consider each pay award by itself and to enunciate no criteria. But at least as much trouble arises because of the absence of any standards to answer doctors' incessant claims that their just needs are still unmet; and the doctors can successfully obtain higher awards without letup.

In practice in public medical schemes, doctors' pay is judged by three criteria: trends in income by other occupations, changes in the cost of living, and effects on recruitment and retention.[33] As we have seen in this

---

Seymour E. Harris, *The Economics of American Medicine* (New York: The Macmillan Co., 1964), pp. 128–64. Planners hope to maintain total expenditures and doctors' incomes in balance with developments in the rest of the economy. Therefore they should plan to raise fees at a pace lower than other indicators of economic growth, since services and productivity rise. But the medical profession in practice often presses successfully to tie fees to the cost of living or other economic indicators, thereby guaranteeing a permanent rise in their incomes *relative* to others. For an example of disagreement over planners' projections about fees, productivity, doctors' incomes, and total medical spending, see Jean Mignon, "Le rapport de la Commission des Prestations Sociales: L'assurance-maladie et son avenir," *Concours médical*, vol. 88, no. 16 (16 April 1966), pp. 2807–8, 2811–12. The complex effects of national economic plans upon determination of fee schedules are discussed in "Les travaux de la Commission de l'Art. 24: Les dispositions tarifaires," ibid., vol. 87, no. 13 (27 March 1965), pp. 2229–32, 2235.

[33] The use of these criteria in discussions about paying the several occupations in the National Health Service is described in, H. A. Clegg and T. E. Chester, *Wage Policy and the Health Service* (Oxford: Basil Blackwell, 1957), pp. 79–91. In practice, none of these

book, application of some of these criteria to medical pay is troublesome and, furthermore, their generalization to all occupations under national wage policy would be self-defeating. For example, as the British and Israeli experiences show, any policy of maintaining existing differentials among occupations often produces a cycle of breakthroughs by individual occupations on special grounds, general pressures by all others to catch up, endless disputes whether the differentials should be proportional or absolute, and unceasing disputes whether the differentials should apply to all sectors of the profession or vary by group.[34] A policy of relativities commits the government to match trends in the private economy, with unpredictable strains upon the budget and tax system. As we saw in a previous paragraph, it is very difficult to plan and manipulate total incomes of doctors by means of methods other than salary. The British experience demonstrates the difficulties of predicting future trends in the incomes of the other occupations used for comparison with medicine. A pledge to raise an occupation's relative position to some undefined level runs the risk of endless demands for even more money by that occupation and appeals for special treatment by all the others.

Basing pay awards on changes in living costs is more difficult to administer than appears at first. To raise medical pay by the same rate as the government's official index of living costs seems easy and self-enacting, but the living costs of doctors may fluctuate differently from those of the average citizen. Doctors' pay awards may be designed to cover practice expenses, but expenses move differently from living costs. If everyone's pay were raised automatically whenever the cost-of-living index rose, permanent inflation of wages and prices might result. If fees were raised in accordance with changes in the cost of living, doctors' incomes would increase considerably more as their productivity rose. The steady gradual rise in income by the successful application of this policy might be too much to discourage overcrowding of medicine in some situations and too little to encourage recruitment when necessary.

In the future, public medical schemes may base more payment decisions on the relation of pay to recruitment, discouraging emigration, and performance. Planners in several Eastern European countries have long been sensitive to the effects of income decisions upon recruitment, and Britain's

---

criteria controlled decisions, which were heavily affected by politics and power-bargaining, but miscellaneous facts about relativities, living costs, and recruitment were considered by the decisionmakers. Ibid., pp. 95–99, 122–23, 126.

[34] The upsetting effects on British national wage policy are described in, Gordon Forsyth, *Doctors and State Medicine* (London: Pitman Medical Publishing Co., 1966), pp. 34–37. For this reason, the National Board for Prices and Incomes refused to adopt a simple policy of relativities when planning the pay of university teachers, and it criticized the use of this criterion by the Review Body when making awards in medicine. *Standing Reference on the Pay of University Teachers in Great Britain: First Report* (London: H. M. Stationery Office, Cmnd. 3866, 1969), pp. 9, 21, 28.

National Health Service during the 1960's tried to substitute the recruitment and retention criteria instead of relativity of income alone. This policy may have more effect on discouraging emigration than on recruitment: doctors can emigrate at any time, but a current shortage can be filled only in the future, after expansion of medical school enrollments. These payment decisions must be combined with correct estimates of future needs, and the numerous nonmonetary variables must also be manipulated.[35] Certain specific incentives and regulations may affect recruitment into medicine and its specialties more efficiently than pay, and manipulating everyone's pay may be too clumsy and may have undesirable consequences.[36]

Textbooks on rational wage determination usually recommend preparing careful job descriptions of the various occupations in an organization and job descriptions of the ranks within each occupation. Then differentials in pay both between and within occupations would correspond to specified differences in responsibility, skill, effort, etc.[37] In practice the rates of each occupation are determined by power-bargaining, although the occupations that fall behind usually catch up again, thereby tending to preserve approximate differentials. Therefore power-bargaining by each occupation tends to press the average money level of wages up against the funds available from employers; but some theory of differential skill and responsibility might be used by planners and bargaining agents in devising the differentials among occupations and among ranks. Perhaps future national wage policies for doctors and other occupations in the public service might be determined with the help of such job investigations and criteria.[38] Needless to say, com-

[35] In social planning, impressive statistics and a careful statement of priorities do not guarantee correct decisions. The generalizations about current facts and future trends may be wrong, and therefore planned allocations may be disastrous. For example, the decision to reduce enrollment in British medical schools on the assumption that trends in population growth and health needs would not require as many doctors as were being produced at that time, in *Report of the Committee to Consider the Future Numbers of Medical Practitioners and the Appropriate Intake of Medical Students* (London: H. M. Stationery Office, 1957).

[36] For this reason, the French commission to study the payment system recommended that "universal mechanisms" like fees not be fixed to influence the recruitment and allocation of doctors. "Rapport de la Commission de l'Article 24 du Décret du 12 Mai 1960," *Notes et documents*, no. 17 (First Trimester 1965), p. 60.

[37] E.g., Belcher, *Wage and Salary* (note 13), esp. part 3. The determination of differential rates according to a theory of measurable differentials in responsibility is proposed by Elliott Jaques, *Equitable Payment* (London: Heinemann, 1961).

[38] I do not argue for a comprehensively planned and controlled national wage policy. The difficulties and the failures in practice are summarized by Benjamin C. Roberts, *National Wages Policy in War and Peace* (London: George Allen & Unwin, 1958), chap. 11; and Martin P. Oettinger, "Nation-Wide Job Evaluation in the Netherlands," *Industrial Relations*, vol. 4, no. 1 (October 1964), pp. 45–59. But pay rates for doctors under national medical care schemes in practice are set in relation to the incomes of other occupations; the growth of public employment and the spread of national private collective bargaining lead to more comparisons of resulting incomes for nationwide occupations; informed decisions are better than guesswork.

plications must be resolved: payment by salary can be determined by these methods far more easily than fee-for-service; some doctors (such as British and Dutch specialists) are employed, while others (such as British and Dutch general practitioners) are self-employed; and doctors' pay must be fixed in the light of the probable consequences for clinical performance and recruitment as well as from the standpoint of recognizing education and skill.[39] However, some tentative job evaluations now are being offered as the basis of pay claims in medicine,[40] and the method might introduce a more objective and dispassionate element into an area that has been one of society's most expensive examples of power-bargaining.

Effective wage administration aims at motivating desired recruitment and performance from the holders of particular jobs. Therefore, we must know the motivations of the people that job is likely to attract. Research should be done on the total motivations of doctors in occupational choice and in work, in order to assess the net effects of various levels and types of payment and in order to fit monetary and nonmonetary rewards together in beneficial combinations.[41] Today many disputes over doctors' pay are conducted and resolved completely by speculation: what the medical associations say may not be identical with the range of individual wants and grievances in the medical profession, and the results of power-bargaining over the publicized issues may omit solution of some essential needs. In pay disputes, the rhetoric usually concentrates attention on the differentials between the higher ranks in medicine and other leading occupations, but research throughout the profession would have the beneficial effect of inducing wage planners to devote more careful attention to the younger and lower-ranking doctors. Payment in an official system cannot be individualized sufficiently to satisfy the great variety of preference schemes that would be revealed by research, but administrators might be able to individualize many of the working conditions that combine with pay to determine each doctor's total satisfaction. Another benefit of regular research about doctors' motivation

[39] It is often said that a further difficulty in setting doctors' pay is that medicine is unique, and no comparable occupation can be found either in public or private employment. But the "unique" occupations are more numerous than is generally supposed, and wage planners are accumulating experience in fixing their salary structures and relative monetary values. For example, see Louis J. Kroeger et al., *Pricing Jobs Unique to Government* (Chicago: Public Personnel Association, 1964).

[40] E.g., *The G.P.A. Report—Part Two: Doctors' Remuneration* (London: General Practitioners' Association, 1965).

[41] On the relations between pay and total motivation at work, see Victor H. Vroom, *Work and Motivation* (New York: John Wiley & Sons, 1964), chap. 5. An example of research identifying the combination of monetary and nonmonetary motivations of professionals is, John W. Riegel, *Administration of Salaries for Engineers and Scientists*, and Riegel, *Intangible Rewards for Engineers and Scientists* (both Ann Arbor: Bureau of Industrial Relations, University of Michigan, 1958).

and performance is to lay the basis for adding another criterion to medical pay awards—one common in other occupations, namely, evidence of increased productivity since the last pay raise. Finally, research is beneficial because infusions of facts—even rival versions of the facts—help convert partisans into realistic negotiators.

Research should be based on more administrative experiments than heretofore. Many national medical care schemes are debated abstractly and then are adopted nationally. But no one can judge how a particular arrangement will work in practice without trials. Cross-national comparisons of entirely different systems—such as this book—are not as good as experimental evidence, since the same scheme may work differently in various national settings. Some fundamental decisions—for example, whether lower income groups should be given direct services or should be given cash and the opportunity to exercise market choices—can be made wisely only after trials.[42]

Future research and experiment should be attentive to variations within the population as well as within the medical profession. A particular payment method may work differently among patients of different classes as well as among doctors of different specialties. The appropriate unit for this economic research—as well as for medical care—is the doctor-patient relationship, classified according to specialty, the doctor's career stage and working situation, the patient's financial and occupational characteristics, the organized setting, and so on. The available evidence about the effects of payment systems on the doctor-patient relationship rarely differentiates among types of patient and usually fails to classify doctors by many important traits. Therefore existing research suggests generalizations about all doctors and all patients in a country—as we have seen in this book—but it does not help plan systems of pay tuned to different types of patients.

Far more research is needed that compares organized national systems of medical care with private payments for comparable patients in the same society. A serious limitation upon my analysis has been the shortage of evidence about private medical transactions: I have compared types of organized payment systems in various countries, but I could not compare adequately the effects of organized and private pay in the same society. During the 1960's, a pessimism has spread in many countries concerning the accomplishments of the once lauded national health insurance schemes and national health services. All countries are experiencing a period of frustration and re-examination, regardless of system: costs rise, utilization

[42] Such administrative experiments are being conducted within American national health insurance for the aged. Wilbur J. Cohen, *Report on Medicare from the Secretary of Health, Education, and Welfare* (Washington: Department of Health, Education, and Welfare, January 1969), pp. 44–48.

increases, no one knows whether "enough" or the "right amount" of care is being given, limited resources are subject to steadily higher demands by doctors, hospitals, and patients.[43] Some critics have recommended shifts from national systems of service benefits with standard pay rates to systems of selective benefits distributed by private purchase in a competitive free market.[44] Others have suggested the revival of private practice in order to keep the official system on its toes. Whether private medical markets can bring their reputed benefits and are free of the defects predicted by defenders of existing national medical systems is completely speculative without research and experimentation.

Despite its changing organization and technology, the mission of medical care remains the same. The patient should receive the proper diagnosis and treatment from the best qualified doctors with the appropriate facilities and ancillary help at the right time. The doctor should have the right combination of technical skill and humane understanding and should do neither more nor less than the patient needs. The payment system should motivate and reward the proper balance between volume and quality of work, between working to one's own limits and referring the patient to better qualified specialists, between psychosomatic support and technical intervention. The payment system should motivate and reward continuing professional education and hard work. But this subtle combination of requirements cannot be met by any payment system alone: standard rates cannot guarantee ideal performance from the great range of individual doctors and individual needs of patients. At best, remuneration can reinforce the beneficial tendencies in the total organization of medical practice. Like other occupations, medicine is expected to do better work because of new trends in social planning and formal nationwide organization adapted to the potentialities of medicine and the needs of patients in each country.[45] Like other professions in the public service, medicine will act in its own self-interest, as well as in society's interest. Despite the tactical rhetoric of momentary controversies to promote self-interest, doctors can also be expected to act according to the philosophy

[43] For example, T. E. Chester, "How Healthy is the National Health Service?", *District Bank Review*, no. 162 (September 1968); Pierre Grandjeat, "L'assurance-maladie en France," *Révue économique*, no. 2 (March 1967), pp. 251–91; and Boris J. Petrovsky, "Sostoianie meditsinskoi pomoshchi naseleniiu i mery po uluchsheniiu zdravookhraneniia v SSSR," *Izvestia*, 26 June 1968, pp. 2–3.

[44] For example, D. S. Lees, "Health through Choice," *Freedom or Free-for-All?* (London: The Institute of Economic Affairs, 2d ed., 1965), pp. 21–94; and Ralph Harris and Arthur Seldon, *Choice in Welfare 1965* (London: The Institute of Economic Affairs, 1965).

[45] For example, Vladimir Dyagilev, "Vrachebnye oshibki i zhiznennye sledstviya," Oktyabr, no. 9 (September 1968), pp. 184–87.

from past centuries that evokes their pledge today during the ceremonies of personal dedication when they join their profession:[46]

> I do solemnly swear by that which I hold most sacred:
>
> That I will be loyal to the profession of medicine and just and generous to its members;
>
> That I will lead my life and practice my art in uprightness and honor;
>
> That into whatsoever house I shall enter, it shall be for the good of the sick to the utmost of my power, I holding myself aloof from wrong, from corruption, from the tempting of others to vice;
>
> That I will exercise my art solely for the cure of my patients, and will give no drug, perform no operation for a criminal purpose, even if solicited, far less suggest it;
>
> That whatsoever I shall see or hear of the lives of men which is not fitting to be spoken, I will keep inviolably secret.
>
> These things I do promise and in proportion as I am faithful to this my oath may happiness and good repute be ever mine—the opposite if I shall be forsworn.

[46] The translation of the Hippocratic Oath was by John G. Curtis and appears in, Peter S. Nagan (editor), *Medical Almanac 1961–62* (Philadelphia: W. B. Saunders Co., 1961), p. 484.

APPENDIX

MY INFORMANTS

This book would not have been possible without the assistance of many people in many countries. The amount of time and hospitality granted an inquisitive foreigner was extraordinary. Following are the persons who generously gave me at least an hour of their time in interviews about doctors' pay or in equivalent help by correspondence. Some directed me through their organizations. Some even acted as social hosts and tourist guides, in addition to our professional shop talk. Many others provided valuable information in shorter conversations, but they are too numerous to list.

ENGLAND. Brian Abel-Smith, George Braithwaite, John L. Burton, Jack H. Carrick, Theodore E. Chester, A. E. Cooper, John Dodd, Dr. Dyce, John R. Ellis, Theodore F. Fox, David Glass, W. P. Gill, William E. Hall, Brian McSwiney, Maurice Orbach, Thomas Rimmer, Arthur Seldon, Robert W. Sharpington.

U.S.S.R. George Antonov, Dr. Bailin, V. Butrov, Dr. Brilantova, Mark G. Field, Nikolai I. Grashchenkov, Dr. Leonienko, Ira Lubell, Josef Vasilovich Melnik, Sergei Nechaev, Elena Pogisantz, Mikhail Sokolowski, Alexander Shevelyov, Dr. Shivanyenko, Alexander Timofeyevski.

FRANCE. Robert Attavi, Louis Justin-Besançon, Jean Bui-Dang-Ha-Doan, Frédéric Choffé, Paul Comet, Pierre A. Debuirre, Guy Forestier, Henry Galant, Jacques Gobinet, Jean Guénézon, François Hoquet, Lucien Jolly, Robert Larmagnac, Alain Laugier, Raymond Lecoq, E. Martin, Paul A. Messerli, Henri Moraud, Jean-Daniel Reynaud, Jean Vatier.

GERMANY. Fritz Beske, Maria Gehrt, Richard Plönes, Heinz Ritter, Dietrich Rüschemeyer, Rolf Schlögell, Rudolf Schütz, Karl Taprogge, Willy Wernick, Mr. Winter, Gerhard Wolff.

NETHERLANDS. Johan Beunder, Jan C. J. Burkens, Gerard Dekker, Johan Fokkema, Menno Klinkenberg, Cornelus Ouwehand, Jacques J. Velthoven, Johan C. M. Hattinga Verschure, Duurt K. Rijkels, G. A. de Ruiter, Jan van der Valk.

SWEDEN. Anders Åberg, Gunnar Biörck, Karl-Fredrick Blom, Kamrer K. Carlberg, Ingvar Ekholm, Sten Floderus, Lennart Hammar, John Henriksson, Carl-Gösta Hesser, Bror Rexed, Ursula Rexed, Malcolm Tottie, Sven Ydén, Ulf Zetterblad.

SWITZERLAND. Emile-Ch. Bonard, Pierre E. Ferrier, Pierre Jaccard, Eric Martin, Jean Maystre, Alex F. Müller, Hal M. Wells, Bernard Wissmer, General Secretariat of the Swiss Medical Institutions (and especially Ulrich Naef).

ITALY. Giuseppe Billiena, Gimo Civai, Oretta Ferrari, Franz Feliciangeli, Elio

Guzzanti, Franco Illuminati, Mario Massini, Innocenzo Moretti, Ignazio Muner, Lucio Nuzzolo, Pietro Omodeo, Luigi Pinelli, Piero Pinna, Vittorio Sabena, Marta Safier, Mimmo Sano, Ugo Siniscalchi, Angelo Tomasini, Sergio Vulterini.

SPAIN. Manuel Alonso Olea, Antonio Bustos Alarcón, Salustiano del Campo Urbano, Gerardo Clavero, Tomás Charlo Dupont, Luis Estella Benudes de Castro, Manuel Jiminez Rueda, Juan Linz, Eduardo Martínez Alonso, Mario de la Mata y de la Barrera-Caro, Francisco Merino Prieto, Alfonso de la Peña, Fernando Enríquez de Salamanca, Antonio Sanchez Dominguez, Mario Zarapico Romero.

POLAND. Jan E. Bielecki, Stanislaus Bylina, Helena Csorba, Wiktor Eychner, Ryszard Jachowicz, Marcin Kacprzak, Nonna Lyzwanska, Tomasz Niedek, Feliks Oledzki, Ksawery Rowicki, Bronislaw Saldak, Adam Sarapata, Magdalena Sokolowska, Walerian Strasewicz, Ludwik Zukowski.

GREECE. Ilias N. Athanasiades, George K. Baritakis, Athanasios Coccalis, Menelaos Germanos, Sofitis Liaticos, John Nicolacopoulos, A. C. Papaioanou, Paul Pavlides, Andreas Placoudas, Anthony Scouloudis, Gregory D. Skalkeas, Constantin Valsamis.

TURKEY. Ihsan Günalp, Aslan Gündaş, Hüsnü A. Ikişnisci, Ekmel Onursal, Omer Ozek, Sabahattin Payzin, Yusuf Tunca.

CYPRUS. Ali Atun, Glafkos Cassoulides, Takis Hadjilambris, Phoebus C. Hadjioannou, George Marangos, Zemon G. Panos, Fikret Rassim, Christos Savvas, Dmitri Souliotis, Charalambos Stamatiades, George T. Strickland.

EGYPT. Mahmoud Abdel Hamud Attiah, Garbis Chemsian, Mohamed Loutfi Dowidar, Abdul Rahman El-Sadr, Nawal El-Saadari, Zoheiv Farid, Paul Jamison, Albert Khalil, Ahmed Kamel Mazen, Moustapha Ramadan, Said Sabon, Ali H. Shaaban, Fathi A. Soliman, Mohamed Talaat.

ISRAEL. Aaron Antonovsky, Tova Yeshurun-Berman, Joseph Ben-David, A. Michael Davies, Fritz Dreyfuss, Peter P. Fleischmann, Shabbetai Ginton, Rafael Gjebin, Haim Sholom Halevi, Ben Zion Harell, Itzhak Kanev, Uri Khassis, Pinchas Koren, Moshe Krieger, Kalman J. Mann, Jack Medalie, Baruch Oren, Ely Presser, Moshe Soroka, Joseph Stern, Nelu Strulovici, Havraham Yarom.

LEBANON. Joseph E. Azar, Charles W. Churchill, Said Dajani, Thomas H. Gray, Farid Sami Haddad, Jamal Karen Harfouche, Father Pierre Madet, Ibrahim Salti, Aida K. Cotran Shammas, LaVand Syverson.

WORLD HEALTH ORGANIZATION. Fawzie S. Bisharah, Simon Btesh, A. C. Eberwein, Edward Grzegorzewski, C. J. Hackett, William Hobson, Leo Kaprio, M. Claude Petitpierre, Gabriel Rifka, T. S. Sze, James M. Vine.

OTHERS. R. A. Amarvi, Salvador Perez Diaz, Craig S. Lichtenwalner, Ananda Shiva Prasad, Cicely Williams.

In addition, I am indebted to several persons who arranged for interviews or for visits to organizations: Mikhail Bruk, Ministry of Health of the U.S.S.R.; Monique Lepeytre, Ministry of Health (now Ministry of Social Affairs) of France; Alphonse Gardie, Assistance Publique à Paris; Mieczyslaw Juchniewicz, Ministry of Health and Social Welfare of Poland; Vassos P. Vassilopoulos, Ministry of Health of Cyprus; Grace Spacht, Eastern Mediterranean Regional Office, World Health Organization; and Miss D. Maitland, International Hospital Federation.

INDEX OF SUBJECTS

INDEX OF NAMES

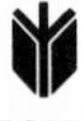

THE JOHNS HOPKINS PRESS

Composed in Baskerville text and display
by Monotype Composition Company, Inc.

Printed on Perkins and Squier, R
by Universal Lithographers, Inc.

Bound in Columbia Riverside Chambray,
by L. H. Jenkins Company, Inc.

302556950Z